The Existential Structure of Substance Misuse

Guilherme Messas

The Existential Structure of Substance Misuse

A Psychopathological Study

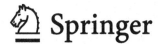 Springer

Guilherme Messas
Department of Mental Health
Santa Casa de São Paulo School of Medical Sciences
São Paulo
Brazil

ISBN 978-3-030-62726-3   ISBN 978-3-030-62724-9   (eBook)
https://doi.org/10.1007/978-3-030-62724-9

This Springer imprint is published by the registered company Springer Nature Switzerland AG
The registered company address is: Gewerbestrasse 11, 6330 Cham, Switzerland

1. The Existential Structure of Substance Misuse – A Psychopathological Study by Guilherme Messas

This book hits the spot! Guilherme Messas combines an in-depth knowledge of contemporary phenomenological psychopathology with extensive clinical and policy experience to provide a uniquely insightful account of the widely diverse experiences of substance misuse. The clear presentation of complex ideas richly illustrated with personal stories of those concerned make for a rare delight.

Professor Bill (KWM) Fulford, St Catherine's College, University of Oxford, UK

2. In this ground-breaking work, full of sophistication and nuance, Guilherme Messas considers the experiential dimensions of substance use and misuse. His book offers a compelling orientation to phenomenological and hermeneutic theory, followed by an original, eye-opening analysis of the ways in which consciousness-altering drugs can foster, but also destroy, a person's sense of meaning and purpose.

–Louis Sass, Distinguished Professor of Clinical Psychology, Rutgers University; author of *Madness and Modernism* and *The Paradoxes of Delusion*.

3. In this wide-ranging volume, the author presents a comprehensive phenomenological conception of mental illness on the basis of the existential conditions of the human being. The concept of anthropological disproportion, which Ludwig Binswanger had already developed to describe mental disorders, is applied here systematically to different forms of illness. For the first time, the author finally drafts an existential phenomenology of substance abuse as a Dionysian form of temporality, spatiality and corporeality. A groundbreaking work that is highly recommended to every psychiatric and psychotherapeutic reader.

Prof. Dr. Thomas Fuchs
Karl Jaspers Professor of Philosophy and Psychiatry
Heidelberg

4. If, in the early days in Europe, phenomenological psychopathology emerged as the phenomenology of psychoses, contemporary Brazilian phenomenology reinvented itself as a phenomenological psychopathology of neuroses and of experiences of pathological suffering in general. The work of Guilherme Messas masterfully addresses the innovative moment in phenomenological

psychopathology, whose framework is the idea that every experience of illness is a form of anthropological disproportion due to the lack of intersubjective anchorage. Through this lens, Messas understands the role of substance misuse as different forms of disproportion. Certainly, this was only possible based on solid clinical experience, daily contact with patients, and a deep knowledge in psychopathology. The intersection between theory and practice allows Guilherme Messas to develop a phenomenological psychopathology of substance misuse addressed in this book; he developed the theory based on his clinical practice, making this book a valuable contribution to clinical practice for treating substance misuse.

Virginia Moreira

Universidade de Fortaleza, Brasil

This book would not come to light without the dedication and competence of its author assistant, my colleague Lívia Fukuda, MD

Foreword

When Karl Jaspers first identified phenomenology as a core method for psycho-pathological research, psychiatry was still gaining a foothold as a major branch of medicine. The systematic description and classification of abnormal experiences provided a necessary foundation for the field. At the time, it was well-understood that without these phenomenological descriptions, clinicians stood little chance of understanding their patients or appreciating their existential predicaments. Yet, the advances made by phenomenological psychopathologists were largely ignored after the 1980 publication of the DSM-III. The rise of operational diagnosis, with its oversimplified diagnostic criteria and inattention to the complexities of abnormal experience, left little if any space for the kind of insights that phenomenological psychopathologists offered.

Yet, today, we're witnessing a new wave of phenomenological psychopathology. On the one hand, this might be cause for concern: A renewed interest in phenome-nological psychopathology, and in philosophical contributions to psychiatry gener-ally, are signs of an ongoing crisis in psychiatry; after decades of failed promises to neurobiologically validate the current diagnostic categories, mental health profes-sionals have become disillusioned with psychiatry's dominant approach to under-standing mental disorders. On the other hand, the renewed interest in phenomenological psychopathology should also be cause for hope and optimism: Mental health professionals now actively seek viable alternatives to superficial symptomatologies provided by the operational approach; as a result, we now find phenomenological psychopathology making its way into major venues for the dis-semination of academic research, including books and articles published by the major academic presses and in the top journals.

However, this new wave of phenomenological psychopathology hasn't simply picked up where the classical figures left off. If one compares much of the recent work in the field with some of the major studies conducted by classical figures such as Ludwig Binswanger or Medard Boss, one is bound to find striking differences of style, presentation, and approach. In particular, the early approaches to phenomeno-logical psychopathology seamlessly blended Freudian psychoanalysis with phe-nomenological and existential philosophy, producing what they called existential analysis. There's a value to this approach that we may find lacking in many contemporary approaches to phenomenological psychopathology. Existential analysis provided immediate clinical value to the therapeutic encounter. The existential analysts sought to understand not only abstract diagnostic categories, but the concrete, historically situated, and constantly unfolding lives of their patients.

Why should we bother to reflect on those aspects of a tradition that we've left behind? Because there's much in these classical works that we should renew, develop, and apply—and this is precisely what we find in Guilherme Messas' book. Messas integrates the abstract, structural analyses of disorders with explorations of the lived, interpersonal dynamics that constitute his patients' personal histories and concrete situations. In this respect, he brings together the best elements of classical and contemporary phenomenological psychopathology, providing us with an approach that illuminates general categories of disorder as well the concrete, day to day lives of those who live with these disorders. To drive home the value of Messas' approach, I want to focus here on two key virtues of his book.

First, Messas does not merely apply phenomenology to the field of mental health or to the topic of substance misuse. Rather, he provides us with a theoretical framework that accommodates and illuminates these ways of being in the world—one that may also be taken up by other researchers and applied to a range of psychopathological conditions. Phenomenological psychopathologists often stress that they're concerned with the "form" or "structure" rather than the "content" of experience. However, while this is more or less true of phenomenology, it's also an oversimplification—not only because the relation between form and content is complex, but because experience takes "form" at many different levels. Messas is careful to distinguish at least two of these levels, highlighting a fundamental difference between what he calls "anthropopathologies," on the one hand, and "structural pathologies" on the other. This should not be understood as a distinction between pathologies that affect the content of experience versus pathologies that affect the form of experience. Rather, the difference is between two levels, or strata, at which the form or structure of experience can be altered.

At the anthropological level, we find disproportions in the relative weight of different poles of existence, such as the poles of self, other, and world. As Messas clarifies, these pathologies—which include personality disorders, phobias, obsessions, and compulsions, among other conditions—do not involve alterations in the most basic structural features of human existence. There's a sense in which these modes of existence, or ways of being, differ from healthy or non-disordered experience only in degree. For example, each of us will experience shifts in the relative weight that we place on how others perceive and understand us. At some points in our lives, our identities will rely heavily on the perception of others—maybe even a particular other. At other points, we may be relatively secure in our sense of identity, granting greater weight to our own self-perceptions. On Messas' account, however, these changes become pathological only when we suffer a reduction in our ability to dynamically shift these relative proportions in response to life circumstances. When we become stuck in a particular distribution of these anthropological proportions, we become existentially vulnerable.

In contrast with anthropopathologies, we can also undergo what Messas calls structural pathologies. Perhaps the best example of such a pathology is schizophrenia, but certain aspects of melancholic and manic experience occur at this level of existence as well. These are pathologies that involve alterations at the most basic or fundamental level of experience—what Messas refers to as the conditions of possibility of existence. These may involve fundamental disturbances in the structures of selfhood, temporality, or affectivity, among other structural features. But it's important to keep in mind that such structural alterations are bound to have ramifications on our anthropological proportions as well. To fully understand a patient with a structural pathology, the clinician must also explore their anthropological situation.

These discussions may at first seem a bit too philosophical for the more clinically minded reader. But Messas is remarkably skilled at tethering these complex and seemingly abstract analyses to the concrete lives of his patients. In fact, the style of Messas' presentation makes the clinical value of his work unmistakable. This brings me to the second virtue of Messas' book. Phenomenological psychopathologists often focus their research on a particular disorder. The diagnostic category establishes the starting point and the scope of the study. But Messas proceeds in a different direction. Rather than start from a particular diagnosis, he starts from a particular behavior: substance misuse. I can't stress enough just how much of a difference this starting point makes. Rather than analyze a broad category of disorder and eventually inquire into how one might behave as the result of having such a disorder, Messas begins from the behavior that leads his patients to the clinic in the first place—only from here does he inquire into the particular pathology, whether anthropological or structural, that may have led his patient to behave in such a way. By moving in this direction, he starts from a position of immediate clinical value. The behavior that his patients want to change is the anchor for his philosophical analyses. And, once he's provided each analysis, the behavior of substance misuse becomes eminently understandable. Substance misuse is among the most stigmatized of behaviors in nearly every culture. Yet, after Messas carefully unpacks the existential predicament of those who engage in such behavior, the reader will find it difficult if not impossible to stigmatize or judge. The behavior no longer seems chaotic or unpredictable; rather, it becomes an obvious way of coping. In this respect, Messas' approach has value not only for patients, but also for the patient's family and friends who want to understand a set of behaviors that, to them, may have seemed beyond comprehension.

The goal of phenomenological psychopathology is to comprehend precisely those experiences and behaviors that, at first, seem incomprehensible. Measured against this standard, Messas' book is an exemplar in the field. It sediments him not only as a leading figure in phenomenological psychopathology, but also as the foremost expert on the phenomenology of substance misuse.

Anthony Vincent Fernandez
Kent State University
Kent, OH, USA
University of Oxford
Oxford, UK

Preface

This book contributes to one of the most challenging areas of mental health: substance misuse. Its focus is on the psychopathological experiences associated with it: both the consequences of substance misuse and the existential vulnerabilities that lead to it, even if such a clear-cut distinction is rarely possible. The work brings an innovative perspective to the issue, as it draws on two scientific fields whose association has not yet been fully explored: phenomenological psychopathology and substance misuse studies. The association of these two perspectives could build a greater understanding of this important topic and be of practical help to a wide array of professionals in their clinical practice.

Substance misuse is a heterogeneous field of existential conditions which range from the free personal decision to modify the state of consciousness to profound changes in the capacity for freedom of existence, passing through various conditions of vulnerability and specific or nonspecific comorbidities. What this heterogeneous group of conditions share, above all, is the uncontrolled use of psychotropic substances, although the exact parameters of the disturbed status of such experiences are not easy to define. Consequently, despite its epidemiological importance, the field of substance misuse studies is still marred by controversies and scientific inaccuracies, which this book seeks to mitigate.

Phenomenological psychopathology is a human science that aims to depict the core characteristics of disturbed experiences, constituting the most comprehensive tool for addressing mental disorders. In recent years, in response to increasing interest in the approach across the world, phenomenological psychopathology has been applied to a variety of mental disorders, especially schizophrenia and depression. More recently, some clinical contributions based on the phenomenological method have been published, pushing the frontiers of the discipline into clinical practice. Although these findings are welcomed as promising for the future of mental health care, the application of the approach to substance misuse is still in its infancy. One goal of this book is to fill this gap, introducing a wider audience to the different ways phenomenological psychopathology can shed light on substance misuse and enable a more informed and targeted offer of clinical care strategies. As a core discipline of psychiatry and clinical psychology, it is the science that delimits the object to which all clinical practice is directed. As such, any clinical training which purports to be comprehensive and coherent should begin with an in-depth introduction to this field. The broad objective of this book is therefore to introduce this understanding, offering a useful instrument for mental health clinicians, psychiatrists, psychologists, nurses, undergraduate students of these disciplines, and all substance abuse workers. The structure of the book is inspired by this overall perspective. Its division into three parts is designed to introduce the reader, in a stepwise manner, to the complexities of the theme, based on the latest advances in the specific literature.

The division of the work into three parts is designed to allow them to stand alone up to a point. As phenomenological psychopathology is based on the conception that all psychopathological understanding is ultimately a general hermeneutic of the human condition, it is impossible to completely divorce it from a philosophical interpretation of human existence. It is this that is presented in the first part of the book, which is recommended for readers who appreciate philosophical reflections and disputes over concepts. The second and third parts are specifically psychopathological. The second examines the topic of substance misuse as a part of general psychopathology, whose fundamental interest lies in the meaning of existential vulnerability and comorbidities with the use and misuse of psychoactive substances. It will be of most interest to those who are keen to acquire a broad and general view of the whole edifice of phenomenological psychopathology. The third part focuses specifically on the psychopathology of substance misuse, observing the ways in which the modifications of consciousness produced by psychotropic drugs gain meaning for existence, while also producing significant changes in the ability of existence to fulfil its dialectical destiny. In this third part, specific psychopathological changes are always seen as modifications that could happen to any of us, as they are fruits of the human condition itself. This part is the most novel and original. It draws the reader into the complex and ambiguous ways in which substance use infiltrates and distorts existence. Throughout the book, clinical examples are given to enrich the psychopathological explanations and show how real people experience the complex interplay of altered experience and substance use.

São Paulo, Brazil   Guilherme Messas

Acknowledgement

This book represents the culmination of an intellectual trajectory which began some 25 years ago almost by chance and now converges in this broad interrogation of the very bedrock of human existence. I am grateful to all the people who have accompanied me in this process, whether through shared readings or in the long years of study groups I have led, giving me the chance to peruse the vast body of classical phenomenological literature. This book would certainly not have been possible without these groups, the hermeneutic rigor of their readings and the temporal breadth of their references, from the earliest contributions to the most recent.

This is a book by a medical doctor who is fascinated by human existence and who in this sense feels like an epigone of the Hippocratic tradition and, in the twentieth century, of Jaspers. Because I am a doctor, the truth is that the greatest contributors to this book were actually the people I have treated over the last 28 years. No literature can surpass in value the deference these people, whom we call patients, paid me in sharing their existential pains. I am profoundly grateful to them all.

Although this short list of acknowledgements cannot include all the people I am grateful to for their intellectual contributions, I will attempt to do so according to the number of hours of intellectual discussion we have shared (in alphabetical order). Initially, my thanks go to Daniela Ceron-Litvoc, Susan Mondoni, Melissa Tamelini and Antonia Tonus, whose meticulous readings of texts in a study group for 17 unbroken years are the very core and lifeblood of this work. In a way, this work belongs to all of us, although it is written by my hand and structured in my thoughts. I also wish to thank all my colleagues from the Brazilian Society of Phenomeno-Structural Psychopathology (SBPFE), who, since 2006, have been divulging and revising phenomenological psychopathology through courses, seminars, lectures and congresses, and especially through the journal *Psicopatologia Fenomenológica Contemporânea*, which it was my honour to co-found and to edit for many years.

The ideas elaborated and developed in this book have been matured over the years at several scientific academic events held in different parts of the world. At all of them, the criticisms and suggestions made by colleagues were indispensable for refining the ideas brought together here. Just as they will continue to be in the future as they are further refined. For their dedication to the discussion of such complex themes, not to mention the boundless passion with which they did and still do so, I extend specific thanks to my partners Mauro Aranha, Claudio Banzato, Georges Charbonneau, John Cutting, Maurício Daker, Thomas Fuchs, Gilberto Di Petta, Otto Dörr-Zoegers, Anthony Fernandez, Bill Fulford, Adriano Holanda, Virginia Moreira, Michael Musalek, Maria Lucrecia Rovaletti, John Sadler, Louis Sass, Giovanni Stanghellini, Pedro Varandas, and both the prefacers of my previous books, the philosophers Alex Moura and Cristiano Rezende

The first part of this book is a synthesis of the didactic material developed and honed over 7 years for the course given as part of the master's program in phenomenological psychopathology at the Santa Casa de São Paulo School of Medical Sciences, my institution, whose courage, intellectual independence and academic ambition were instrumental in bringing this topic to prominence in the country. I am most grateful not only to this institution, but also to all the students have who shared their lives with me over these years and helped me mature these ideas. They have each left their own mark on the work.

Thanks also to the Collaborating Centre for Values-Based Practice in Health and Social Care, St. Catherine's College, Oxford, coordinated by Bill Fulford, from which I have received great support and of which I have the honour of being a member, and to the International Network of Philosophy and Psychiatry (INPP), which keeps alive the flame of philosophical thinking in psychiatry and psychology.

A small portion of the ideas presented here have been published elsewhere in peer-reviewed scientific publications. To their reviewers, whose attentive reading and careful suggestions influenced this work diffusely, I also express my gratitude.

I would also like to express my thanks:

To the two reviewers who approved the proposal of this book.

To my colleagues Melissa Tamelini and Livia Fukuda, for their detailed and painstaking reading of the drafts of this work – and for their sharp, relentless and generous criticism. Especially to Livia, the associate author of this work, for her detailed, competent and tireless support in discussing all the intellectual details that I expose here and presenting solutions to all the editorial and bibliographical difficulties. Literally, this work is ours.

To my editor, Erica Ferraz at Springer Nature, whose dedication, courteousness and competence (and patience) were instrumental in bringing this work to light.

To my proofreader Rebecca Atkinson, whose meticulous reading, discussion and post-editing of the manuscript gave it a new voice in English.

To Valentim Gentil, my friend and Master, who, despite never having devoted himself to phenomenological psychopathology, has in various ways enabled me to successfully pursue this life course.

To Tadeu Andrade, for kindly offering all his professional expertise in Ancient Greek, so fundamental for the linguistic precision of all the neologisms created here.

Finally, the people to whom this book is dedicated. To Cris, Pedro and Mari, the eternal loves of my life. And to my parents: I am nothing but proud of incarnating your spirits, which already inhabit the ether; a link in the chain between you and those who will come... it has been a great honour.

Contents

Chapter 1
Introduction

Wine, teach me the art of seeing my own past
As if it were already memory's ash
(Wine Sonnet, Jorge Luis Borges)

Phenomenological psychopathology is a core discipline of psychiatry and clinical psychology, as it is the science that delimits the object to which all clinical practice is directed. As such, any clinical training that purports to be comprehensive and coherent should begin with an in-depth introduction to this field. The first person to postulate an association between phenomenology and psychopathology was Karl Jaspers (1968). However, this young German psychiatrist and future philosopher saw phenomenology as no more than a descriptive stage in an intellectual procedure geared primarily towards the epistemological organisation of methods that already existed in psychiatry. In his conception of a general psychopathology, Jaspers saw the role of phenomenology as being restricted to a first-person description of distorted experiences (Messas 2014a). Despite this limited conception, it was precisely this procedure that marked the birth of psychopathology as an autonomous science, validated by its own internal criteria and with its own categories for apprehending reality.

However, it was when the scientific scope expanded to more than just a description of psychopathological experiences that a truly phenomenological psychopathology came into existence (Fuchs et al. 2019). Its origins date back to 1922, when figures such as Minkowski and Binswanger, attending a symposium in Zurich, set the founding stone of what is today known as phenomenological psychopathology (Tatossian 2002). From then on, phenomenological psychopathology started to be understood not just as a description of the subjective experiences of persons suffering mental disorders but also a search for their conditions of possibility – the structures that underpin the experience of reality, which, when modified, determine psychopathological experiences. The results of a phenomenological comprehension of the conditions of possibility serve to reconstruct the whole structure of

© Springer Nature Switzerland AG 2021
G. Messas, *The Existential Structure of Substance Misuse*,
https://doi.org/10.1007/978-3-030-62724-9_1

existence[1] of some afflicted persons, whom I refer to here as patients. Although throughout the history of the discipline there has been considerable variation in the names and perspectives of the conditions of possibility, it is possible to argue that their identification and study is what unifies the science of phenomenological psychopathology. The wealth of scientific writings produced after 1922 is characterised by analyses of modifications in these conditions of possibility and their correlated distorted experiences. Similarly, in the wealth of contemporary contributions to phenomenological psychopathology, as demonstrated by a recent edition of the *Oxford Handbook of Phenomenological Psychopathology*, the study of the conditions of possibility of existence is of primary interest (Stanghellini et al. 2019).

The fact that phenomenological psychopathology operates on the level of the conditions of possibility calls for two further explanations of how they interrelate to patients' subjective experiences. First, a condition of possibility is not an experience but a zone of determinations and restrictions within which experiences may emerge. It is therefore beyond the field of experience but is responsible for setting the limits and defining the features of experiences. It is like a mould that provides the contours of a sculpture but is not present in the final work. As it is beyond the layer of subjective experience, it is called transcendental. The best example of this property is perspective. When we look at an object, our perceptual experience identifies it as something that exists in the world, independent from us and at a certain distance from our body. Nonetheless, for there to be such a perception, there must be a prior world design that enables the object to be appropriated by our gaze. This prior field of vision is perspective, which delimits and determines the way the subjective apprehension of the object is endowed to us. As such, its transcendental action is fundamental in determining the way the world is transformed into visuality for us. Due to this interest, the scope of phenomenological psychopathology is different from that of descriptive psychopathology, the mainstream of psychiatric training. Descriptive psychopathology focuses on examining subjective and objectively measurable experiences (Oyebode 2018), whereas the ultimate field of knowledge of phenomenological psychopathology is the study of whatever preconditions and preconfigures these experiences. Its overarching interest encompasses the whole structure of existence.

Second, subjective experiences stem from the organic articulation of these conditions of possibility amongst themselves, which brings about the manifestation of a structured existence. So, any subjective experience must be understood from its

---

[1] Although the whole of existence as an object of study in phenomenological psychopathology is also known as "lived world", I gave, in this book, preference for this more somewhat philosophical concept of structure of existence due to its more overarching meaning, since it comprehends not only the self, but also the other, and the world, as we will see throughout the book. On the other hand, "lived world" unjustifiably highlights only the worldly aspect of existing. In addition, I tend to agree with Charbonneau that it is not easy to determine what lived world means, because it has to do with the "indeterminate background" (Charbonneau 2010, tome 1, p. 69, note 12) in which the mysteries of human existence occur.

articulation with the whole of existence, constituting a dialectic relationship. It is dialectic because it is based on the idea that each specific experience (sadness, fear, hope, delusion, etc.) gains its own meaning from its relationship with the significant whole of existence. There is no such thing as a specific experience endowed with an inherent meaning without reference to its relative position in the circle of intersubjective and worldly relations in which existence is rooted.

In order to operationalise this enlarged conception of psychopathology, a specific two-step epistemological procedure is required. First, from the direct description of the subjective experiences of some patients, the psychopathologist is able to gain a first-person perspective on the psychopathological object. This procedure is not, however, enough to gain access to the conditions of possibility of existence, for which a second-person perspective must be added. This is gained through the exercise of phenomenological comprehension, in which the psychopathologist penetrates the material contained in the subjective description of the patient and, by an act of hermeneutical comprehension, comprehends the meaning of their experiences (Messas and Fukuda 2018). This search for meaning penetrates the very structure by which the unity of existence is organised and assured. The methodological strategy of this book adopts this mixture of first- and second-person perspectives. The many clinical examples it offers serve to two purposes. First, they give us access to some self-reported experiences of patients: the first-person perspective. Simultaneously, they are articulated in such a way as to bring forth their respective psychopathological structured experiences, constituting a second-person perspective. It follows from this procedure that the reconstruction of these structured existences – that is the epistemological result of phenomenological psychopathology – is a composite of subjective self-descriptions and phenomenological comprehension.[2]

Phenomenological psychopathology is based on the conception that all psychopathological understanding is ultimately a general hermeneutic of the human condition. It is therefore impossible to completely divorce it from a philosophical interpretation of human existence. Although the core interest of this volume is limited to psychopathology, it also inevitably evokes an anthropological bedrock. In other words, there is a theory of human existence underpinning each category of phenomenological psychopathology and each clinical act or therapeutic decision. Accordingly, the first part of this book sets forth the anthropological roots of my conception of phenomenological psychopathology. This defence of a fundamental anthropology makes this work auctorial in nature. Science and auctoriality are not mutually exclusive. Indeed, evidence acquired in scientific research is enriched by the incorporation of the values of the researcher who applies them to specific cases. Every psychopathology is the application of the humanities, which makes it a

---

[2] It is worth noting that although the psychopathological positions expressed here always employ this two-step approach, the first part is sometimes not included and the phenomenological comprehension is proposed without any accompanying subjective account. This is done simply because of space limitations.

values-based science (Fulford et al. 2012; Messas et al. 2017a). An auctorial work in the field of psychopathology is thus not so much an exercise in academic erudition – although at no point is its rigor abdicated – as an exploration of new frontiers that the empirical application of a body of personal values may lead to. Its language is therefore inevitably essay-esque, insofar as an essay, like music, permits improvisations on themes already examined, synthesised and acknowledged. Or insofar as an essay, in the classical sense given by Montaigne, is an indication of dialogue with a consolidated tradition. A values-based essay is a personal contribution to a heterogeneous but unified body of work.

The anthropology that underpins this undertaking is expressed in the conditions of possibility of experience. Every experience is based on and rooted in the world through these conditions. They are the a priori foundations of existence, which provide the conditions for any personal biography to be developed and expressed. For the purposes of this book, the fundamental conditions of possibility of existence will be given technical terms designed to distinguish them from the acceptation of the words in non-specialised language. For example, I use temporality rather than time, spatiality rather than space, embodiment rather than body. These terms serve to indicate transcendental and non-experiential categories that have to do with the conditions of possibility, rather than the time, space or body we experience subjectively. The reader may notice, in the dynamics of the book, the relevance of this decision.

But the notion of condition of possibility is not exhausted with this preliminary delineation. Presented one by one, linearly articulated as if they were isolated points to be checked off for a diagnosis, they reveal little about any one existence. Investigated in isolation as elements, they would serve no more than a first step towards psychopathological understanding. Elementarism as the endpoint of an investigation is an epistemological position refuted by phenomenological psychopathology (Tamelini and Messas 2017). A deeper understanding of existential reality calls for us to define conditions of possibility as participants in the dialectical relations that constitute existence, which converge towards a notion of whole, existential totality. Therefore, this first part is complemented by an overview of the structure of existence. The part-whole dialectic between the conditions of possibility of existence as an ontological-epistemological option is what distinguishes the approach offered in this work. I call this procedure dialectical-proportional phenomenological psychopathology. By *dialectic* I mean the examination of the reciprocal relationships of the components of human existence, which interact in oppositions, tensions, absorptions and ambiguities. It is precisely because it is essentially dialectic that human existence can be enriched and modified over its biographical trajectory. In line with Jaspers, I argue that these dialectical movements, always in often irreconcilable tension and opposition, are responsible for the emergence of the existential movement (1997, p. 341).

The empirical results of this branch of phenomenological psychopathology will be presented throughout the work. In this introduction, I would just like to mention the epistemological contributions the notion of proportional dialectic brings to the science of psychopathology and person-centred psychiatric and psychological clinical practice. Due to its ability to articulate different existential tendencies in a simultaneous regime of proportionality, dialectical-proportional phenomenological psychopathology (i) enables the accurate apprehension of the complexities of psychopathological experiences; (ii) helps offer a more refined scientific observation of the movements and transformations existences undergo in their life course by introducing pre-reflexive conceptual elements for apprehending the kinetics of existence; (iii) equips the psychopathologist to identify the ambiguities contained in existence and in each psychopathological experience and (iv) provides conceptual instruments for the expansion of the science of phenomenological psychopathology to territories as yet little explored, such as substance misuse, the specific object of this work.

Although phenomenological psychopathology has been applied to a vast array of topics, the field of substance misuse is largely unexplored by this empirical science. One of the possible explanations for this is the degree of complexity required to address it. Substance misuse is a heterogeneous field of conditions which range from the free personal decision to modify the state of consciousness to profound changes in the capacity for freedom of existence, passing through various conditions of vulnerability and specific or nonspecific comorbidities. The complexity required for a comprehensive approach to such a topic stems, I would argue, from the fact that the psychopathology of substance misuse cannot be approached from a single investigative perspective. The psychopathological approaches must therefore be organised methodologically. Two perspectives will be placed side by side, although it would be erroneous to imagine they are completely independent of one another. In the first of these, substance misuse should be understood as part of existential vulnerabilities, the main result of which are the comorbidities of mental disorders and substance misuse. The second part of this book examines the topic of substance misuse as a by-product of general psychopathology, whose fundamental interest lies in the meaning of existential vulnerability and comorbidities with the use and abuse of psychoactive substances. This part should therefore be understood as a miniature general psychopathology tailored to the understanding of substance misuse. All the phenomenological analyses conducted in this part are based on empirical evidence of the conditions of vulnerability and comorbidities that are most epidemiologically relevant for the understanding of substance misuse. In this sense, substance misuse is a secondary product in this approach despite being the ultimate purpose of this whole section on general psychopathology. To my mind, no coherent approach to substance misuse is possible without first having a general comprehension of the alterations of existence. Given its more general nature, this second part is called psychopathology *and* substance misuse. The third part of the work focuses specifically on the psychopathology of substance misuse, observing the existential meanings by which the modifications of consciousness produced by psychotropic drugs gain meaning for existence while also producing significant changes in the ability of existence to fulfil its dialectical destiny. In this third part, specific psychopathological changes are always seen as modifications that could happen to any of us, as they are fruits of the human condition itself. This third part is entitled the psychopathology *of* substance misuse.

The fact that there are two simultaneous phenomenological psychopathological approaches to the same topic has its pros and cons. On the plus side, I intend to bridge the gap in the psychopathological literature on substance misuse without oversimplifying it. This dual apprehension of reality prevents any psychopathological understanding of substance misuse from calcifying into a rigid system of thought that would ultimately close itself off to intellectual renewal. The downside of this dual epistemological perspective is that it leads to a certain overlapping of themes. Some repetition will be inevitable to ensure coherence to the text. However, the overlapping does not imply an *ipsis litteris* reproduction of certain concepts; rather, it means observing similar subjective and intersubjective experiences from different perspectives, with the same experience gaining a different name according to the epistemological perspective to which it is linked.

The division of the work into three parts is designed to allow them to stand alone up to a point. The first part can be read separately as an anthropological proposal on the foundations of existence and also, to some extent, a glossary for the two subsequent parts. It is recommended for readers who appreciate philosophical reflections and disputes over concepts. The second part can be read as a dialectical-proportional contribution to phenomenological psychopathology. It will be of most interest to those who are keen to acquire a broad and general view of the whole edifice of phenomenological psychopathology. The third part is the most novel and original. It draws the reader into the complex and ambiguous ways in which substance use infiltrates and distorts existence. However, while each part is relatively independent, full understanding can only be achieved by delving into all three. I therefore provide cross-references wherever appropriate to help enrich the reading experience, and by so doing make the work more reader-friendly.

This book is the final volume in a trilogy devoted entirely to the examination of the main dialectics of existence. The first focused on the dialectic between permanence and stability in existence, using clinical cases as illustrations to examine the contradictions inherent to a being that is transformed over time and yet never ceases to be identical to itself (Messas 2010b). The second work in this trilogy contributed to reflections on the human antinomy that is particularity-generality. Through clinical cases, I indicated how the science of psychopathology can and should access human existences as simultaneously singular and representative of a general type (Messas 2014c). Finally, in this work, I return to the dialectical relations studied in the previous two works, synthesising them with the examination of the internal relationships and reality-constituting relationships implied in each psychopathological experience. From the perspective of psychopathological science, it is the most comprehensive work of the three. It consists of the dialectical and synthetic maturation of the previous two, building on and lending new meaning to their contents.

This effort of synthesis takes form in an immersion in the structured existences of substance misusers. The notion of substance misuse goes beyond the operational sense with which substance-use disorders are catalogued in the latest mainstream classifications of mental disorders, the World Health Organisation's International Classification of the Diseases (ICD-11) and the American Psychiatric Association's

Diagnostic and Statistical Manual of Mental Disorders, fifth edition (DSM-5). This distance between the conception developed here and the mainstream classifications does not imply a denial of their worth, as will be indicated – albeit briefly – in the third part of this book. Rather, what this volume offers the community of psychiatrists and clinical psychologists is an in-depth reflection on the integral existential meanings that underlie these operational criteria. The destiny of phenomenology is to go beyond the evident manifestations of reality without ever denying them. It is an attitude that is profoundly anchored in admiring respect for the infinite complexity contained in the ineffable fact that we exist.

Part I
The Anthropological Roots of Phenomenological Psychopathology: Core Concepts

Chapter 2
The Conditions of Possibility of Existence

I will start by presenting the conditions of possibility as elements, that is, apprehended from an isolated perspective. This separate investigation, covering the first five sections of this part, will allow a detailed assessment to be made of the essential properties of each of the conditions of possibility. While such a detailed analysis takes us into the depths of the bedrock of existence, it does have a somewhat idealised fictional overtone, insofar as it separates out what actually happens between the different conditions of possibility in relationships of articulation and simultaneity. Any psychopathological comprehension will only be complete once an examination supplementing this isolated view of the conditions of possibility has been done (Fukuda and Tamelini 2016). For the purposes of psychopathology, the importance of identifying each condition of possibility separately is matched by the importance of examining how they are articulated dialectically among their own intrinsic components and among themselves in a regime of anthropological proportions. After this, I will show how these conditions of possibility are unified in the existential whole, constituting a structure. This will be the theme of the sixth section of this part.

Once the conditions of possibility of existence and its structural unity are presented, I will conclude this first part of the book with reflections of an ontological and epistemological nature about the psychopathological object. These considerations serve as a final clarification so that the contents presented in Parts II and III can be understood by the reader to their full extent.

2.1 Temporality

Temporality is the condition of possibility that has received the most attention in classical phenomenological psychopathology. Several of the early authors sought to understand pathological mental experiences from the perspective of alterations in temporality (Minkowski 1995; von Gebsattel 1966b; Straus 1935; Binswanger

© Springer Nature Switzerland AG 2021
G. Messas, *The Existential Structure of Substance Misuse*,
https://doi.org/10.1007/978-3-030-62724-9_2

1957, 2000). Whether in the importing of philosophical concepts[1] or in the direct observation of patients, temporality is the fundamental condition of possibility that constitutes and enables the historicity of existence. Important contemporary contributions of phenomenological psychopathology continue to sustain the capital value of temporality as the anthropological foundation of psychopathology (Charbonneau 2010; Fuchs 2013; Messas 2014c; Moskalewicz and Schwartz 2020a, b). To exist is to unfold over time, allowing existence to reveal itself. Ultimately, every existence and every disorder is lent a peculiar timbre of temporality, which provides the best guide for the phenomenological psychopathologist for both diagnosis and therapeutic management. But first, I shall explain how I understand this notion.

There are two simultaneous perspectives from which I will observe temporality in terms of phenomenological psychopathology. The need to understand a particular clinical case will always be what dictates which perspective is best for a given patient in a determined period of observation.

2.1.1   Transversal Temporality

All human experience is conditioned by a prior temporal articulation. This is so primordial that we do not always realise it. For example, at this very moment, as I write, there is the direct, physical presence of the computer screen in front of my eyes. At the same time, there is a flow of ideas in my mind which I record on this computer. These are the most direct experiences of my consciousness at this moment; they are part of the *present* of my consciousness. But I am in front of the computer typing with a clear purpose, namely, to write a work of phenomenological psychopathology. There is a tacit assumption here that other people will read it, which will generate discussion, interest or repudiation. The whole field of purposes to which my activity is directed – and which is therefore virtual and not directly experienced now – is conditioned and enabled by the *protention* of my consciousness. I could also name this temporal dimension "the future", but I prefer protention, with its roots in Husserlian philosophy (Husserl 1991). However, just because I am borrowing terms from works of philosophy, such as protention (and later, retention), this does not mean I will necessarily use them as they were originally conceived. In the case of protention, Husserl was guided by a remarkably specific interest, focused on the examination of temporal consciousness.[2] The example he uses is of music. As a melody evolves, we expect it to continue in a particular style. This expectation is protention. At the same time, we apprehend the sounds we hear separately as belonging to a melody. This maintenance in our mind of previous sounds, lending them unity in the form of melody, is retention. This focus on the temporal forms of

---

[1] Heidegger stresses the value of temporality for being (Heidegger 2006); Bergson proposes it as fundamental to life (Bergson 1889).

[2] For Husserl, protention is the future to which an immediate state of consciousness is directed, while retention is the web of themes which sustains that state.

human consciousness is not what I am interested in here. However, it seems to me that these categories can be used to convey a specific phenomenological sense, justifying their use in this psychopathological work. The choice of the word protention is justified by the fact that its meaning covers not only what is to come, in a broad and generic way – as is implied in the notion of future – but also indicates the internal connection of this future to the present structural state. Protention is the future that is by definition connected to the direct presence of whatever is or exists now. In other words, protention is everything that is part of the specific future restricted to the field of possibility of this present in which my existence is embedded. Protention is the future of my circumstances. Therefore, protention is also mobile, because it depends on the current conditions of the present. For example, if I am going through a deep existential crisis because I am dissatisfied with my work, but I cannot give it up, my protention is restricted to wondering how I might inject some pleasure into something that does not motivate me. My imagination and my affects are restricted by this protentive range. If, however, I suddenly lose this job, my protention enlarges to encompass wider concerns about how I will manage to survive and support my children.

As I continue to write, I recover ideas and thoughts that were already sedimented in my memory. They flow ceaselessly through the present towards a purpose, conjuring up subject matter and emotional states lodged in my memory. This restoration is permitted by the *retention* of my temporal experience. At first glance, it may seem that retention is memory, but we should not equate the two terms. Memory is the cognitive–affective portion of retention and, in a way, the most voluntary part of it – the part which may arise as a representation in present time (in images, abstract thoughts and feelings) of something that has already occurred. But we should not forget that the choice of these ideas and the value some have in relation to others stem from my experiences as a psychopathologist over the years. Even if (as is usually the case) I am unaware of all these experiences at the moment of my flow of thoughts, they are still active, as it were, giving involuntary support to my present consciousness and its protention, much like geological layers support the outer face of the Earth's crust. This sedimentary support is retention. Equally, it should not be confused with the past, for much the same reasons that we chose not to use the term *future*. Retention has the characteristics of implicit memory; however, in the conception I want to use here, it precedes implicit memory, because it does not just include the incorporation and automation of values and behaviours in apprehending the world. My concept of retention also includes the way in which these values and behaviours given in implicit memory are recruited in the instantaneous state of existence. Thus, retention is the implicit and explicit memory of *this* present, with which it has a dialectic relationship. Not only does it limit the possibilities of the present, but it is the portion of sedimentary experiences that is recruited pre-reflectively to sustain it. Retention is ontologically prior to implicit memory; it is the mould that provides the specific framework for the actualisation of experiences sedimented in existence (including memory), which are linked to the current state of existence. Because it is dependent on the current existential moment, as is protention, retention is also mobile. It is like the pattern a dressmaker uses to cut out the fabric for a dress, retaining only the parts of the fabric which serve their present purpose. There is, then, an umbilical relationship between retention and protention, because both depend on and are subordinated to the current state of the anthropological proportions of existence, as will be explored throughout this work. For example, a melancholic person tends to retain, from the total experiences of their life, the ones that have more to do with their social responsibilities. This hierarchy of priorities in the accommodation of experiences is a condition of possibility for memories per se, both explicit and implicit, as well as for imaginations concerning future life plans. This means that the concept of retention itself encompasses other conditions of possibility of existence, such as identity, which I will examine later (Sect. 2.5).

From an essential point of view, in a broad, preliminary simplification, we could say that the present is continuous actuality, protention is indetermination and the horizon of experiences relative to this actuality, and retention is its sedimentation and determination. It is also important to emphasise three aspects. The first refers to the inevitable co-activity of retention and protention in each conscious experience. Except in very serious psychopathological configurations, every experience of existence is constituted by this transversal trinity of temporality. Because of this inevitable intertwining, I will refer to retention and protention as two dimensions of temporality. Since experience is always present (even when we have a mnemonic representation, we actually have a present that experiences something with the typical intentionality of the past), I will treat the "virtual" dimensions as extensions which involve, enable and sustain the whole of the present, even if they are forward-oriented (protentive) or backward-oriented (retentive); hence, the term "dimensions". We should not, however, be mistaken by the metaphorical "virtuality" of these dimensions (given the unavoidable presence of existence in the world to oneself and to otherness): they should nonetheless be taken as active constituents of conscious experience. All present experience is only given by the non-present activity of retention and protention. They are indispensable even though they are transcendental, in that they are not experienced directly.

The second aspect to be indicated is the proportionality that inevitably exists between the three dimensions of temporality. Present, retention and protention co-occur actively in every act or experience. However, their internal relative participation varies enormously, and this variation is of great value, psychopathologically speaking. At this point, suffice it to indicate tangentially, with an everyday example, what this proportionality of the temporal dimensions means. When we are at a family gathering, we have psychological experiences and a general state of mind that are different from when we start working at a new job. From the point of view of transversal temporality, this happens because when we are with our family, the relative participation of retention is increased, giving greater stability to the emotions that arise there (for good and for bad), while in a new, formal setting, retention is minimal and the relative participation of protention is increased.

Third, it should be pointed out that these temporal dimensions have internal components whose differentiation is important for the progress of a psychopathology. Both retention and protention have one immediate and one remote components. The immediate portion of the dimensions generally refers to the needs of daily life, the mundane operations of the present. Working memory (in retention) and restlessness and anxiety (in protention) are cognitive instruments or typical experiences of immediacy. They are marked by a limited distinction between facts that are important and facts that are irrelevant to the whole of existence, since they are apprehended in crude terms. In contrast, the remote portion of the dimensions is what retains the core of each experience, reducing the unit value of each experience and giving it a broader meaning to the whole of existence. It is precisely because the structure of existence participates in an extended remote temporality that can give some meaning to life (Blankenburg 2007b). The loss or impaired development of the remote portion leaves the whole of existence at the mercy of immediate facts or experiences, culminating in typical conditions of anxiety or agitation. In a simplified way, we might say that when faced with a patient suffering from anxiety, agitation or restlessness (including some attention disorders), the psychopathologist should always try to identify whether these symptoms have their roots in remote or immediate temporality. In the former case, the disorder will be more severe, since existence does not move to any specific point, nor is it sustained by any guiding personal value. In the latter, although this may also occur in more serious conditions, the clinical finding is usually less relevant, given the solid footing existence has in temporality and thus the greater strength of the existential project.

2.1.2 Longitudinal Temporality

The notion of longitudinal temporality is intertwined with the classical notion of development, adopted in both Jaspersian psychopathology (Jaspers 1997) and phenomenological psychopathology (Lanteri-Laura 1962). Longitudinality is temporality par excellence, the line along which existence unfolds in movements of expansion and retraction, with experiences succeeding one another in a flow of time. Even a pathological existence that does not change over time – severe schizophrenia, for example – is not immune to the notion of longitudinal flow, as it registers its immobility as an addition to its biographical sedimentation, which therefore becomes retention. All existence is based on the sedimentation of the biography, so ultimately the effectiveness of all therapeutics derives from their capacity to offer new layers of sedimentation which have the effect of attenuating the activity of the previous ones, more prone to suffering or mental disorder. In Jaspers' words, the psychopathologist's supreme knowledge is the "bios" of his/her patient (Jaspers 1997). As every experience is inevitably present, longitudinal temporality is nothing more than the articulation of the successive stream of different transversal temporalities. As a consequence, longitudinal temporality can only be reconstructed from an understanding of transverse temporality, whose ontological (and heuristic) value is greater as it is always present and actualised. However, the condition for the possibility of any sustained modification in the proportions of temporal dimensions is longitudinal temporality, typically acting quietly and steadily on existence.

A simple example could serve to clarify this point, which is key for any psycho-pathological diagnostic assessment. Let us say that at a given moment, we experience a particular situation that leaves us stunned, shaken in every fibre of our being, as if the ground had disappeared from under our feet; yet at another time, we may be far less upset by circumstances which are even more complex or intolerable and may even have a far worse outcome. From the point of view of longitudinal temporality, this may occur because our transverse temporality, on the first occasion, was too present-oriented, making us susceptible to the acute distresses of life, while on the second, it was more rooted in retention, giving us a stable basis from which to withstand the ordeal. Stages of life, mental disorders or contingent existential states change the proportions of our temporal dimensions, making us more or less resilient to the challenges of existence and expanding or reducing our capacity to pursue an existential project. Whatever the reason, it is essential for the phenomenological psychopathologist to bear in mind the notion that each style or moment of longitudinal temporality has a typical proportional configuration of the dimensions of temporality. Generally, youth is more protentive and old age is more retentive. A hyperthymic person is more protentive, while a melancholic one is more retentive (as we will see in Sects. 3.3 and 3.4). A very interesting and enlightening experience of these typical dimensions of transversal temporality is to investigate how moments of existential anxiety appear in different personality types. A melancholic personality – even when going through a very healthy state – will tend to experience their existential anxiety as anguish, lack or indebtedness, focusing their consciousness on what they should have done in the past. Their anguish pursues them from retention, showing its relatively greater participation in existence (Tellenbach 1983; Dörr-Zegers 1995; Ratcliffe 2015). Meanwhile, a schizoid personality will experience their anxiety as a risk of rupture, an imminent threat to their life plans and a derailment of their existential course (see Sect. 3.7).

The most intense longitudinal structural movements of transformation in the proportions of transversal temporality are known as existential crises. Although they may be triggered for reasons that are sometimes relevant, what matters for their diagnosis is the recognition of a change in the anthropological proportions that constitute temporality. Continuous suffering, even if it takes on the magnitude of a mental disorder, does not constitute a crisis provided it occurs without the impetus of change in the proportions of temporality, although the re-accommodation of the proportions may occur as scarring in consequence of a pathological condition. For there to be a crisis, some transformation in the typical configuration must take place from within. For this reason, psychological reactions are not existential crises, since they have the purpose, on the structural level, of rebalancing proportions that have lost their equilibrium (Messas 2007). Nonetheless, an initially reactive phenomenon may turn into a crisis if it meets the conditions described earlier.

In summary, we have to identify a duplicity in the temporal condition of possibility of existence. On the one hand, every existence is flow and therefore continuous transformation, endowed by the very constitutive transversal nature of protention. But, simultaneously, it is continuity and permanence, endowed by the transversal constituent of retention. Anthropologically speaking, existence is therefore determined by a dialectic tension between stability and transformation (Messas 2010b). Given that the temporality of development is constituted by a chain of transversal temporalities, this means that from an existential point of view each characteristic style of transformation is relatively stable. This knowledge is crucial for the psychopathologist. Respect for this core of the structure of existence is synonymous for deep respect for the possibilities, values and expectations of the patient. Therapeutic success depends on it. I will deal with this subject in Parts II and III of this work.

Longitudinal temporality can be divided into different characteristic styles of personal experience, according to their basic forms of temporal proportion. They may mark a specific period of life, such as childhood, adulthood or old age, and they may mark certain fields of vital experience, such as marriage or professional roles. Sets of experiences can also be understood from these categories of longitudinal temporality, like membership of a group of friends or interest in a topic. Existential crises are marked by transformations that affect the whole of existence. In general, when resolved, these crises bring about a complete change in the basic style. The disproportions typical of each mental disorder, which are its transverse essence (Parts II and III), can be combined in all manner of ways with these longitudinal styles, giving each clinical case its unique overtones. Anxiety during adolescence will be different from the same anxiety in old age, not just because of its clinical presentation (Rubio and López-Ibor 2007) but primarily because of the longitudinal temporal orientation of the person in question.

Broadly speaking, there are six basic forms of longitudinal temporalisation, each associated with a typical transversal proportion. They will be presented here as existential phases: dawning, flourishing, maturity, twilight, exhaustion and iconisation.

- *The basic forms of longitudinal temporalisation*

(a) **Dawning** This phase often emerges in the person's consciousness intermittently, although often very intensely. This intermittence is the capital fact the psychopathologist must recognise; it is due to a significant diminishment of the dimension of retention with a concomitant elevation of protention. While retention loses strength at some of its most solid points, protention opens up at these points as an almost infinite field of as yet undetermined possibilities. The indeterminacy of this field of protention is propitious, in the most solid existences, for enabling creative imagination about oneself in the future. Of all normal experiences, adolescence is the field where this form of longitudinal temporalisation tends to occur. Experiences are intermittent and intense and marked by great passions tinged more with imaginative force than with the density of their real feasibility. Adolescent imagination is the fruit of a structure in which protention is the fundamental guiding thread, since the adolescent needs to progress and has as yet no thickly sedimented layers of retention.

However, in the most fragile existences or at times of greater existential vulnerability, this expanded protention can produce frightening phenomena in the affective domain. The most typical example of this situation is the emergence of panic attacks in early stages of existence, such as marriage, the birth of children, promotion at work or graduation, and heralding a new life. In the phase of dawning, the connection between protection and retention in transversal temporality is weak. The protentive movements are so wide that they are not always able to invoke enough retention for their execution, leading to an oscillation in the present dimension. In such a situation, the psychopathologist should recognise the importance of offering the patient present support. This serves not only to prevent the danger of this instability being augmented (which could lead to a deeper crisis, forcing an existence to recede) but also to help the patient not lose touch with the protentive elements which may begin to guide their existence. Going back to the example of panic attacks, this assistance, seen from an experiential perspective, means helping the patient remain aware of what their chosen life plan is – the new job, the marriage, etc. – and what elements in their biography give them the power to succeed in that endeavour.

(b) Flourishing   This is the continuation of dawning, but now with a solid enough grounding for the present to be articulated coherently and relatively consistently with protention and retention. This incremental connection with protention and retention in the existential structure produces a paradoxically enriching restriction of protention. Infinite, absolute, frightening protention is replaced by a protention that is broad but has defined edges and is sustained at specific points by retention. The transversal result of this new arrangement is the prominence of protention along with the simultaneous stability of the present and its retention. It is the existential period in which life becomes exciting and hopeful for future achievements, but without the hesitations typical of dawning. If we return to our example of our patient who suffered panic attacks in the longitudinal phase of dawning,[3] they are now at a stable point in their lives, taking the appropriate form for their new existential function, to which they can devote themselves fully. The existential atmosphere of flourishing is unsaturated, because the existential structure is constituted of a stabilised protention in search of fulfilment, with all the dimensions of temporality focused on one primary project. Existence is now ready to execute a life project. It is a time of greater subjective well-being, and one during which psychopathologists are rarely called upon to act. When they are, it will usually be for ad hoc adjustments to a life project or when the capacity to envisage such a project is temporarily blurred. In a way, this is when humanistic psychotherapy in its strict sense, which is to help in the implementation of an existential project, is most suited. The protentive orientation during flourishing means the present is involved with and attracted to protention, but is already solid enough to offer resistance in the face of any obstacles hampering the existential project. Imagining oneself in relation to the future is still more important than its effective experience actualised in the present, which makes the experiences in this period less solid, but makes it a period with more excitement

---

[3] Sometimes, panic attacks will disappear without therapeutic intervention, although in many others they will become dangerously chronified if they are not treated, obstructing the transition to the subsequent stage, flourishing.

and psychological impetus (although it may also lead to disappointment in the face of failure). This relationship changes in the next stage.

(c) **Maturity** As the name denotes, this is the period of maturity of experience. Maturity here refers not necessarily to the whole of existence, but perhaps to some key project that has reached its culmination, even if the overall meaning of life has not yet matured. Its distinctive mark is solidity and articulatory balance between the present and its temporal dimensions, which attain a stable configuration. Unlike in the previous period, there is a balance of power between retention and protention, giving rise to a plateau for the present that affords the safest of presences. Phenomenologically speaking, existence is immersed in an assured life project, in which experience has the same value as future imaginings of oneself. (For example, when asked about her dreams, a patient says, "why would I have any if I have every-thing I ever wished for? A happy family and all the material conditions to live?") Existence knows what it wants, it already knows how to do it and it has already acquired some security from its achievements. Although there are still protentive experiences, they are organised in coherence with the corresponding retention, rarely leading to oscillations in present consciousness. The scarcity of oscillations is not down to any restriction of the temporal flexibility of existence, but to an expansive equilibrium capable of accommodating many new facts without produc-ing turbulence. Sometimes, truly new experiences are even rejected because they make no sense to an existence immersed in the security of a project. Life is perme-ated by security, such that rarely will the psychopathologist be sought out at such a stage unless it is to help tolerate the pains inherent to this phase (such as loneliness). Rather, it is the psychopathologist's role to lead his patient to such a longitudinal configuration, which usually corresponds to the successful end of treatment.

Maturity favours the confrontation of radical themes. In the previous stage, flour-ishing, as the main project is not yet concluded, existence oscillates between opti-mism at what it feels it will accomplish and discouragement at any obstacles faced along the way – obstacles which will always constitute a threat to the execution of the project. This fundamental oscillation is produced by the horizon of indetermi-nacy in which it occurs and ends up vetoing any direct confrontation with the capital theme of existence: its finitude. Meanwhile, during maturity, this temporality of maximum equilibrium of the structure of existence, the project, now clearly defined and mature, is no longer capable of drawing an affective curtain across the horizon. Existence is faced with the clear consequences of fundamental decisions taken along the life cycle. In the absence of the obstacles generated by the affective oscil-lations of immaturity, existence starts to face the fact that it is itself the realisation of previous decisions made and the incorporation of values over time. The most serene reflections about the irreversible decisions of existence are the exclusive fruit of the phase of existential maturity, with its sense of satisfaction and clarity of vision. They are experienced with a minimum of emotion and a minimum of volun-tary effort, for retention now receives, processes and acts on the world pre-reflexively with maximum effectiveness. This is what enables a mature professional to make many of their technical decisions without even knowing clearly why they are right.

It is because of this sedimentation that acts during maturity that existence becomes distanced enough to take an interest in its continuation through transindividuality: its legacy, its life's work, which are the only perennial offerings human beings can give themselves and others. During maturity, a theme reaches its peak expression in the individual to such a point that the individual is distinguished from the theme. Having developed a theme to the full, the individual is absorbed by the totality of existence. For analogous reasons (and precisely the opposite of the ones seen in flourishing and twilight, which we will see below), this is propitious for opening up a magnificent clearing in finite existence. Only occasional moments of dense anguish overshadow the clarity required by the mystery of existence in order to be evident.

(d) Twilight Existential decline can only be defined by reference to the period of maturity which precedes it. It is the dusk that follows the fullness of maturity. It is revealed in phenomenological terms by the relative saturation of experiences; in structural terms, by an atrophy of protention in conjunction with an absence of any loosening of its link with the equivalent retention. This means that the existential project no longer moves existence as much as it once did, but remains its focus, even if existence will not normally find opportunities to reconfigure itself in the dimension of protention (not least because if this occurs, it will by definition be a crisis). The experience of sedimentation exceeds that of renewal or stimuli for the incorporation of new fecund experiences, transforming existence into a numbness of value, boredom or monotony. The thickness of the sedimentation of experience, which during maturity freed existence to concern itself with its legacy, now becomes automatism, where the doors of existential renewal are closed. During twilight, pre-reflexive professional experience may remain competent, irrespective of any clear support from rational will, but it can no longer mobilise existence. The structural expression of this condition is the relative supremacy of retention, accompanied by a lengthening of the present. What lengthens the present is the lack of protentive traction, since there is no loss of retention. Although this does not prevent sedimented experience from continuing to endow existence with value, it lacks the colours and lightness of before. The general atmosphere is one of the saturations. Some lighter, less tradition-oriented temperaments may withstand the twilight period better than others that are already very dense and naturally more retention-oriented.

In psychopathological terms, it is important to stress that the relationships between the period of maturity and its subsequent twilight are of considerable value. Twilight may occur after a state of maturity that is already rarefied in itself. This rarefaction means the present puts down quite superficial roots in retention, so when it enters twilight, it may quickly lose its articulation with retention. Given that protention is now also in decline, the loss of retention can push the present into a dangerous articulatory void, foreshadowing the style we will see next. In theory, such a situation could be indicative of the emergence of a serious disorder in a patient who is still very close to their period of maturity, as if the disorders were presenting anomalously, out of the blue, as it were. Sometimes, supposed maturity hides a structural flaw that is very vulnerable but is barely visible in everyday life and only recognisable with hindsight. In general, all that therapy can hope for at such times is the expectant maintenance of the status quo, offering support until such a time as a new phase of dawning can be glimpsed and preventing any vertiginous falls, which would culminate in more serious, potentially psychotic scenarios.

(e) Exhaustion This is the longitudinal style typical of severe mental illness. Transversally, its hallmark is the isolation of the present from the other temporal dimensions. Protention virtually disappears: existence loses its fundamental direction or even, in more severe cases, the capacity to experience any meaning. Retention is devalued to the extreme: there is nothing in the layers of existence that justifies it or even gives it a minimum of sustenance. Existence is crushed and restricted to a petrified present, null and void. This disconnection of the present from the other temporal dimensions forces all existence to attach to it. It is a state of extreme constriction of the present and extreme elevation of its participation. To exist is to be present to oneself and to the world all the time, with no path to follow or points of repair to go to. Phenomenologically, there is a tendency for affective experiences to be intense and disruptive, or else a need to produce extremes of affective experiences, even if by artificial means. An example of the former is the acute experience of anxiety and agitation in schizophrenia (Roberts et al. 2018 LF); the latter includes drug abuse by people who have reached exhaustion (the whole Part III will devote itself to this subject). Senile dementia with neurological roots is also an existential expression of exhaustion.

Exhaustion may appear after any of the aforementioned phases. Similarly, it may run into a new phase of dawning. However, exhaustion can affect a whole life, as in the case of schizophrenia or dementia. It is the style that psychopathologists have to deal with most of the time, or, at the very least, they will be their most serious cases.

(f) Iconisation In the general successive movement of longitudinal temporality, exhaustion follows twilight, which itself follows maturity. However, from the perspective of the totality of human existence, there is another evolutionary path from maturity to be found in the old age of certain particularly fulfilled biographies. This is iconisation, when the characteristics of maturity take on a particular structural hue without entering the downward slope of exhaustion. As I said earlier, during maturity, the existential project is based on a balance between retention and protention, which leads the present to broad, calm stability, where imagination of the future and incorporated experience have equal worth. When it evolves into twilight, this balance is lost and the experience of sedimentation overcomes that of renewal, draining the existential tonus. However, this biographically inevitable imbalance may take another course: while protention will still be lost, existence is not dragged down into retention. Ageing does not lead to twilight, but to iconisation. In this stage, existence is identified with a single theme, which is revealed as the maximum expression of the biographical opus. Protention recedes, and existence gradually loses interest in the pain of the world and becomes pre-reflexively desensitised to its variation and multiplicity. The present is assimilated into retention, and both engage in the continuous actualisation of a life project that can no longer be renewed, a project that represents complete fulfilment. All new experiences are rejected, but this does not mean life is exhausted or enters decline. On the contrary, it enters a sustained phase of maturity that is no longer disfigured by temporality. If in the phase of existential twilight, emphasis is on the accumulated layers of experience which densify the present; in iconisation, the emphasis is on the existential result (Dörr-Zegers 2005). The functional losses of ageing should not be mistaken for existential decline (Minkowski 1999b). While any deficits do express a measurable impairment of performance, they also reveal the structural transformation of all temporality: they are the adjustments of a cognitive instrument that must now serve an existence devoted exclusively to the maintenance of its own history, to contact with a self identified with a theme, to a specific value sense (Note: I explain this term in detail in Sect. 2.6.1) imprinted on and represented in the world. The protentive horizon is assimilated into retention and the present in a spiral of time that contemplates eternity. And the affect that eternity gently brings forth in consciousness is love, the objects of which are so assured that they allow for the almost absolute serenity of fulfilled old age. The perennial love of a fulfilled existence does not cease to envisage its continuation in other works, in epigones, in children and grandchildren, in the resonance of a name into a future in which the individual will no longer participate physically. In a way, this sensing of presence outside time is still a type of protention; however, rather than arising from the unsaturated openness of life, it arises from the penetration of spiritual sight and the serene experience of completeness of life.[4]

2.2   Spatiality

In its plurality of perspectives, spatiality is a condition of possibility that offers an original framework from which all manifestations of existence in relation to themselves, otherness and the world emerge. The following proposal does not exhaust all the ways in which the dimensions of spatiality may be framed, but is based on the understanding that spatiality encompasses some fundamental aspects for understanding existence (Straus 1935; Minkowski 1995; Binswanger 1999; Figal 2015; Silverstein et al. 2017). Some phenomena are understood through one dimension and others through another. But spatiality as a whole is a condition of possibility of every experience. Likewise, it is worth pointing out that only for didactic purposes can we separate spatiality and its dimensions from the totality of experience. The special problems arising from the projection of the other conditions of possibility on spatiality will be treated in the categories themselves, since they are modifications of spatiality problems and presuppose it. Nevertheless, it is not always clear when a particular theme belongs to spatiality or to another condition of possibility, nor is

---

[4] Completeness of life should not be mistaken for anthropological plenitude, which I will examine in the second and especially third part. The completeness of the phase of iconisation is an experience of fulfilment which does not reject the dialectics of existence, as occurs in plenitude.

there a clear dividing line between one dimension of spatiality and another: sometimes the choice is dictated by habit, the psychopathologist's experience or the need to elucidate a phenomenon more clearly.

Spatial Polarities The concept of proportionality, which I have already used in temporality to indicate the relationships between the temporal dimensions, is more self-evident in spatiality. Spatiality manifests more clearly the dialectics of its constituent proportions than temporality, which is useful not only for the presentation of its dimensions but also for their simultaneous investigation. For example, it is easier to perceive the proportion between the height and width of a building – since both appear simultaneously before our eyes – than the parts of a symphony, since in music the passages stored in retention are no longer before us when we have to articulate them with their meaning as a whole. Simultaneity is helpful for the identification of proportion; succession hampers it.

For this reason, spatiality is a prime perspective for the proportional dialectic comprehension of existence. Through this comprehension, the characteristics of spatiality are understood from the simultaneous observation of polar relations of components. Dialectic-proportional psychopathology focuses on spatial polarities (Messas et al. 2018). When we identify a spatial polarity, we immediately have the two ends of a continuum. Although there is an infinity of intermediate points, there are just two ends. For example, the geographical relationship between two cities can be examined in terms of poles. If we know their respective coordinates, we can measure the distance between them, which constitutes their maximum degree of opposition. However, if we go by car from one distance to the other, we will always be in a relationship of proportionality between them. We will always be closer to one than the other (except at the midpoint), which will give us a different perspective of the city we are leaving – which is becoming further away – and the city we are approaching. From the point of view of spatiality, existence is this car, which is sometimes closer to one pole, sometimes to the other. Similarly, spatiality is propitious for the reciprocal dialectics of multiple, simultaneous perspectives. As we will see, most of the time, the categories chosen differ from each other and are relevant primarily because of the polarities they encompass. It is the capacity of polarity to elucidate certain regions of existence that gives epistemological substance to their analysis.

2.2.1 Distance–Proximity

This is perhaps the only component of spatiality that could be reduced to a single term, namely *distance*. That is why it is the most generic polarity and the one which in a way contains all the others. Distance is the essence of everything that appears and which, by so doing already refers to something else. Only in an abstract composition of the world could we contemplate the idea of a phenomenal manifestation devoid of distance: an absolute being enclosed in itself and unrelated to anything other than its own identity. Since phenomenological psychopathology is not interested in the investigation of this ideal being, every manifestation is related to something in the world, linked to a network of other beings that have a position relative to it. The world of existence will always need a point of reference.

Distance from a particular point of reference is what enables the polarity of distance–proximity. This in turn rests on the conception of a point of reference which is not absolute, but is chosen to be central in the act of determining issues of distance and proximity. The experience of the self – which will be examined later (Sect. 2.5) – is this central point of distance. For example, we can feel the affectivity of a loved one as being very close to us, even if their body is at a considerable distance. The self can also modify its distance from its own centre through the necessities imposed by spatiality. In this sense, the self can be conceived as a sphere. For example, if we lose our balance as we are climbing a ladder and have to grab onto something so we do not fall off, our hand becomes the field of attention from which all distance is measured, while our previous centre – the experiential centre of the self – moves to the background. The ways in which distance and proximity are expressed are infinite, but their endpoints are fusion and vanishing.

But it is not only at the centre of the self that this spatial polarity is revealed; moods are also experienced through distance and closeness. Mood is the atmospheric texture that colours the relationship of the self with the world (Heidegger 2006). Mood can be more or less in tune with the naturalness of the cosmic world, more or less in harmony with it. There are some people, for example, who get nostalgic when the weather is fine or agitated when it is stormy, and then there are some whose mood is practically unaffected by changes around them. This spatial attunement develops into expansion or restriction of the participation of the world in the totality of existence. Psychopathological science benefits from the observation of this polarity, as we will see in the second and third parts of this study.

2.2.2   Centrality–Peripherality

This component is directly related to the previous one, but enables a distinction to be made that will be capital in diagnostic differentials. If the distance experienced allows two extreme points to be delimited, it says little about the way these two extremes relate to each other. The polarity that we are now investigating specifically concerns one way the poles can relate to each other. Every distance can be structured from an organising and irradiating centre. The relationship between this emanating centre of distance and its opposite pole determines a dialectic between centrality and peripherality. In the spatiality of *centrality*, the phenomenon being manifested appears in focus. The objects phenomenalised in centrality appear as if in the middle of a stage, constraining the other phenomenal manifestations to a less determined, less important background, which I call peripherality.

The most obvious example of centrality is shyness. When in the company of others, a shy person will feel uncomfortable simply because they exist with these others, even before the appearance of any subject matter or situation that might constitute a cause of vexation. The shy person's self is too centred in relation to otherness; they cannot help but feel they are attracting an excessive amount of attention by the human collectivity. It is worth noting, however, that centrality is not necessarily distressing. The performing arts are totally based on centrality, taking it as a source of inspiration and personal expansion.

Centrality can also focus on the objects of the world. In this case, the world-pole (the world that appears to the subject) appears in strong figure-ground contrast, where only the core of the object attracts the subject and everything else goes unnoticed. The romantic souls of certain people experience spatiality in this way. Their objects of infatuation enchantment appear in a passionate, idealised form, flawless and untainted by concrete existential circumstances. They are capable of acts that might be seen as unthinking, but most of the time there is no lack of reflection. Actually, they are resolute acts that come from a firm, lucid determination based on an object endowed with excessive centrality and focus.[5]

Centrality should not be taken for proximity. Proximity seeks to reduce the distance between the self-pole and the world-pole,[6] while this relationship is irrelevant for centrality. Indeed, more often than not, centrality shows a preference for distance, because it allows a much wider range of gazes to behold it. Attention-seeking behaviours, for example, tend to prefer a multiplicity of gazes, which requires distance. However, centrality may be linked to closeness, as is seen in the love relationships of immature people, who need the beloved pole to be nearby to remain as such.

In peripherality, the opposite occurs. Here, the presence of objects is faded and they are stripped of value and clarity. The figure-ground contrast is flattened in a lack of differentiation whose counterpoint, centrality, is located at the other extreme of spatiality. This is commonly found in mild melancholic depression or in some melancholic or low self-esteem temperaments. Melancholic people never experience themselves as the focus of an experience of inter-human interest, turning in on themselves and "disappearing", even against their will, in the eyes of otherness. Just as they feel they are unimportant, their fields of interests will also be peripheral, sometimes containing nothing attractive enough to be central, even if they never lose the ability to recognise the existence of some centrality. As one patient puts it, "sometimes I'm excited about my work, which I like, but there are times when every taste disappears, as if nothing was worthwhile any more". Whenever her "taste" disappears, the pole which her life is geared towards, her work, appears spatially as peripheral.

---

[5] The endowment of objects means the way the self-pole experiences objects. Endowment is a common philosophical term. Although it may be unfamiliar to the reader, I have decided to keep it because it is still the best way to indicate that what we perceive is "given" by the conditions of possibility that structure us pre-reflexively.

[6] In order to highlight the essentially dialectic and interdependent relationship between self, other and world, I have added the suffix "pole" to the three nouns whenever this interdependence is central to a precise comprehension of the meaning I wish to express.

However, in its relationship with the objects of the world, the most dramatic examples of peripherality are to be seen in attention deficits. This is a heterogeneous experience, an outcome that combines a diversity of psychopathological conditions whose use here as a homogeneous category would be a gross oversimplification. People with attention disorders find themselves in a world whose centre they are, a priori, unable to find. They grope for reality, experience its attractions here and there, but find no point at which to tether themselves. They jump from one point to another, from periphery to periphery, always looking for the centre. Every phenomenon of peripherality is a yearning for a centre around which to gravitate. This peripheralisation of the world therefore tends to be accompanied by different attempts to create a fictitious, temporary centre, especially by using psychoactive substances, or, in more serious cases, in the formation of delusions, about which I will speak later (Parts II and III). But peripheralisation is not all bad. Although the impossibility of centrality rocks and weakens existence, it also removes the weight of an overcentralised world, which can become an intolerable burden and lead to existential paralysis.

One specific mode of centrality–peripherality is spatial orientation. Here, the self emerges as the focal point for all movements in space. The centrality assured by spatial orientation functions like a safety jacket, bringing clarity and sharpness to all experience. With this orientation, the meaning of all experience is absolutely determined and is constituted by a self situated geometrically in a space in which objects are located according to the significance of their relationship to it. Spatial orientation is, so to speak, the fixing of the clarity of the self-pole in a world that is also clear and defined. It is no wonder, then, that disorders involving a lowering of consciousness (mainly of a neurological origin, but also in some mental illnesses and withdrawal syndromes), marked by a loss of spatial orientation, tend to trigger non-delusionary hallucinatory manifestations in a world experienced by the self as having no clear outlines. A patient may see and talk to spectres of long-dead relatives or see terrifying ghostly figures. Although the self-pole manages to remain intact, within certain limits, it is assailed by an indeterminacy of spatiality which produces these frightening overtones and an inability to put together any meaning, even if delusional. Where there is delusion, there is already some oriented mode of spatiality.

2.2.3 Integrity–Fragmentation

With the concept of integrity, I want to indicate every phenomenal manifestation that offers the entirety of its content or the object to which it relates,[7] both at the self-pole and at the world-pole. When at the self-pole, it indicates that the self is

---

[7]This wholeness does not exclude the typical indeterminacy of the endowments of temporality. When referring to the integrity of temporal things, we should understand that everything that can be actualised in a given period of time is endowed.

fully immersed in its experiences and in the reception of the objects it comes into contact with. Similarly, at the world-pole, the appearance of an object – otherness, material world, whatever the phenomenon – is integral and complete. This yields a relationship between a cohesive self and a cohesive world. The most dramatic example of this integrity of spatiality is melancholic psychosis, where not even severe psychosis is capable of shaking the integrity of the self-pole (Sect. 4.2).

In order to grasp the wealth of understandings this integrity–fragmentation polarity offers, we need to investigate the notion of integrity further. Essentially, it refers directly to the idea of plenitude of meaning. All meaning relates in some way to a whole, whatever dimension it is being observed by. When we see a human profile, for example, we immediately recognise its typical form as a figure and associate it with humankind. Even if this human is deprived of some limb, we still apprehend it in its entirety as "human" and only then will we "see" what it lacks. This is also clear in written language. It is normal, when we read a text in our most familiar language, for us not even to notice a simple typographical error, like a switched letter. This is because we are so attracted to the entire meaning of the word or what the text is about that we fail to notice a trivial shift in meaning. Integrity is meaning and meaning is integrity. This definition itself gives us grounds for a differentiation of enormous value for psychopathology, both in helping reach a diagnosis and in capturing existence as a whole. The integrity–fragmentation dialectic unfolds in two ways, depending on how spatiality relates to the preservation of existential meaning.

Integrity–Fragmentation Dialectics, with a Fully Preserved Meaning It was precisely this mode of polar spatiality that was revealed to us by the psychoanalytic view of hysteria and went down in the history of psychopathology. From the perspective of fragmentation, the self-pole or the world-pole is shattered, but it maintains a hidden relationship with a totality of meaning. Precisely because it is hidden but still exists, this pregnancy of meaning can be recovered by a hermeneutic act. Examples of this condition are classic cases of hysterical dissociation, in which the dissociative symptoms can be traced back in their biographical genesis and even cured through psychotherapy. When a fragile existence is faced with an experience whose biographical meaning is intolerable, it breaks this experience down into fragments, spreading the intensity of its meaning into smaller parts which are more bearable to the consciousness or lodging them in places – such as the body or otherness – to which consciousness has no access. Clearly, the existence of meaning is a prerequisite for it to be fragmented. So in fact, none of the integrity of the meaning is lost; rather, it is displaced and masked in a superficial movement of compensation. As such, there is no actual impairment of the completeness of meaning, which would consist in a peripheralisation of spatiality. In fact, the meaning is so powerful and intact that existence needs to fragment itself to tolerate it. Clinically, this fragmentation arises as hysterical indifference (Messas et al. 2019a): a special form of indifference hounded by meanings on every front.

If we turn back to integrity, what we have is meaning appearing in its absolute fullness, leaving no room for peripheral indeterminacy. It is all or nothing: either the manifestation makes sense or it is scotomised from the field of consciousness. This is typical of paranoia, where all things, all words, all personal interactions overflow in an uncomfortable excess of meanings. In this case, the typical polarity is not lost either, although it is reduced to a minimum. The only fragmentation that the paranoid person bears is a strong division of the world between friends – with whom they practically merge – and foes – whose great cohesion makes them so threatening they have to be kept away. In any case, integrity with preserved meaning always entails a certain relational tension which the psychopathologist can latch onto for diagnostic recognition.

Integrity–Fragmentation Dialectics, with Loss of Meaning The distinction between this and the previous mode of spatiality is fundamental for avoiding one of the most common misunderstandings in psychopathology: biographical hyperhermeneutics. In this case, a wide range of biographical meanings are read into every experience, even in those where mental disorders prevent them. For example, hyperhermeneutics treats hysterical experiences existentially in the same way and through the same categories as it treats schizophrenia. As I have suggested, if we want to track down biographical meanings hidden in hysterical experiences, we may find them. However, there is no reason to assume that meanings of the same nature can be found in schizophrenic psychosis (I will return to this in Sect. 4.1). It is clear that general anthropological meanings can be addressed, as Binswanger does (Binswanger 1957, case Suzanne Urban; Tamelini and Messas 2016), but in no sense does the content of a chronic delusion have the same existential value as the content of a hysterical psychotic dissociation in terms of its biographical origin and meaning to the whole of existence (Sigmund 1997; Messas et al. 2019a).

The archetypal case of the annulment of meaning is schizophrenia, especially its negative forms. Here, isolated fragments disconnected from existential totality multiply in the consciousness. Although they may be the remnants of something that once made some sense to the self, it can no longer be said to maintain any internal living relationship with any integrity. The field in which this form of spatiality is most evident is motricity, leading to repetitive, disjointed movements of limbs or the trunk with no particular objective. Even if the observer is able to see something in these stereotypes that resembles ordered movement, disharmony is actually what motivates them. In delusions, on the other hand, the level of confusion is exacerbated and the chance of hyperhermeneutics is greater, since many delusions contain subject matter that derives from the theme of the whole existence. Nonetheless, it is important to pay attention to the way these delusional ideas are manifested spatially. More often than not, especially in chronic schizophrenia, these delusions reveal a shattering of the dimensions of spatiality.

In these extreme cases, even the relational polarity between fragmentation and integrity is lost, with fragmentation taking precedence. Even in those cases where zones of integrity are retained in the structure of existence, a loss of polarity can still be observed. In most such cases, all that is preserved is some relationship between fragmentary annulment and the rest of the structure of existence. The most typical case of this is the relationship between a chronic schizophrenic and their delusion. Although this is devoid of biographical meaning, the fact that it attends existence chronically transforms it, dialectically, into an object of existence. Finally, I should point out that in the annulment of meaning, there is also no zone of gravitational indeterminacy, as seen in the centrality–peripherality dialectic. The world and the self are fragments lost in an existential vacuum, incapable of engaging mutually and meaningfully.

2.2.4 Compression–Relaxation

This dialectic is a subcategory of proximity distance, in which the emphasis is on a perspective that is useful for understanding the psychopathology of substance misuse. There is a formation of spatiality in which phenomena are endowed in such a compressed way that the very emergence of meaning is altered. I do not mean that it is lost or even fragmented; on the contrary, what happens in an excessive expression of meaning. Excessive integrity is implied here, since every meaning is totality. In this spatiality, the self-pole and the world-pole are so close that they tend towards fusion. The self-pole tends to be immersed in intersubjectivity and in the world and its components, especially materiality, with which it merges. Kimura (2005) calls the radical form of this spatiality *intrafestum*, a kind of banquet where the dividing lines between the world and the self are lost due to excessive compression. The paradigmatic case of this condition is intoxication by psychoactive substances. In this, the self is "freed from itself" and dissolves, Dionysian-like, approaching the inter-human world through eroticism and violence or in collective-inspired celebrations. Dionysian phenomena are par excellence structured by the spatiality of compression, the absorption of individual consciousness by a kind of ecstatic collective consciousness (I will return to this in Part III).

In spatial compression, there is a suppression of phenomenal plurality. In other words, whatever is being experienced overpowers the field of consciousness, hindering the natural human dialectics of part–whole relationships in favour of the whole. Other competing experiences are banished, which itself is also a phenomenon of integrity. In reality, it is the most radical form of integrity. The preferred temporality of compression is the present, which becomes a total present, in which absolute emphasis is placed on the manifestations of the object, which appears as absolute actualised presence. The compressed present functions like music heard too loud: the meaning is not lost, but the self is harmed by the excess of materiality through which it is conveyed.

The polarity that is dialectised with compression is relaxation, the simultaneous endowment of multiple experiences in consciousness. Relaxation is the spatiality of deep reflection and the healthy dialectics of existence. In it, there is a central theme that organises the subjective contents, attracting them to its course. However, as the contents take their course, other ideas, associations, more distant connections, unexpected metaphors, and syntheses all come to light, enriching the central theme. This fringe of indeterminacy that can be added to the central path is the hallmark of the spatiality of relaxation. Something that sets it apart from the other polarities is that where there is relaxation, there is no compression and vice versa. There is therefore no active polarity between compression and relaxation. Their dialectic is only of principles, not of simultaneity and proportion. An experience within the spatiality of compression cannot contain anything from the realm of relaxation. By definition, compression restricts dialectics, making the transition to the pole of relaxation difficult. The main example of this is the difficulty people have in giving up an addiction, which is the equivalent of replacing compression with relaxation (I will deal with this in more detail in Sect. 7.2). However, relaxation can be problematic in schizotypal or abulic personalities. In the former, the thought style or affect style encapsulates plurality to such an extent that no central meaning is capable of imbuing the totality of existence, which remains lost in a universe of polysemic but ultimately unproductive mental richness. In abulia, the absence of the pressure of meaning acts more on the will. In excessive relaxation, the self-pole is brought into play only weakly; in compression, it is an absolute presence.

2.2.5   Collectivity–Individuality

Classically, an essential anthropological distinction is observed between two forms of lived space: light space and dark space (Minkowski 1995). The former is responsible for the human experience of breadth, distance, freedom and range. But also, precisely because of its "daylight" brightness, it is the space of maximum evidence of objects, of defined borders; the space that conveys our similarities to our fellow human beings, making everything appear in a similar way to all. While still permitting the burgeoning of reflective introspection, light space is fundamentally the space of the collective, of the public domain, whose prime sensory expression is visuality.

But humans also live in dark space. Marked by indeterminacy and mystery, the self-pole is enshrouded in and directly touched by the surrounding atmosphere. It is the space of sonority, of music and of perceptive individuality. This individuality should not be mistaken for solipsistic subjectivism. Rather, it designates the singular proximity of contact between the world and the self, meaning objects are given in a configuration that is not shared. This is the spatiality of the individual, idiosyncrasy, introspection and experiential depth.

The dialectic polarity that fundamentally determines these opposites is collectivity–individuality. Phenomena can appear in space in two extremes. In collectivity, all experiences bear the mark of public similarity, of shared certainties and experiences, and of harmony with social values and themes; the preservation of the forms of phenomena; and also the presumed objective unity of phenomenon and object (whatever appears "is" the thing). In superficial, purely descriptive terms, it is the field of low subjectivity. To travel through collectivity is to reside in a world identical to the one inhabited by one's peers. It is the world of the *polis*.

The other extreme that of individuality is the spatiality of the individual, irreproducible involvement, resonant penetration, idiosyncratic interpretation and a particular frame of objects in existence and in the depth of their presentation to the self-pole. The emphasis is on the way the object endows the self, not the object per se. It is a world of blurred senses. Superficially, it is a world of subjectivity. It is important to emphasise here that this subjectivity does not override the value of the world and its "objectivity", it merely changes its emphasis. The importance of this observation stems from the fact that in the dialectic relationship examined here, each experience, while still conveying reality, can sometimes put more emphasis on the way it is singularised in an individual's consciousness or at others on how similarly it appears to individual consciousnesses. If we take an example from the arts, we might say that the spatiality of portraiture is aligned with the pole of collectivity, seeking to portray figures in precisely the way they are seen by everyone. Meanwhile, in impressionism, the spatiality of individuality means a figure may be portrayed in a single aspect; it is subjectivised by the painter's gaze, gaining new proportions and reliefs to become, so to speak, unique.

Thus, even under normal conditions, there is an asymmetry of the dialectic relationship between the two poles. The spatiality of individuality has access to the spatiality of collectivity, since this is common to all. Meanwhile, collectivity has a harder time translating individuality empathically, since it stems from a unique formulation. For the collectivity to gain access to individuality, it must make patient endeavours to gain familiarity with it. This asymmetry is the hallmark of this polarity, as it is this that sets it apart, in terms of reciprocal relations, from the others, where emphasis on one pole implies a corresponding weakening of the other. In collectivity–individuality, although there is also a relationship of proportionality (structures that are more collective tend to be less individual and vice versa), the two extremes have to interact and even overlap. Only in the most serious pathologies is this channel of interaction lost. In severe schizophrenia, for example, individuality can be dominated and drained by collectivity (which is actually a pseudo-collectivity, to which I will return in Sect. 4.1.2), and in certain schizoid disorders, individuality loses its place in the collective (Sect. 3.7.1).

The observation of existence through the dialectic notion of collectivity–individuality allows the experiences contained in the notions of light and dark to be extended to sentimental and ideational-representational experiences. A feeling can be enlightened by the collectivity; for example, at a party political congress, when everyone is shouting out the same slogans, it is fair to assume that their emotional experience is similar. All become one. This is also the spatial face of patriotism, although here – except in extreme conditions, such as war – the compression is experienced less intensely. It can even be said that feelings are the most effective way of transmitting collective spatiality. Although feelings are also engaged in individual spatiality, ideas and representations are the closest experiential elements of this pole. Every idea is ultimately an individual manifestation, even when it is cognitively shared by all. It is for this reason that ideational interpretations of the world, appearing in an individual intellectual consciousness, are not always received by the collective world as intended by their creator. After all, the mundane reception of a worldview depends more on sentimental rootedness than on intellectual conviction, since this, in its "pure" form, is the fruit of dialogue between inaccessible experiential intimacies (except in the case of the abstract sciences, such as mathematics, which are more like convincement and intellection).

2.2.6 Horizontality–Verticality

The introduction of this dialectical polarity to phenomenological psychopathology comes from Binswanger's classic paper on the anthropology of extravagance in schizoid and schizophrenic disorders (Binswanger 1992a), although his work did not completely exhaust this rich analytical vein (Blankenburg 2007c). He had explored verticality previously in "Dream and existence" (1992b), and applied it empirically to the Ellen West case (Binswanger 1957, case Ellen West). This polarity bears some similarity to the opposition identified above, except that it adds the directions of meaning in which existence moves (Chamond 2005). Also, I would contend, even though it is extremely helpful and applicable in everyday psychopathology, it is one of the broadest categories, indicating anthropological conditions of possibility that are so general that they sometimes mix elements of temporality and spatiality.

Verticality is the axis through which existence finds its particular differentiation. The two points of this axis are height and depth. In height, existence aspires to its most distinct values; in depth, it falls into the underground chasms of a material, mineral nature. But depth also has a productive face, indicative of a radical immersion of the self-pole in some object, which, by increasingly attracting the self-pole, fosters an experiential enlargement of existence. Verticality presupposes, on the one hand, an upward route by which the self is raised, gradually attaining and embodying its spiritual values, while at the same time obtaining a broad view of mundane reality. This element of ascension actually already belongs to the field of longitudinal temporality, as it shows how necessary repeated existential effort is to reach the stratum of existential values. An element of Aristotelian ethics can also be identified in this space–time synthesis described by verticality. The quest for happiness, the ultimate goal of existence (as Aristotle puts it in his *Nicomachean and Eudemian Ethics*) for the Greek philosopher, is fruit of the continuous, repeated effort to attain a form which is never definitive, always escapes the individual and can only be maintained by an act of unshakable ethical will.

However, verticality is also a movement of crumbling, loss of ascendant capacity and thus defeat in the face of the gravity of the world. This transfigures existence into solid matter, sucked into mud, swamp, hell or primitive animal instinct. We might say that the human vocation is upward, and for this very reason, existential failure, in extreme conditions, is referred to as the opposite of vocation, or a fall. The end of the world experience (*Weltuntergangerlebnis* – Callieri 2001) therefore reflects the shattered existential condition of some schizophrenic persons. Rise and fall provide the atmospheric backdrop for the whole of existence, from the conscious imaginary of wakefulness to the unconsciousness of dreams, passing through the whole realm of metaphors (Binswanger 1992b).

Horizontality is the axis of the world on which existence is projected and, through this interplay, configured. Moving horizontally, existence interacts directly with the rules of the game of the world, partially renouncing its authenticity in order to merge with the collective. Horizontality and verticality have a proportional dialectic relationship, with pathology being a paralysing overemphasis on one of the poles, as I will explore in Parts II and III of this work.

2.3 Interpersonality and Intersubjectivity

The name of this anthropological dimension reveals the difficulty language has to face in overcoming its long cultural roots. There is no term in English[8] to denote exactly what I want to indicate.[9] Our dualistic Western tradition is barren of concise terms that describe an intermediate human region that predates the distinction between two empirical and thus interrelated selves. The linguistic way out to indicate this region of existence is the use of a prefix indicating dialogue and transit between non-autonomous parts which are inevitably organised in seamless totality; parts that are as radically interconnected as life and oxygen in the atmosphere. The prefix "inter" is designed here to indicate that the object to be studied is not on either side of a polarity, but in its integration. It is a type of dialectic proportion of the poles of an experience, and the form of this proportion is what should interest the scientist. As we will see later (Parts II and III), this conception will serve as an important aid both in comprehending altered psychological experiences and in constructing therapeutic strategies. But the inclusion of the prefix is not enough to resolve the difficulties of this region of existence, because the linguistic gap which prevents access to this intermediate zone ends up warping the way the poles are united with each other. In writing the categories self, identity, embodiment or even individual historical self, I am drawing on the tacit assumption that these entities can subsist autonomously, and that only secondarily do they relate to each other in the world. In our semantic and lexical universe, there is no way to avoid these mental divisions. All we can do is point them out and try to mitigate them, because we have to coexist with language and the creation of new concepts would lead us to a level of scientific hermeticism that I feel is unjustified and unnecessary. What an empirical science needs is the capacity to illuminate sectors of reality and to transmit this illumination to a corps of practitioners, building a tradition.

---

[8] Nor, indeed, is there in the main languages in which psychopathology and phenomenological philosophy developed.

[9] Writing in Japanese, Kimura (1982, 2000) called this region of existence which ails in schizophrenia aida: a space which does not only concern the in-between, but the intersubjective in the broadest sense, as a principle of encounter between individuals.

Bearing this in mind, I have chosen the term *person* to synthesise the poles of this co-active relationship between two historically situated existences. A person is the all-encompassing wholeness of each individual existence, which makes it an indeterminate concept. Its merit as a term lies more in what it does not define and what it can encompass virtually than by what it does define. However, I do not mean with this choice to remain in the field of conceptual indeterminacy; on the contrary, I want to indicate that the notion of person brings together all possibilities of existence: its structural conditions of possibility as well as the set of values and rational experiences of any human being. This is consistent with the understanding that the person is more than subjectivity and its partial identities. A person is a unique whole that results from the conditions given by existence and refined by our free actions which shape this totality and are guided by a set of pre-reflexive or explicit values (Cusinato 2017). The person is a limit concept of singular human existence, encompassing all the attributes and possibilities of an individuality.

This is how the notion of *interpersonality* is constituted, referring to the widest and most mature manifestation of existence and its implantation in the world of equals, of other people. However, this concept does not serve to help us understand something that, contained within it, is its own condition of possibility and that of all other experiences. It is also a basic and pre-reflexive interrelationship, which functions as a transcendental foundation that enables the relationships between integral people. This foundation ontologically predates consciousness and its personal relations and is therefore transcendental. It underlies and determines each personal and interpersonal experience. For this reason, it is the original subject – or intersubject, to be more precise – that makes all experience possible. We will refer to this foundation as *intersubjectivity*: the condition of possibility of all interpersonal experience (Sass 2019). For example, a very shy person can relate quite well with other people in their world. Their interpersonality is mature and skilled enough to carry out their life projects. However, they experience an inexplicable tension every time they come into contact with another person, as if that person was always bothering them and scrutinising them. Although the shy person knows this discomfort is irrational, they are unable to overcome it. This is because the intersubjectivity of the shy person produces a relational form in which the other-pole's proportion outweighs that of the self-pole. In spatial terms, the self-pole is very close to the other-pole and centred in relation to it. This prior, tacit spatiality which precedes interpersonal contact and which is so important in shaping it is what defines the specific intersubjectivity. In anthropological terms, we have to bear in mind that the relationship with the other appears twice in us, like Russian dolls. In the deepest, transcendental layer, the other appears as a condition of possibility of the proportion of the intersubjective spatialities and temporalities that constitute the subject itself. Subsequently, more clearly and consciously, the other appears as a constituted historical person. Every time I use interpersonality, I am focusing on the complete singular individual, the person, in his/her relationship with his/her peers. When I want to emphasise the conditions of possibility of such encounters, I use the term intersubjectivity. It is important to stress at this point that more often than not, the most serious mental disorders affect the intersubjective dimension, subsequently causing changes in the interpersonal dimension. A personality disorder will manifest in the sphere of interpersonality, but its roots lie in the constitution (generally during childhood) of intersubjectivity.

2.3.1 The Fragmentary Nature of Intersubjectivity and the Limitations of Absolute Anthropological Knowledge

If, in ontological terms, existence has a structural integrity composed of intersubjectivity, epistemologically speaking it can only be accessed by a perspectivism situated in the duality between the cognised pole (patient) and the cognising pole (psychopathologist). The unavoidable perspectivism of intersubjectivity itself annuls the possibility of completely knowing another as a person. To us, the other is a totality that has a part that exists in us and vice versa; only by this symbiotic connection, we can illuminate it. The knowledge of this other radiates from this maximum core of evidence, intersubjectivity (Messas and Fukuda 2018). However, as soon as we perceive otherness, we already sense it as totality: we know we are in the presence of a unique person with a unique biography, although at that very moment all we know of it, through our senses and through affective resonance and memory, is a part. That part is also part of us in the other.

This contradiction inherent to existence reveals a fundamental constituent of intersubjectivity: its fragmentary nature. We will only ever experience a fragment of the meaning-filled totality of another – their individual biography – which allows us to engage in an experience – inevitably incomplete – of this otherness. Others have the same experience of us. This theme will be taken up again later, but it should be mentioned here that this fragmentary nature of intersubjectivity is responsible for the multiplicity of ways in which a psychopathology is actualised, often defying definitive diagnostic knowledge (Messas and Tamelini 2018). To know someone definitively is to fix the perspective from which that other reveals him/herself to us. Such a fixed perspective is only seen in extremely severe psychopathological conditions. In most cases, otherness is a secret that can be glimpsed furtively between the lights and shadows of uncertainty. Psychopathological science will always be a hermeneutical art.

Intersubjectivity is fragmentary at both of its personal poles. The cognising (psychopathologist) and the cognised (patient) are actualised in an infinite diversity of forms. There are as many forms as there are anthropological possibilities of existence and intersubjectivity. However, the contextual attitudes by which intersubjectivity is defined restrict the field of this inexhaustible potentiality. If, for example, we are in a religious cult, the a priori intersubjectivities will evoke segments of the personalities that are appropriate to the situation. It will be the cult, actualised in its members, that frames the perspective of intersubjectivity. These modes by which the two poles of intersubjectivity are actualised therefore constitute integrities of meaning, total forms whose primary fragmentation is intersubjectivity itself. As such, the characteristic styles by which the poles of intersubjectivity participate in human interpersonal relational integrity are also of great relevance to psychopathological observation. The science of psychopathology must define what fragments of intersubjectivity it will identify as objects of analysis from a whole host of possibilities. Therefore, the anthropology that develops from it and its fundamental attitude is a limited anthropology, just as all anthropology is inevitably limited, since it is based on some fundamental attitude. Even philosophical anthropology, which generally aims to encompass the whole of human existence, fails to take account of its own perspectivism. If it insists on this approach, it will inevitably veer into abstract, spurious absolutisation. Any reflection on existence in general, when pursued in abstraction, always has some point of reference, even if it is not declared. Therefore, no philosophical anthropology can claim to attain absolute knowledge of human existence.[10]

2.3.2   Integrity and Intersubjectivity: Visuality and Empathy

The inherently fragmentary nature of intersubjectivity cannot, however, deny the integral existence of a singular historical individual. We always observe from the perspective of a part, but are fully able to grasp the totality. If in visual perception we only need to see one aspect of a house to apprehend it as a whole, we can be even surer of our original, pre-reflexive conviction of the presence of an individual person when we first make contact with that other. It is as primal a certainty as the identification of ourselves as unity. The unity of my structure and the unit of the other are mutually validated. Intersubjectivity is, therefore, also integrity.

The two main forms of access to this integrity are of great importance in phenomenological psychopathology: visuality and empathy. The former is based on the spatiality of distance and collectivity and the latter on proximity and individuality. The first and safest way in which otherness presents itself to us is by visual contact.[11] With it, the cognising pole acknowledges the presence of the cognised pole with the utmost evidence: we are sure, when we stand before someone, that this is a single person, an integral existence, not just an inanimate mass of matter. The focus of the recognition of this biographical unity is the face and its gestures and expressions. Meanwhile, the totality of the body is lent singularity through its gesticulations and habitual demeanour in movement and repose. Yet, it is in the face that the difference between individuals of the species is most marked. Likewise, facial

---

[10] We are indebted to Hippocrates and Jaspers (especially his existential philosophy) for, refusing an abstract generalisation of anthropology, reminding us that the human can only be known partially and in a mutating perspective that never ends.

[11] I will disregard here, due to its rarity, the case of amaurosis, in which the other makes their presence and integrity felt by other sensory means, where collectivity is smaller and therefore individuality is greater.

expressions enable great clarity in the apprehension of psychopathological phenomena. The omega expression of a melancholic person, the fixed stare of a phobic person in a state of panic, and the almost metaphysical dread of certain schizophrenic people are examples of the clarity and evidence that the face offers as access to human integrity. As we move away from the other to get the best perspective to access it, we allow the public, collective experience of visuality. The other presented through visuality is the one whose comprehension is most easily shared by others. In the field of psychopathology, the above examples are accessible to all who observe the patient at this moment. Usually, the interpretations will tend to be similar, but this is not the case in the empathetic form of approach.

Empathy is the expression of intersubjectivity as proximity; that is, of the fact that an experience – a pathos – is sustained simultaneously in the space of the two poles of intersubjectivity. Hence, a feeling, an idea or an emotion is neither in one person nor in another, but in both. In this sense, visuality reveals only the most superficial and unipolar face of an experience that is in essence dual. The idea that a feeling is the isolated patrimony of an individual is inaccurate, a simplification born from everyday language. Each individual obviously experiences feelings directed towards and centred in their self.[12] However, these feelings have their roots in a pre-reflexive spatiality which enables and marks their emergence. The primordial spatiality in which experiences occur is, then, an interspatiality (Messas 2004): a spatiality constituted by the dialectic composition of two subjective poles. As a consequence, one important element of any psychopathological diagnosis is the investigation of the interspatiality in which some experiences happen. Interspatiality is also governed by the principle of proportionality. Some patients experience their feelings as more grounded in their individual consciousness: they have low interspatiality as a condition of possibility. (From the psychopathologist's point of view, this is evidence of a lack of resonance of the patient's affects in their own consciousness.) Others have experiences as if they were totally produced in the simultaneity of intersubjective relations, constituting high interspatiality. Schizophrenic people, for example, have low interspatiality, while manic people's interspatiality is high.

Interspatiality is phenomenalised in affective resonance; that is, in the way some affection at one pole resonates and synchronises with the other, so they both enter in harmony, becoming one, as if they were musically attuned. The way this happens is unique for each intersubjectivity. Affective resonance gives ultimate access to the other as a whole, even if it is hard to define how it is understood and defies expression in rational language. In this sense, empathy and resonance differ from visuality, which is marked by definition and clarity. This principle is the root of the classic notion of praecox feeling, which in everyday practice is not to be ignored. It is through this that the psychopathologist picks up through intuition (which precedes any linguistic formulation) the whole of the other and, by contrast, accesses the essence of the pathology. The praecox feeling gained notoriety in its use for the

---

[12] Later in the text, I designate this the historical self. As this concept has not yet been presented, I use it only in its trivial sense.

diagnosis of schizophrenia (Rümke 1990) and remains a valid diagnostic strategy to this day (Gozé and Naudin 2017; Pallagrosi and Fonzi 2018).

The other as integral existence cannot be reached through words, given that it is ineffable and unattainable, but it can be sensed intuitively twofold. The intuition of the whole is an act of identification of an individual potential which, when actualised in existence, can only be endowed in parts. The whole can be grasped intuitively, while the parts can be objectified as science (Jaspers 1968, 1997). The condition of perspectivism in which intersubjectivity takes place – and psychopathological science – hinders knowledge about the whole, but does not stop it from being sensed as a mystery of individual existence.

2.3.3   Modes of Intersubjectivity: Singularity, Collectivity and Anonymity

Intersubjectivity is the foundation of existence and is therefore an indispensable constituent of individuality. Individuality is differentiated and established through a dialectic relationship with a pre-reflexive intersubjectivity. Thus, every individual existence is, in different proportions, a balance between subjectivity and intersubjectivity. Intersubjectivity is therefore a constituent of individual existence. The way in which one of the poles of the intersubjective relationship behaves exerts an influence on the anthropological proportions of the other. There is therefore activity in the reciprocal constitution of the intersubjective poles: we, as a person, are shaped by the mode of pre-reflexive relationship that others propose or impose on us, and vice versa. However, the constitution of intersubjectivity (as a condition of possibility) between biographies occurs passively, which means we cannot control the fact that we are codetermined by someone else. The passive synthesis of intersubjectivity is, in turn, the precondition for the various anthropological proportions that a single human existence produces, with all its highways and byways. The fact that intersubjectivity is not static and definitive makes the examination of the modes of reciprocal constitution of intersubjectivity all the more important.

Intersubjectivity is also constituted reciprocally in poles, from which extremes must first be identified (Zahavi 2018). First of all, intersubjectivity can be singular. The paradigm of the singular relationship is the I–thou duality, raised to a higher category in existential philosophy in the work of Martin Buber (1971). His fundamental assumption is that two historically unique individuals are in dynamic dialectical counterpoint. They enable each other existentially, meaning that one pole opens up to all the complexities of the other singular existence, which is at once fragmentary and integral. The singular mode of psychopathological anthropology is therefore the one that best fosters the expansion of the potentialities of an integral life. Although this integrity is never achieved, it is presupposed as a possibility throughout the entire course of the *singular intersubjectivity*. This is the source of all its existential vitality: it is the differentiating element par excellence of its biographical development. What distinguishes it is the simultaneous presence of historical singularity at both the related dialectic poles. Thus, the temporal experiences of singularity are fluid, protentive and expansive. The subjective contents of individuality become propitious for successions of themes, which are accommodated in the midst of other subject matter – individual and collective – and rarely reach a dominant proportion. The spatiality of singularity is therefore porous, ductile and multifarious. Singularity is the mode of democracy, gradual maturation, dialogue, concessions and fertile syntheses between individual and culture. Mutually constituted, the relational interplay of the two poles opens a channel for the themes of culture to gradually settle in individuality, being able to take root with depth and serenity without trampling individual aspirations. By the same token, the experiences of singularity are stained by doubt, uncertainty and the long route to the formation of conviction.

Although the I–thou relationship is the most typical form of singular intersubjectivity, we should not forget that this is a condition of possibility and not a factual description. Singular intersubjectivity can also be achieved in family relationships, in groups (a psychotherapeutic group is strongly singular) and even in work relationships. Every time a relationship or a system of interpersonal relationships is based on an intersubjectivity which does not fix the temporality of the biography at a single point, be it an idea, a personality trait or a social identity, a singular mode can be established.

It is precisely the fixing of individuality at a specific proportion of its parts that characterises *collective intersubjectivity*. Here, one of the poles of the relationship (e.g. the religious or political leader, the head of a group or the guru of some movement) becomes dominant and thus fixes the identity of the dominated pole, unifying it into a homogeneous, collective identity (a member of a particular faith, a political activist, a group or a cult member). While the unification of the identity of one of the poles through rigid intersubjective polarity hampers the various anthropological dialectic movements of the led pole, it nonetheless offers stability and density for its existence. Collective intersubjectivity takes place when the capacity for transformation and creative pluralisation based on temporality is replaced by the fixing of existence in a rigid identity stripped of personal creativity. It is the intersubjectivity of fascination, impact, exuberance, identity security, faith, blind trust, but also of imposition, violence, tyranny, dictatorship, fear and absolute power. We might wonder what the anthropological sense of the possibility of such intersubjectivity is, if it embalms precisely the noblest core of existence. The reason for the frequency and scope of this mode of intersubjectivity lies in the depths of human constitution. The protentive temporal nature of existence calls for support in some safe haven the whole time, which is usually found in retention. Yet, historical retention is limited and may not be enough to grant a minimum of stability to existence, especially at times of particular fragility: in the phases of dawning and twilight, in individual crises or in periods of social upheaval. At such times, the dissolution contained in the fragmentary nature of existence seems intolerable. This is when the unifying force provided by collective intersubjectivity comes to the rescue. The existential

solidity introduced by the deshistoricisation contained in intersubjective collectivisation is quite unique, and to many seems the only crutch available. The individual
biography identifies security for itself in a rigid, coercive and often invasive identity,
taking on the power of a conviction it cannot create for itself and that it receives,
with the pressure of direct contact, as an order it cannot resist. The solid convictions
that burgeon from collective intersubjectivity are not built and sedimented historically; they operate as a foreign body, serving to give adherence to reality for some
fragile individualities. Although biographically they are sometimes fictitious, they
should be considered in their structural value.[13]

Finally, there is a third mode of intersubjectivity, which is essentially a pathological variant of collective intersubjectivity. Let us look at the difference between
this pathological form of intersubjectivity and its collective counterpart. Collective
intersubjectivity presupposes the possibility of individual integrity in the dialectic
relations of the self-pole and the other-pole. A football supporter who cheers on his
team and shouts abuse at everything and everyone from its rival still apprehends the
individuals who support that rival team. In a battle between fans, it is the collectives
who battle, but the individuals who commit and sustain the offenses and injuries.
This constituent presence of individual integrity is distorted in the anonymous version of collective intersubjectivity. Here, even if otherness can be experienced in the
human form of a specific persecutor (or, for example, one who leads an attack
against a specific individual), it is constituted in such a way that this supposed persecutor can never have the pre-reflexive characteristics of an individual, like a personal history or the capacity to have other partial identities besides their collective
one. (Returning to the football supporter scenario, if, for example, individuals from
the two different camps happen to be co-workers, they will likely be able to strike
up some form of friendly interaction after the match.) Anonymity is therefore a
constituent of this pathological intersubjectivity, which takes the form of a diffuse
human personality, the persecutor, who never effectively becomes a whole human
being. That is why the anonymous persecutor often takes the form of a mysterious
organisation – potentially extra-terrestrial – or some entity far away from the individual's history (being pursued by the CIA, for example). *Anonymous intersubjectivity* is the basis of schizophrenia (Binswanger 1957, case Jurg Zund).

Collective intersubjectivity is above all thematic. As the flow of protentive temporality (responsible for the succession of different themes and their dialectical
interaction) is hindered, it becomes overwhelmingly difficult to include new themes;
when intersubjectivity is anonymous, this can be completely devastating. The consciousness of individuals is dominated by the themes of the collective intersubjectivity; it is not the individuals themselves who receive and elaborate them.
Accordingly, rituals, reverence for traditions and rules, and transcendental absolut-
ism abound, while in pathological forms, we see the single monstrous theme that
pursues the schizophrenic paranoid person wherever they go. Although the human

[13]This support rendered for existence by collective intersubjectivity will be explained in more
detail in Parts II (Sect. 3.5.6) and III (Sect. 8.3).

formations most grounded in the collectivity are great mass movements, it is also perfectly possible for there to be collective intersubjectivity in a two-way relationship, such as occurs in the jealous delusions of alcoholics, where one of the poles no longer sees the other as anything but as a threatening medusa.

2.4 Embodiment

The integral unity of an existence is embedded in the world as intersubjectivity. It is through this that the self-pole and other-pole are constituted and, in so doing, are enabled to know each other. The other is perceived immediately, through visuality, empathy and language, as a totality. These three channels all need a carnal foundation for them to be materialised and recognisable as existence. This primordial materialisation is embodiment, and this is why others are initially accessible to us in embodied form. Embodiment is not just the physiological soma hidden within and behind each experience – with which internal medicine concerns itself – but also the most stable and evident experience of presence, position, permanence, movement, sensation and interaction with the world. The body (Körper), pure and simple, exists as a biological mass; embodiment (Leib or lived body), as a dwelling place in a world full of levels of significance, ranging from the general level of the species to the particular of the individual (Zutt 1963c; Blankenburg 2007d). Therefore, just as occurs in temporality, all embodiment is, strictly speaking, accessible only through intercorporeality, since we access the significant embodiment of the other through the limitations and conditions imposed by our own embodiment. Both poles of intersubjectivity are in the same antepredicative world circumscribed by the embodiment of the human species. Because we have eyes to search the world, we know that the other's gaze also searches the world; because we have touch, we know how the other explores the intimacies of the world and humans and so on. So whenever we address embodiment, we are actually expressing it, first and foremost, from an intercorporeal perspective.

A vertical stance is typical of the human species. Even in those who cannot balance on their legs, verticality is maintained: reason inhabits the apical pole of embodiment. The gaze, in turn, reveals more of the plurality contained in an individual than, for example, clothing, which has more to do with social status and roles in culture. The gaze is the most intense moment of encounter through embodiment. Tone of voice, body language and mannerisms are all situated at some point in the triangle of species collectivity–individuality. In short, all the characteristics examined above regarding spatiality are actualised in inter-corporeality, now at its peak of cognoscibility, position (spatiality) and fixation (temporality). It is the point of maximum apprehension of the other. However, for the very fact that it is the maximum presence of the present, it is limited in terms of retention and protention. The price of knowing someone with maximum clarity and evidence is knowing the very least of them. This maximum clarity and evidence does not mean interpreting facial expressions, or demeanour is not without its difficulties. Often, a manifestation of embodiment may be dubious. However, what I want to stress here is that *all* manifestation is contained in this time interval, since embodiment does not extend to the other dimensions of temporality. Admittedly, a particular gaze and bearing do express an existential trajectory, the yearnings and frustrations of a life or a social identity. But in doing so, precisely because they are fixed in the present, they present to the onlooker only one facet of their wealth as existence, the face that is most easily compressed in the solidity of embodiment. The totality inherent to embodiment inevitably reduces the range of significance that is given in the temporality of existence. This takes us directly to a reflection on individual embodiment.

The temporality of the existential structure is extended by memories, representations from the imagination, language and values. These, in turn, are invariably revealed in embodiment; however, the passage from the range of the temporal dimensions to the total presence of embodiment is limiting, thereby restricting, in my view, the role of embodiment in the manifestation of the complexities of human temporal existence. The price paid for clarity of embodiment is its ontological deficiency. Existence is much more than its embodiment. Embodiment is the necessary material condition of possibility for the biography and its movements of expansion. In embodiment, spatiality is prominent and so is stability. Embodiment is the most solid point at which sufficient stability can be obtained for the existential structure not to be dissolved by temporality. It ties materiality to temporality, and in doing so allows existence to take the form of a dialectic between stability and change.

But embodiment is not only a constricting material support of temporality but also an instrument for the pursuit of projects in the world. Through the movements of embodiment, we draw in the world the paths by which it is constituted as an individual plan stratified and endowed with meaning. And, as embodiment moves and criss-crosses the world, its reception of the world – perception – inevitably acts in conjunction with this movement (von Weizsäcker 1950; Fuchs 2018). A body that touches is also a body that is touched, if we are to stay within Merleau-Ponty's classic example of touch (1945). The hands are the centre of clarity of touch and the point of reference against which other ways of apprehending objects – with different, decreasing levels of clarity – are measured. The hands of the self are also the core of its most substantial intercorporal relationship with the world: apprehension. We apprehend the world so we can deal with it (Heidegger 2006). The act of apprehending precedes cognition and gives form to our intentions. It allows us to bring into relief, from the fluidity and diffuse interpenetration of reality, certain objects which become instruments for our construction of the world and its modification to our image and likeness. For this very reason, emotional situations that prevent some experience of existential solidity, such as fear or anger, weaken the fine movements of the hands. In the grip of fear, we become so small before the dangerous world that we no longer experience our body as an instrument of resolute personal intention. Our hands become trembling instruments of self-defence. In anger, too, we are so absorbed by the importance given to the interpersonal object that this is all we focus on. Losing sight of the other as an integral individual, we also lose the fine instrument to explore it with finesse. We are left with thick, clenched fists, before which the other can only appear as a wall to be attacked. The finesse that is so important to hands can only be born from open and integral intersubjectivity. The arms, together with the hands, determine the size of the diameter that can be inhabited by the embodied self in the world. The length of our arms is what delimits what is within (mine) and what is beyond (the other's). In other words, movement and perception are no more than polarities of a form of dwelling in the world (Fuchs 2018). As an instrument of pre-reflexive and species-related significance and of a social or individual project, embodiment can also become an obstacle, as in somatic diseases. Embodiment impaired in its capacity to constitute a project or to execute it is misshapen into an afflicted mass; it deteriorates from body–material–condition of possibility into a burden, a handicap and a hindrance.

Embodiment is also implied in the singularity–collectivity polarity. The experience of a scream of pain, imprinted on the gaze and in the expression, is situated in the field of the collective. The transformation of the body into a burden during a mild depression or a strong bout of flu is manifested in the space of intimacy, insofar as it can often only be accessed by a third party through a direct report. Embodiment can be fragmented. In the case of anguish, it may lodge itself in the chest or the throat, or, in the insularity of certain schizophrenic people, it may be experienced as alien. It can also integralise itself, as in depressive or schizophrenic asthenia, where the whole body is experienced as devoid of vital energy.

2.5   Identity, Historical Self and Ipseity

Identity stems directly and exclusively from temporality. Only through the flow of time do we acquire the capacity to retain a similarity to ourselves. If we were to create a fictional human being who was only transversal in time, unaffected by the chain of temporal accumulation, they would have no identity, since they would be completely contained in one time interval and could totally free themselves from the next. The complete rupture of temporality seen in some catatonic-like psychoses is indicative of an eradication of identity and reveals how intimately it is linked to temporality. It is because we are essentially retained as existence, because we insist pre-reflexively on a certain style of being, that we have identity. For this reason, identity is also comparison. When something comes into our consciousness, we first try to register whether it belongs to some chain of continuities. We compare this object or image with previous moments of our experience, and by so doing, we identify and confirm its identity. Or else, we do not find it and therefore reject it. It therefore follows that the negative of identity, or non-identity, which is manifested as deviation from the chain of existential retentions and ultimately refers to the dissolutive temporality of the biography, is itself constitutive of identity. Every identity possesses its dissolution, its opposite, which is pure potential and negation of the self, dialectically within itself. As identity is temporal, it is potentially open to new additions and thus to changes in the proportions of its own composition. If what was potential becomes part of identity, a new negative identity (or non-identity) will appear on the horizon of experience, tracing a new path for the ever-temporal, ever-open identity.

But the fundamental anthropological dimension of identity and its dialectic negative do not transit freely through existence. Identity is constituted through a dialectic relationship with a coalescing centre of reception, which is the *experience of the self* (Zahavi 2019). There is no such thing as pure, autonomous identity; it needs a self to constitute it transcendently in the act of its presence. Identity belongs to a self that affirms and enables its existence. It is heralded as a gravitational field around an ego axis, to which it directs its intentionality. Its spatiality is therefore also constituted in a special radial kind of centrality–peripherality relationship, whose focus is the self. This focus of the self is, however, ex-centric, since it tends to concentrate at the apical pole of embodiment, at some virtual spot behind the eyes. There is an infinity of regional spatialities in the radial circle of the identity's relations with the self that constitutes it. Our lower limbs, for example, are part of our identity, but they are positioned at a localisable point in space far from the centre of the self. This is made clear by everyday language, when we say that we "have" a foot, not that we "are" a foot. Bodily sensations are focused, but they can still "touch" the self directly in a way, more than the limbs can, which are always at a distance. An example of this is the feeling of hunger: although it is located somewhere in the upper abdomen, it has the power to directly mobilise the self. This closeness is already expressed in the expression "I'm hungry" (rather than "I feel hunger", for example). When it comes to feelings, this dispersion is complete: the whole identity is tinged by them, and they cannot be attributed to any one point. This is expressed linguistically in "being" happy (rather than "having happiness"); it imbues the whole of the self.

The spatiality of identity is limited by the identity of the otherness, be it human or the inanimate objects from the material world. We experience that there are other selves with their own identities and that they are not ours. However, the experience of the identity of others is also an experience of our own identity: we are the ones who experience that there is an other or that there are objects of and in the world. The experience of the identity of otherness is not therefore an experience of non-identity, which is only capable of interacting with its own identity and its self. Some schizophrenic people experience their thoughts as if coming from other selves. In this case, the spatiality of identity is compromised and invaded by some external spatiality. This is one phenomenon of the fragmentary nature of spatiality. Yet, in this case, the temporal matrix is still intact because the patient continues to know how to recognise their own identity. Only in cases of complete pathological substitution of the identity could we say that there is an alteration of the identity, even if incomplete. An example would be a patient who suddenly experiences themselves as Jesus Christ and behaves as such, with all its consequences. In this case, the centre of the self is compromised, preventing the biographical identity from being contrasted with the new pathological identity. Yet, even so, much of the historical identity remains, allowing some logic for behaviour and expression. Given the space constraints here, I will not examine the sedimentation of this new pathological identity into the totality of existence.

The experience of the self and identity are not assimilated reciprocally, insofar as they do not completely overlap one another. To explain this better, I should develop the distinctions further. If identity needs a self to which to relate, then there will always be a self present in identity. If I know who I am, if I feel my body as my own and my history as my own, I always have a minimal self (in this case, mine) that is present (Sass 2014b). This will be my identity self. This self, which embodies and actualises the temporal retentions of identity, is a *historical self*[14] (i.e. it exists and unfolds in the world, of which identity partakes, in a radial dialectic central–peripheral relationship). This historical self and its identity are permanently bound together in a dialectical relationship.[15] However, the temporality of the web of identity has greater historical breadth than the temporality of the historical self. We find elements, overtones or tendencies in our own and our peers' identities that come from the sedimentation of other generations. Not infrequently, in cultures with many immigrants, we perceive in our peers' manifestations whose roots lie in experiential behaviours that permeate the personal history in the culture in which they live, revealing other times, other places and other hues. Similarly, certain representations of partial social identities determined by the social classes to which we belong reveal times other than the particularity they are given by the individual. Identity is therefore temporally transgenerational. It is continuity across generations referring to a historical self incarnated perforce in a single biological generation. Melancholic people are transgenerational par excellence.

The historical self also transcends identity. The aforementioned non-identity is announced to a historical self actualised in identity. The historical self becomes the guarantor of identity. A panic attack where the historical self no longer recognises itself in relation to the identity that belongs to it (depersonalisation) is an experience of non-identity by a historical self. Only the historical self is able to translate, by the temporality it has retained from the identity to which it is dialectically linked, the sense of an identity negativity. Additionally, the historical self is responsible for identifying the moment when non-identity becomes part of identity. This occurs either by assimilation of the non-identity (learning a new skill, for example) or by the co-presence of both modes of identity (a new way of executing an acquired skill). The first case is typical of most experiences. What initially appears as external to identity gradually becomes commonplace for the historical self, turning into implicit identity. The second case, in the case of pathologies, is peculiar to schizophrenic processes, although not exclusive to them. Certain patients continuously

---

[14] Up to this point, I have treated the notion of self non-specifically, sometimes indicating it as a pole (self-pole), sometimes only pronominally, like myself. From now on, with the introduction of the historical self, every mention of the pronoun self will receive a technical meaning.

[15] The historical self is the owner of its own narrative, constituting its own narrative self (Parnas and Zahavi 2002). The narrativity of the historical self is, however, secondary to its constitution as a dimension of existence and I do not see how it can be considered an autonomous variant of self. Narrativity serves an identity that is previously embodied constituted, pre-reflexively, and which guides its articulation as narrative (Køster 2017, p. 163), although narrativity also has value as a regulator of one's own identity experience.

experience their historical self as being accosted by non-identity. For example, a patient may experience a sense of defamiliarisation in the world (derealisation) or in themselves (like aliens controlling their thoughts or not possessing parts of their own body) that does not belong either to their historical identity or to the identities of others (which, because they are part of their life, ultimately come from their own identity). This non-identity experience may not be assimilated into the identity, remaining as negativity. However, unassimilated repeated negativity becomes identity through sheer familiarity, becoming, in Jaspersian language, development within a process. The most acute conditions in which non-identity appears only as negativity and is not incorporated into historicity also show how the historical self transcends identity: even without any identity, a proto-experience remits primordially to a historical self, which thereby becomes a centre that generates temporality relatively and transiently. In this case, even though it is not possible to accommodate the proto-experience in identity, the historical self remains capable of tolerating and maintaining this dialectical state of tension between meaning and absence of meaning. But these conditions are not lasting. The tendency of existence – and this at the structural level, as I will explain in Sect. 2.6 – is to resolve negativity into identity positivity, thereby turning strangeness into delusion, for example, and putting an end to the dialectic tension. Formless strangeness is taken on by identity as a historical persecutor or implicit mysticism is reworked as a divine manifestation. In this sense, delusion is the inclusion in the historical identity of an absolute negativity that can be sustained by the historical self for a limited period of time, a period during which the weak autonomy of the psychotic historical self is able to operate. It is important to stress that for an experience to be included as delusion in identity, this experience must be prepared in advance by the structure of existence. It is by taking on a pathological configuration that existence offers a form for identity to process some subject matter as part of itself. We shall see more about this in the section on schizophrenia (Sect. 4.1).

The historical self nonetheless relies on a spatiality that cannot be restricted to a focal point. The centralising self of identity is usually experienced only as a centre and therefore a point of attraction for identity and the activity of the existence. However, this focal nature should not be misapprehended as a complete absence of spatiality. The historical self also possesses a virtual spatiality, whose framework becomes visible whenever it becomes distorted. One example would be a schizophrenic experience of delusional influence, where something or someone else controls the voluntary activity of the historical self. In this situation, the very limits of the historical self are broken (Minkowski 1995), a finding that can only be justified if there is a minimum of dynamic spatiality, implicit in the focal nature of the self; a spatiality which is itself fragmented in schizophrenic experiences (Sect. 4.1), even affecting the limits of the supposedly focused historical self. I conceive the focused nature of the historical self as being endowed with a pre-reflexive virtual spatiality which can also expand, as in mania, for example (Sect. 4.2). In essence, then, although the historical self is focused, it reveals its spatiality when it is affected by fragmentation or expansion. As such, when we are dealing with the historical self or the self-pole (when the self is viewed in its relations with the world-pole), we cannot but conceive of it as a focal point that is sometimes surrounded by an elastic zone of penumbra.

As the historical self is sustained by spatiality, it is able to modalise itself into parts without losing its unity. These parts are *identity roles*. Each role, in turn, also constitutes a unit in itself. If in the morning at home I act as a father, and in the afternoon I act as a doctor, although it is always me and my identity that in action, I actualise something different in each situation. Different sectors of my existence, with their own coherence and dynamics, are invoked at each time. I know it is always me, but I am not wholly the same all the time. Identity is capable of modalising itself because of its *ipseity*. Ipseity is the potential of the historical self to multiply in partial identities. It is the condition of possibility responsible for enabling the creativity of each identity part. It is the virtuality that lends the historical identity flexibility, allowing each part of the historical self to be exercised. There is an inversely proportional dialectic relationship between identity and ipseity: the more differentiated the identity is, the less ipseity it has, and thus the more pliable it becomes; the more ipseity there is in an identity, the more creative it is, but the less differentiated and mature. It is through ipseity, for example, that social and gender identities are possible, sculpted by family relationships and social classes. The richer ipseity is, the richer normal human life becomes, although stronger ipseity reduces the unit value and cohesion of each partial identity to existence, lending it an existential instability that is often psychopathologically significant (Messas et al. 2018). The virtual presence of ipseity, allowing sectors of identity to be actualised, is responsible for the contrasts experienced by identity. Then, when in the presence of someone from another family, another gender or another social class, we experience them as not ours, not belonging to us, as belonging to someone else, even though they will inevitably interact with us and may even influence us.

Identity also follows a dialectic regime between singularity and collectivity. At one end of the spectrum, each partial, sociologically determined identity receives singular treatment, being exercised in a creative and particular manner (Ballerini 2008). In this regime of proportions, originality supplants normativity, bringing gains and losses to the person. The individual gains from the deeper involvement of their own characteristics in their social actualisation. The richness of conducts and the experience of authenticity subjectively mark this form of disproportion. However, they are not supported by the strength of group cohesion that a collective identity provides. If we behave and feel the world in the same way as our fellow human beings, we are more solidly united with them. Correspondingly, the dominance of the collectivity in the exercise of social identities fosters unification, which enhances intergroup solidity, but it reduces the experience and vivacity of originality in the actualisation of each social identity. In a disproportion of collective identity, creativity is sacrificed for the sake of ontological security. The psychopathological importance of this dialectic of proportions will become clearer in Parts II and III.

2.5.1 Otherness as a Source of Ipseity: The Dialectic Relations Between Identity and Ipseity

As I set forth above, identity is unsaturated and is therefore capable of transformation. This ability is derived from the ipseity it contains. In its action over existence, ipseity needs an aspirational force to call forth the negativity of identity, always in potential, to actively flourish in creative novelty. This force comes from otherness. Existential ipseity comes from relationships with others. Whenever we are in someone else's presence, the contact of our unsaturated identities activates our ipseities. I will not return here to the text about intersubjectivity (what was said there – Sect. 2.3 – is still valid here), but it is important to also indicate that from the perspective of identity, otherness is an indispensable point of analysis, since it is the pivot of ipseity. An imaginary state of complete solitude would lead to an identity deprived of ipseity, impoverished by its incapacity to be distanced from itself. Identity is expanded by calling on ipseity, which is essentially a dialogue with otherness, summoning the negative potential of our identity and actualising it.

In the dimension of identity–ipseity, there is a dialectic of authenticity–inauthenticity in the Sartrean sense (Kraus 1991b). We actualise only a part of ourselves in each relationship, and this means we are inauthentic. But in order to modify ourselves as life demands, we have to take advantage of this inauthenticity temporarily in order to find a new authenticity downstream. Some clinical examples may help us understand this human dialectic. A hysterical person loses themselves in excessive inauthenticity, so that their partial identities are not sedimented in their historical self. They play roles that are very far from being incorporated into their identity. They therefore have a surplus of ipseity. At the other end of the scale, a melancholic person refuses any healthy inauthenticity, leaving little room for new incorporations to their identity. Their ipseity is curtailed. As ipseity is activated by otherness, in a hysterical person, otherness is extremely valuable for summoning identity negatives; in melancholia, otherness is circumscribed to an interpersonal game closed to creation.

The force of ipseity varies in the different expressions of social identities. I will give some examples in decreasing degrees of ipseistic power. Ipseity is more important in diffuse social roles and in personal friendships. An example of a diffuse social identity with high ipseity is the consumer identity. Although this partial identity is widespread in contemporary societies and in most Western countries, it is endowed with formally regulated rights, and it is not unified into a single or homogeneous form of conduct. There are many personal ways of performing it. Similarly, the social identities of friendship are organised loosely and very differently from each other, leaving plenty of scope for personal creativity. These partial identities are more distant from the identity centre of the historical self, so they are less stable and more creative. Biographically, they are incorporated later and lost faster. Precisely because of its more creative nature, the friend identity is propitious for the expansion of existence. Professional identities are also more distant from the identity centre of the historical self. They are sedimented later and are guided by more rigidly prescribed conduct, meaning they often provide existential solidity. Evidently, the variety of work-related identities offers a spectrum in which ipseity is fostered to different degrees. By contrast, social class offers less ipseic capacity, since it is incorporated early and is limited in number within a society. The family identity is the one that has the least ipseic power, while lending identity greater stability. We have the least opportunity for creativity in the family. As a result, melancholic people will tend to maintain proximity to the nuclear family throughout their biographical trajectory, while schizoid people will only maintain it if the family operates as a support for their unique existential pretensions. Within family roles, however, there is one important specificity: the role of father/mother is assimilated late in life, which gives it some resemblance to a professional role. However, once acquired, it confers the most solid attachment to the identity, since intrinsic to its constitution is the offer of stability directly to third parties, namely, children. Its late acquisition and the high demands it makes on existential ipseity contrast with the reduced ipseity that it encompasses in its mature expression, generating an existential tension that makes several pathologies unable to attain it (Tellenbach 1968; Schrank et al. 2016). It is the identity that calls for the greatest range of temporal variability in the identity–ipseity relationships of existence.

All biographical development is thus, from an identity perspective, a reciprocal interplay of ipseic expansion and retraction. In moments of existential expansion and innovation, where some instability is needed, ipseity is called for, generally resulting in some distancing from less ipseic identities, such as family relations. (One example would be the adolescent who no longer shares intimate experiences with their parents.) In moments of existential retraction, where stability is salutary, the familiar identities of social class are given precedence over ipseity. The density of the sedimentation of longitudinal temporality has a great influence on the expression of these movements. For example, a mature adult with a consolidated professional role may, at a time of existential crisis, lean heavily on their professional identity and experience a corresponding retraction of ipseity. A young adult may gain greater ipseity through a restricted group identity (e.g. a group of social activists), since although this is of limited creativity, it still contrasts with their family identity and may lend them enough stability for their identity not to collapse when they are moving away from the family. Paradoxically, a young adult may even use an incipient professional identity to gain some stability when moving out of the family circle. The professional role reduces ipseity, since it has set rules of action and invocation of identity. One of my young patients, after serious psychotic episodes that prevented any student activity, found a way to start his adult life by going directly into a professional role, saying that as it was "all determined, it gives me more security".

The right choice of partial identities to predominate in the totality of existence is determined by the dialectic exchange with otherness. So it is that during an event of national significance – say, the football World Cup – the contrasts between class identities may become blurred, giving way to a national identity that is at the same time unifying and reductive of the differences between individuals of the same nation. Identities and ipseities are therefore movable, shifting in response to the totality of relations with otherness in an inversely proportional ratio. The greater the ipseity, the lower the relative value of each partial identity in the existential whole, while restricted ipseity will reveal and empower partial identities, which can come to assimilate the whole personal identity (e.g. in the way a war between two countries will unify the individuals' partial identities). If we have one rigid identity, we will be more trapped in narrow existential boundaries and therefore more structurally stable. Increased ipseity in interpersonal relationships also reduces the contrast between identities. For example, in a culture where gender identities are not prescribed clearly or rigidly, their relative differences will be smaller and their boundaries looser. As a consequence, each partial identity becomes more creative. Conversely, a scarcity of ipseity between the poles sets identities, amplifying the differences between them. However, even in intersubjective compositions where there is little ipseity, existence may find ways to take it beyond the imposition of social habits, as we see in individuals who are able to transcend the precepts imposed by their social, professional or class determinations.

Partial identities are organised in concentric hierarchical circles according to their othernesses. For example, in a way, class identity is an expansion of family identity. A family identity is recognised in contrast with other families, and similarly a class identity is identified in contrast with other classes. As families exist within classes, then in terms of temporal retention and stability, belonging to a class identity means belonging to a large family. Therefore, it is more effective for a person to sustain their identity either in a family or in a class.

2.6   The Structure of Existence

This presentation of the conditions of possibility of existence, from which phenomenological psychopathology is derived as an empirical science, ends with a description of the *structure of existence*. It is a notion that represents a synthesis of all the proportional dialectics of existence. The notion of the structure of existence[16] gives rise to the most classic and fundamental of the dialectics of psychopathology, the relationship between parts and a whole (Dilthey 1977; Jaspers 1997; Gadamer 1988). Phenomenological psychopathology is interested in totality, existence, in its altered forms. But totality can only be grasped through its parts. To examine the structure of existence is then, ultimately, to enter into a total synthetic category which coordinates all the conditions of possibility described above in a significant unit. It is time to define this total notion conceptually, even if complete conceptual precision is not possible, given that total notions can only be grasped intuitively. However, the degree of conceptual imprecision we may face is not, in my view, a cause for intellectual concern. Ultimately, for any worldview to be expressed meaningfully, the way its concepts are used and what meaning they are given is arguably

---

[16] I use "existential structure" and "structure of existence" interchangeably.

worth more than any categorical definition. In science, pragmatics supersedes abstract conceptuality. If definitions restrict the inevitable polysemy of a concept, their tacit use defines and specifies them (Banzato and Zorzanelli 2017; Zorzanelli et al. 2016).

What I understand by structure of existence is a configuration of the fundamental conditions of possibility of existence – temporality and spatiality and their ramifications in intersubjectivity, identity and embodiment – which I shall call *position*. As this position is an articulation of conditions of possibility, it is a pre-reflexive structure of existence and is marked by the proportional relations between these dimensions. A position is thus a style of dialectical proportionality between conditions of possibility of existence. There is no fixed position throughout the longitudinal temporality of a biography, although it tends towards permanence and only gradual changes in the relationships between its conditions of possibility. One of the goals of psychopathology is precisely to empirically examine the internal dialectical tensions of a structure that simultaneously changes and remains immobile (Messas 2010b). Strictly speaking, this means that what in fact exists originally is a transversal implantation of existence in the world. The biography is a consequence of the maintenance or alteration of this continuous transversality, projected on existence and gathered by a historical self. There is no biography inscribed originally in the structure of existence. The biography is endowed by the sedimentation of the experiences enabled by the retentive and protentive dimensions of transversal temporality. It is the structure that leaves a trace we call biography, because it is this that has continuous retentions and protentions (Tamelini 2008). This trace is then gathered up by identity and its historical self. Existential structure is thus eccentric in relation to identity and prior to the constitution of the historical self; it is the condition of possibility for the incarnation of both. As a consequence, an existential structure that has been overtransformed, whatever the reason, during the course of its biography may, at an advanced stage of life, have nothing in common with its initial moments, in terms of the proportional composition of its partial elements. The identity is maintained, in this case, by the continuity retained in the historical self.

The reciprocal articulation of the conditions of possibility of existence in a dialectic regime of proportions is a necessary precondition, but not enough for existence to be structured in a single unit. The whole of existence is greater than and qualitatively different from the inorganic sum of its parts. For the composition of the conditions of possibility to take on the ontological status of existence, this arrangement of heterogeneous conditions of possibility must be integrated and unified organically. Existence is a structured unitary organism, made possible by the union of distinct and interdependent conditions of possibility based on specific synthetic conditions, which lend its original and distinctive qualitative nature. The creation of this structured unity is its constitution. I understand constitution here to mean the passive process by which experiences become possible in existence, just as existence itself becomes possible (Gallagher and Zahavi 2008, p. 26). The integrity of the structural unity of existence depends on there being a self-pole, a world-pole and an other-pole that are themselves whole and able to organise themselves in terms of anthropological proportions. The constitution of the structure of existence has two essential characteristics. In the first place, it is *transcendental*; that is, it depends on factors external to subjective experiences.[17] Existential personhood therefore depends on an impersonality immanent to all experience. This impersonality has a dual function in the empirical emergence of the person. First, it allows its emergence (through its constitution), and second, it limits the ways in which the conditions of possibility configure personal existences. Changes in the two functions of impersonality will be addressed in this work. The changes in the constitutive function will be called structural changes, and changes in the forms of configuration of the conditions of possibility are referred to as anthropopathological.

The second essential characteristic of impersonality is *ambiguity*. Although the constitution of existence determines a single person, its constitution is intersubjective (Husserl 2003), that is, for us to be existence, we must already pre-reflexively be coexistence. The constitution of existence – and simultaneously of reality – is therefore, in its essence, co-constitution. Therefore, every time I refer to the original passive process that makes the structure of existence organic, I will use either *intersubjective constitution* or *co-constitution* of existence. Multiple unity is the ultimate foundation that allows a single existence to be synthesised and developed as a personal project in history.

The structure of existence is also individual, meaning that each existence takes on a particular configuration for its structure, although the general notion of structure falls within the scope of anthropology. So, every human existence is constituted, *in abstracto*, as structure, but this structure exists only when instantiated individually in its participative dependence on the surrounding world. All structural knowledge is therefore individual and idiographic. This does not mean it is impossible to know instantiated experiential generalities, the essence of which is the object of nomothetic empirical science of psychopathology. In his *Metaphysics*, Aristotle says there is only science of the universal, since the particular may refuse to take on a permanent form, which is a prerequisite for it to be an object of science. Although my perspective is not exactly Aristotelian, since as a clinician I always have my sights on the individual, I still align myself in part with his notion, as I believe the ultimate object of psychopathology, the individual, cannot be fully apprehended by the general science I am developing here. The nomothetic science of psychopathology seeks to recognise the essential typical pathological forms that are manifested in different ways individually (Messas 2014c). More specifically, psychopathological science seeks to identify and analyse the essence of the anthropological disproportions that make the potentiality of individual existences vulnerable. This is the limit of psychopathology and thus of the scientific ambitions of the psychopathologist.

---

[17] These factors external to consciousness, responsible for its delimitation and final form, are not covered in this book, as ultimately they fall within the realm of philosophy. The transcendentality of the constitution of the structure of existence should not be confused with the neurological mechanisms on which consciousness depends. These are merely its physiological basis. For more details on the relationships between the neurological bases and the structure of consciousness, I refer to the work of Fuchs (2018).

The individual forms of this existential structure can only be recognised through an immediate, intuitive, total act; the identification of the essences of psychopathological experiences is partial, positive and scientific. There is a general anthropological intuition of the meaning of the existential structure and a direct intuition of it in its individual actualisations, but there is no science of them. The science stops at the revelation of the general in the particular. The individual extends beyond the scientific. Knowing one existence does not enable knowledge of the next, but knowing the essences of psychopathological entities enables their identification in another existence. Only clinical experience, a mixture of science and experience acquired in the pragmatic application of anthropological intuition, provides the conditions for the genuine application of psychopathological knowledge. The complete approach to phenomenological clinical practice is to merge scientific knowledge of pathological existential formations with intuitive experience in managing individual biographies. This complete form exceeds the objectives of this work. Thus, all psychopathology that is applied to the individual structure transcends science and passes to the extra-scientific terrain of pathography, inaugurated and developed by Jaspers (Jaspers 1970; Minkowski 2002).

2.6.1   Structure of Existence, Positional Sense, Value Sense and Individual Freedom

The structure of existence, as the primal pre-reflexive position of existence, is itself already an ordering of the importance of the world and is thus a source of meaning. As it is mobile and endowed with proportionality, its meaning is open and springs forth whenever the dialectic articulations of the various conditions of possibility intermingle. However, this is not the only meaning existence can be endowed with, since existence is also free to deliberate on its own meanings. There are therefore two ways of understanding existential meaning. In one, the *positional sense*, the emphasis is on the way the primal articulations of the self-pole, the other-pole and the world-pole are given. The positional sense is the primary framework for the meanings of existence, inescapable and independent of the action of consciousness, but essentially incomplete, insofar as it can be complemented by decisions of free will. The existential structure itself generates meaning continuously and spontaneously, even before it is expressed in consciousness. Although the positional sense is mutable, it is not a freedom; rather, it is the delimitation of the possible field in which freedom acts. Let us suppose that someone was born with a temperament whose anthropological proportions are propitious for them to apprehend the world sensorially. Accordingly, they will sense the world mainly through colours, sounds and shapes and less through abstract ideas, for example. Their basic experiences will be tempered by a material density that precedes the deliberations of their free will. Freedom, as an act of the historical self, decides how to frame these ways of apprehending, but always while immersed in an endowed world that precedes it and over which it has no decision-making control. Freedom can only act on pre-reflexive choices (Kraus 2014) which are imposed on it.

The structure of existence gives the world an original meaning, pre-reflexively stratifies an order and hierarchy of ways to access the world and itself, and designs and flattens the reliefs of reality, powerfully delimiting the frontiers for existence. It gives a positional sense to existence in the world. However, it does not circumscribe everything that will be assimilated by the historical self. It offers a framework, but, except in the psychopathological situations to which I will return, it does not carry with itself all determination of existence. Rather, the positional sense is the architecture of the anthropological proportions of the stage on which a single existence develops its epic. I can, for example, have a wide protention which offers my historical self a vast array of themes for me to investigate. Or else, my protention may be structurally narrow, making the range of themes that present themselves pre-reflexively restricted to one or two. These are the conditions in which my free will acts.

In parallel, there is also an explicit or implicit value in each act or representation of the historical self, endowed with subjective affectivity. We feel and manifest in thoughts and ideas a hierarchy of principles of conduct and experiences by which we guide our life (Fulford and Stanghellini 2019). This is our *value sense*. Here, we are already further away from the primal nature of the positional sense and therefore closer to the action of the will. This kind of action chooses, up to a point, what values we live by. Or, even if it does not choose them, it is guided by a hierarchy of values on which it is capable of reflecting. The value sense is secondary in relation to the positional sense, but it is the first object accessible to the historical self, which experiences it directly. We are enthusiastic, for example, about a subject we freely decide to be drawn towards and on which we base our lives. This theme becomes our value. Here, in this secondary circle, the action of freedom (always partial) is limited by the positional sense. Even on topics where free will is able to assess its values, the twists and turns of the primal positional sense can never be circumvented. Freedom chooses its values, but it depends on a prior, primal sense for them to become incarnate. Every individual existence is a positional concession to an insistent and in a way visionary free will. An existence that assimilates and unifies the positional sense and the value sense develops into authentic existence.

The positional sense and the value sense strive for harmony so that existence can be perceived as authentic and fulfilled – the subjective experience of happiness – although, by the very dialectic and contradictory nature of existence, neither can avoid some passing dissonance. This dissonance, rendered by the actual maturing of the positional senses throughout life, is what allows the refinement and readjustment of values to the real situation of existence. We may value social justice, for example; however, the way we instantiate this value in the web of reality will change throughout our trajectory. More mature, we see through the windows of positional sense that what we always understood as value should be introduced into society in a different way than we thought in our youth; that it requires points of social articulation which the youthful position did not let us see and that in fact made it harder for our value to be realised in society.

In the same way, our value sense may change over time and the restrictions of the positional sense may hinder its instantiation. In many cases, now nearer to psychopathology or extreme temperaments, the positional and value senses may enter into discord. For example, a patient who is structurally phobic (we will still see the definition of this in Sect. 3.2) and impulsive puts great value on social justice. His imagination and free action are effectively geared towards the construction of an institutional apparatus to protect his fellow men. However, his phobic position restricts a priori the potential for the actualisation of his genuine vocation based on his value sense. Certain forms of otherness which, from a value-oriented perspective, should be encompassed in his action, appear pre-reflexively to his consciousness as immersed in such an atmosphere of risk that his existence excludes them from his field of action. This does not make his existence unauthentic, but it does restrict it in terms of the experience of happiness.

The mismatch between the positional and value senses can also be experienced as existential conflict. A certain markedly schizoid section (see Sect. 3.7) has the constitution of a family – wife and children – as an ingrained value for his life. However, the original position of his existential structure, which is extremely fragmented, does not offer him an affective definition of how and with whom to realise this value. The patient is incapable of liking anyone enough to form a bond of matrimony. His existence is guided by a value which cannot be harmonised with the positionality of his existential structure, making it empty and unproductive ideation. The will alone cannot make its main value become a reality in the interpersonal world. His consciousness is ceaselessly tormented, wearing itself out in anguished observation of a life slipping by without a decision being taken. Here, we have a dissonance between a positional sense (the inability to experience the value of the otherness of the opposite sex) and a value sense absolutely dependent on a valued other for it to be exercised (to constitute a family). In this existence, it is the historical self who seeks to force the original positionality to adjust pre-reflexively towards the expression of a value.

2.7   The Ontological Sense of Phenomenological Diagnosis: Existential Types and Moderate Realism

One founding conception of phenomenological psychopathology is that every human experience, pathological or not, can be reduced to its essences, which can then be apprehended scientifically (Cutting 2012; Dahlberg 2006; Basso 2009; Messas et al. 2017b). And, as it is devoted to comprehending how these essences are manifested in existence, it understands that the essences of psychopathological objects are typical anthropological formations. As these psychopathological types are actualised in existential forms that are lived and constituted intersubjectively, they are, from an ontological point of view, *real*. By this, I mean that regardless of the different interpretations a psychopathologist may make of a psychopathological phenomenon, it will be based on some basic style of anthropological disproportion or of fracture in the intersubjective co-constitution of reality (see Chaps. 3 and 4), which are the two existential modes of disorders. These alterations modify the way in which the structure of existence is constituted and articulated proportionally, and so they are ultimately rooted in the most real foundations of existence. As they are based on the roots of existence, they constitute *existential types* of psychopathologies (Kraus 1991a; Dörr-Zegers 2008; Messas and Tamelini 2018). The reality that underlies the psychopathological object should not, however, be mistaken for biological or chemical realism (Kendler 2016), derived from a third-person approach, whose actualisation does not depend on the participation of an observer. The reality of existential types, depending as it does on the participation of the other to be accessed, inevitably constitutes second-person knowledge.

The objects of phenomenological psychopathology do not exist as absolute essences (Platonic absolute realism) or as mere provisional clusters of operational descriptions (nominalistic operationalism). The reality of their intersubjective existential incarnation can be defined in terms of ontological autonomy as *moderate realism* (Oulis 2008). This form of realism understands that the psychopathological object is a typical style of dialectical involvement of the pre-reflexive anthropological proportions of existence in reality. Each style has an essence and can therefore be known in its generality, but this general reality can only be apprehended validly at the moment it appears in a concrete interpersonal relationship, which is why it is called moderate.[18] If existence is expansion and mobility and the essences of the pathological modes of existence are typified and fixed,[19] phenomenological moderate realism proceeds along the tortuous paths by which mobility and stability interact, giving rise to dialectical relations in which interpersonality plays a primordial role from an epistemological and an ontological point of view. Diagnostic knowledge that stems from moderate realistic ontology thus enables a psychopathological essence to be identified in the context in which it can be apprehended. A phenomenological diagnosis simultaneously intuits the essence and apprehends its singular characteristics in its presentation in an individual history, always in transformation.[20] The essential characteristics of each psychopathological experience are therefore dispersed due to the personality of each individual in which it emerges. Dispersion is the individual shape the typical essential form takes when it is

---

[18] In the ontological philosophical tradition (especially in medieval thinking), the essence of an object that appears as such only in its concrete reality (*in re*) is called *moderate*; it is different from an essence that can be grasped irrespective of reality, which is said to be *absolute*, as occurs, for example, in geometry (*ante rem*). This contrasts with nominalism, which is the knowledge that, sceptical as to the possibility of identifying the essence of reality, grants the status of reality only to the names that represent it (*post rem*).

[19] This concept will be demonstrated in detail in Parts II and III, given over to pathologies.

[20] It is important to highlight that this apprehension of the essential in the particular, which will be seen in Parts II and III of this study in several clinical examples and in patients' own words, should not be confused with the original intuition of an individual existence, which is outside the scope of a science, as stated above (Sect. 2.6). The act of apprehending the essence of a pathology through its existential examples is in fact the only genuine way of practising the nomothetic science of psychopathology without resorting to nominalist abstraction.

actualised in each existence and the root cause of most of the difficulties psychopathologists face in elaborating a diagnosis. The phenomenological endeavour is thus uncertain and dubious, although it investigates a full, accessible reality. It must simultaneously recognise psychopathological experience as a fact of reality and investigate the ways in which this typical psychopathological reality is customised in each individual existence. The essences of psychopathological entities and their modes of manifestation in existences are inseparable in phenomenological psychopathology (Abettan 2015; Fernandez and Køster 2019). This inherent difficulty of existential reality leads to epistemological imprecision, which I now examine. The fact that there is imprecision in any psychopathological diagnosis has led some authors of phenomenological psychopathology, inspired by Jaspers, to argue that the psychopathological object is, in essence, an ideal type or a prototype (Schwartz and Wiggins 1987; Parnas et al. 2013; Fernandez 2016; Schäfer 2001). The ideal type is not an empirical reality that exists in the world as such, but an intellectual tool for accessing a reality that is deemed inaccessible or inevitably biased by the examiner's value options. The same is true of the notion of prototype, despite the supposed differences between these concepts, as analysed meticulously by Fernandez (2019). Jaspers went so far as to state that ideal types represent the limit of knowledge of the great psychopathological syndromes (Jaspers 1997). My position is that there is a clear confusion between ontological status and epistemological conditions of access to reality itself. In this confusion, difficulties of access (epistemological) are taken as indications of the impossibility of any real definition of the object (ontological), leading to an unnecessary and unjustified narrowing of the potential scope of psychopathological science. A real ontology may perfectly well coexist with a pragmatic epistemology, which takes from it what can be instituted as science, without denying that the object exists as such, in reality (Zorzanelli et al. 2016). I refute this restricted and even timid view of psychopathology and do so literally in Binswanger's words (Binswanger 1922, p. 297): "if comprehensible relationships are ideal types, this means that in psychology we should work with concepts that, on the one hand, do not correspond to nothing in reality, which are nothing other than images coming from thought … Psychology is not an abstract theory or a simple intellectual construct; it intends to address reality and inscribe this reality in concepts that can 'be valid' for reality…". This is the phenomenological psychopathology that I defend and intend to develop in this work.

2.8 Imprecision and Objectivity: Second-Person Knowledge

It has been said that the phenomenologist is a person without certainty (Di Petta 2012). This could not be more correct, for it reveals the state of the soul of a dialectic scientist who knows that confronting the reality of his/her object of study – human existence itself – produces great challenges due to its ambiguity. The contradictory nature of this reality calls for the psychopathologist to adopt a correspondingly prudent approach to scientific certainties. Specifically, I would say that

the search for knowledge by this certainty-less human comes up against a fundamental difficulty: the dialectics between diagnostic imprecision and diagnostic
objectivity (Rossi 2008; Keil et al. 2016).

The individual variability of the essential manifestations of disorders makes the
meaning of any diagnosis *imprecise*; that is, on many occasions, it is impossible to
establish the essential nature of a pathology. This imprecision is manifested in both
the transverse and the longitudinal aspects of phenomenological psychopathology.
Transversely, clinical daily life shows us *ad nauseam* how often experienced psychopathologists will diverge in their diagnosis of the same patient, each basing their
hypothesis on sensible arguments. From a longitudinal point of view, clinical evolu-
tions show us how phenomenological manifestations change in the same patient
over time, forcing diagnoses made previously with presumed assurance to be
reviewed (Baca-Garcia et al. 2007). This weakness of diagnostic accuracy should
not, however, be confused with subjectivity, understood as the expression of an
individual impressionistic judgement by a psychopathologist without the necessary
correlation with factual reality. On the contrary, phenomenological diagnosis postu-
lates total objectivity for everything it claims (Blankenburg 2012). This objectivity,
supported by the elements of empathy, language and visuality, is not inconsistent
with imprecision. Objectivity comes from the full experience of contact with the
patient, an experience which, as it takes on board the descriptions of the simultaneous subjective experiences of patient and observer and examines them exhaustively,
reaches the level of objectivity (Gabbani and Stanghellini 2008). This is structural
objectivity, situated in the pre-reflexive form of intersubjectivity. It is therefore a
truth obtained in the second person (Stanghellini 2007; Fuchs 2010; Dörr-Zegers
2013; Nordgaard et al. 2013; Galbusera and Fellin 2014), which synthesises dialectically the knowledge obtained by the subjective description of the patient – first-
person perspective (Leal and Serpa Junior 2013) – with the reflective understanding
offered by the scientist from their participative relationship with the patient (Messas
and Fukuda 2018).

It is true that this objectivity gives rise to various subjectivities and is only accessible through them. However, the transcendental structure of experiences is objective and can be studied empirically with reproducible results (Giorgi 2009). Any
clinical disagreements regarding diagnostic objectivity originate in the multiplicity
of intersubjective points of access to objectivity. This multiplicity is more epistemologically decisive than any supposed diagnostic subjectivity.[21]

Let us take here an example in which a supposed excess of subjectivity tends to
cloud the notion of objectivity of the phenomenological diagnosis. Let us imagine a

---

[21] Depraz et al. (2011, p. 139) describe definitively this relationship between intersubjective imprecision and access to objectivity: "therefore the presence of contradictory or opposing descriptions
may very well be indicative not of any theoretical aporia as to the nature of the universal truth of
experience, but of an invitation to produce a more nuanced description, one that is more fine-tuned,
more differentiated, taking into account additional dimensions. In other words, the conflict of validation in the intersubjectivity of the act of descriptive practice leads to a deepening of both the
description and the quality of validation".

schizophrenic patient before us; he expresses disconnected ideas that are not directly attuned to our affective experiences. The psychopathologist has the clear (subjective) impression that they do not understand the patient's experience and that there is something minimally human lacking for it to be comprehended. The only thing sustaining the researcher's attitude is perplexity. The interpersonal distance blocks the affective vibration of the patient–psychopathologist relationship. And there is no direct access to the patient's psychism by empathic means except by using interpretative resources. This state of inaccessibility between two psychisms is strongly objective, irreducible, reproducible in other situations with other evaluators, and the expression of the maximum possible reality a situation of duality (Pallagrosi and Fonzi 2018). It will be the psychopathologist's reflections, in conjunction with the patient's account, that will reconstruct, at the level of transcendental comprehension, the details of this crystalline objectivity. After all, the absence of affective resonance is itself an irrefutable case of phenomenological objectivity (Pallagrosi et al. 2016). After all, objectivity arises when a patient's experiences are included generally in every dimension of existence, which never ceases to be manifested in interpersonal relationships – one of the cornerstones of the fundamental validity of phenomenological psychopathology (Giorgi 1994, 2009).

The variability of manifestation of the essence of each pathological experience in the totality of existence makes the diagnosis imprecise, but objective. Nevertheless, a diagnosis is still subject to greater or lesser degrees of validity (or access to objectivity). I suggest that there are two reasons for this. The first arises from the fact that the anthropological disproportion itself responsible for the pathological experience may be more distant from the intersubjective relationship, where it would gain maximum evidence. Melancholia, for example, when relatively mild, may only occupy embodiment, leaving its manifestation in the dimension of intersubjectivity relatively intact. Physical pain, malaise or general fears of illness may be the expression of an existential restriction typical of melancholia (see Sect. 4.2), which still resonates weakly in the psychism of the observer. In this case, the observer's access to the experiential essence of melancholia would be limited. Only in later stages, as the experience expanded, could one begin to envision the pathological core intersubjectively by means, for example, of a fixed, heavy or laborious intersubjectivity.

Another situation where the degree of imprecision may be greater is longitudinal diagnosis. Recognising, for example, the difference between mild melancholia and a limited existential crisis presupposes detailed knowledge of the patient's biography, which only a long clinical–patient relationship would allow; a relationship that enabled the clinician to have an overview of their patient's entire biographical development. Longitudinal diagnoses are therefore less valid, although they can still be valid and objective. In them, the comprehensive evaluation of pathological experiences over longitudinal temporality is the reason for the imprecision. By contrast, transversal diagnoses are more objective and therefore less imprecise.

2.9   The Existential Meaning of Psychopathology Experiences

In order to understand the existential sense of psychopathological experiences, it is fundamental to remember how crucial temporality is in the constitution of existence. To exist is to define oneself over time in a pre-reflexive movement out of oneself towards a future that is indefinite and largely impossible to control. As temporal beings, we are always having to deal with the need to take on new existential forms, whether we like it or not. The development of the biography thus involves a dynamic regime of creation, extinction and recreation of the reciprocal proportions of the existential conditions of possibility. The fact that we are projected in temporality means the modes of proportion on which we depend pre-reflectively in the world, in ourselves and in our intersubjective relationships change throughout life. Our existential substrates are articulated in different anthropological proportions over time. This general statement becomes clearer if we set their extremes in contrast. A baby bases its existence only on the intersubjective relationship with its mother (Ceron-Litvoc 2020), without which its actual biological life would be impossible. Its existence is restricted to a transversal temporality of the immediate instant and to a spatiality circumscribed to direct bodily contact with the mother and with nourishment. The adult, on the other hand, is constituted by an extended transversal temporality and a spatiality marked by distance, perspective and the capacity to form multiple intersubjective relationships.

The continuous changes in the anthropological proportions of each individual never happen in isolation. There is an intimate connection between the conditions of possibility that sparks a dialectic relationship between them. Every change in the relative participation of one condition of possibility implies a corresponding change or reproportioning of the others. An existence may advance at a certain moment (spontaneous existential maturation, for example), expanding the proportional importance of protention and reducing the importance of retention. Such a state or condition initially leads to an existential imbalance, but this is necessary for existence to open up to the future and thereby mature. In order to maintain a minimum of equilibrium for its sanity, the structure of existence spontaneously sets about rebalancing the other conditions of possibility, increasing the participation of some of them. It might seek to broaden its support in intersubjectivity (e.g. meeting up with a group of like-minded peers) or in its own values (reminding itself what its life goals are), or its own embodiment. (At times when our projects are under significant threat or uncertainty, we may increase the participation of our body, doing more physical exercise, for example.) There is no shortage of examples, but all have in common the idea that the anthropological proportions of the structure of existence are mutable and that this inevitably affects all the dimensions of its own constitution. All existence operates in a dialectical regime of balance and imbalance, symmetry and asymmetry. This dialectical regime between transitory instability and stability is of the utmost importance for understanding the emergence of pathological existential experiences (Messas 2010b).

Strong biographical development depends on it having multiple supports in intersubjectivity, the self-pole and the world-pole, which oscillate in terms of their relative participation. This makes it less likely for the whole existential structure to be dominated by dependence on just one condition of possibility. An adult in good existential shape has more than one point of support to keep their existential form open to protention: in the meaning of their professional projects, their family commitments, their ethical values, their close friends and relations, their contribution to society, etc. This ensures the points of articulation in the dialectics of their existential proportions never condense into one disproportional form. In a way, launching oneself into the moving flow of life distributes the partial participations of each single condition of possibility. The health of existence depends on a certain pluralism, on a refusal to focus too much on one of the foundations of existence. In health, the whole of existence is more relevant than the parts that constitute it dialectically. All these parts are called on in turn, serving to maintain the typical human existential form: forward-oriented and open to the complexity of the simultaneity of elements in contrast and composition. When different supports in the conditions of possibility are leant on, the "weight" is shared among them, making existence better able to handle the challenges of personal expansion. This whole thematic field will be clearer when we deal specifically with the essences of psychopathological experiences.

In situations other than full health, temporality is weakened (in mild cases) or shattered (in severe ones).[22] In these conditions, this primordial constituent of temporality is restricted and so existence tends to be fixed in one anthropological disproportion. The pathological nature of such a disproportion is given by its duration and thus the dominance of the existential structure. Temporality is, then, the first citadel to tumble on the path to the desolation of existence. A mental disorder is primarily an obstacle to the accomplishment, on the part of existence, of the movements necessary for the synchronic and harmonic superimposition of the positional and value senses. An everyday example, far from pathological, serves to illustrate this relationship between temporality and existential immobility. Let us imagine that we get a headache precisely on the day of an important business meeting where we plan to propose an important new project. During the meeting, the headache disappears as if behind our urge to try to get the best results from it. We are focused on the future, where we want to get to. Later, when the temporal stimulus disappears, we are at the mercy of the relaxed body, which the headache is accosting. The reduction of protentive temporality, which occurred when the meeting and its associated stimuli came to an end, increases the participation of embodiment in existence and becomes, due to the intensity of the pain, its main point of support (the previous point was the ideal of life, when the body served mainly as a means to enable it). This illustrates the general principle that the loss of the moving force that temporality brings into existence leads to a tendency for the dialectic relations

---

[22] We will see the conditions of possibility of this shattering in the section on structural disorders (Chap. 4).

among the pre-reflexive dimensions to condense at some point, tending to immobil-
ise existence. This immobilisation comes in many forms. Indeed, the various ways
in which the dialectics of existential proportions are immobilised are the basis of the
matrix of psychopathological experiences, as we will see below. The structure of
existence is like a dynamic three-dimensional geometrical figure which depends for
its health on its capacity to dissolve its forms. For example, sadness is a state in
which a fault or frustration takes hegemony over the momentary whole of existence.
It can only be overcome if it is extinguished in the indefinite horizon of protentive
temporality. It is only through the stiffening of this continuous dialectic movement
that psychopathological experiences emerge. However, the stiffening or even paralysis of the transformative capacity of existence is only a general definition of its
form as mental disorder. Mental disorders manifest differently and with different
degrees of severity. This severity depends on where the core of the disorder affecting the whole of existence is located. Essentially, mental disorders can be divided
into two groups according to the severity of the impairment of the dialectic capacity
of existence. This is what we will study in the next section. For didactic purposes, I
will first present the less serious pathological experiences and then the more serious ones.

The experiences of the first sense, called *anthropopathological* experiences, are
closer to the daily experiences of all humans; they are therefore, in a certain degree,
easier to be apprehended by the reader. The ones affecting the second level, *structural*, originate in deeper regions of the constitution of existence, making them less
easy to access. From an existential point of view, however, structural disorders pre-
cede and are hierarchically superior to anthropopathological ones, which means
every time there is a structural pathology, there will be consequences on the anthropological level. Meanwhile, pure anthropopathologies do not lead to structural rup-
tures. A descriptive analysis of the essence of each psychopathological experience,
structural or anthropological, includes the presentation of their typical anthropological disproportions and their constituent dialectics. The explanation will involve
three modes of dialectical understanding. The main one, *dialectics of anthropological proportions*, aims at identifying the main tensions in the existential conditions
of possibility underlying each psychopathological experience. This form of dialectic merits attention, since it is the one that provides the best potential for observing
existential movements. Given that anthropological proportions rearrange themselves all the time, knowing them is the best way to help existential movement
resume, which is the primary objective of clinical care. The second dialectic explores
the *ambiguities* present in each psychopathological experience, identifying favourable and unfavourable aspects in them. Although a psychopathological entity is
defined by its unfavourable elements, the ambiguity inherent to human life allows a
window to be opened to favourable elements contained in the essence of these experiences. From these, it is possible to envisage ways to conduct the clinical case that
takes the favourable face of each psychopathology into account. The third dialectic
will only be outlined in this work, since it is not strictly a psychopathology. It refers
directly to the theme of the construction of clinical care: the *dialectics of decisions*.
Through this, the typical positional and value senses put into play in each

psychopathological experience must be seen in their relations with the decisions the clinician has to take. It is by examining the pre-reflexive positions and values in tension in each pathological form that the clinician and patient freely choose the paths along which they should orient their therapeutic choices. The dialectics of decisions foregrounds and provides inputs to foster the rationality contained in clinical decisions.

2.10   The Nosographic and Nosological Meaning of Phenomenological Diagnosis

The particularities of a phenomenological diagnosis mean that it cannot be immediately used in psychiatric nosography. Phenomenological diagnostics and semiological diagnostics are not synonyms (Gorostiza and Manes 2011). The function of phenomenological diagnostics is to collaborate with the nosography and nosology of mental disorders, without, however, any immediate translation of what is apprehended by phenomenological psychopathology in the psychopathological entities of a nosographic system. Phenomenological psychopathological diagnoses describe and enable a profound comprehension of typical existential situations, which can be part of a mental semiological picture, according to the intensity and pervasiveness with which they affect the whole of existence. I shall give two examples, for clarification. We will see below that the essence of manic experience is the reduction of existence to a total temporality, the present, which is apprehended by the spatiality of intersubjective proximity. However, this essential experience can also describe the high of moderate alcoholic intoxication or an experience of very intense mood swings, for whatever reason. In this case, whatever is described and understood in its constituent existential structures on a phenomenological level becomes a nosological entity – in this case, mania – only if it is very long-lasting or invades existence to the point of compromising the person's capacity for sociability (and, in the case of mania, is not caused by acute intoxication by some psychoactive substance). In this case, the nosological diagnosis of mania would be understood as the complete subjugation of existence to a typical phenomenologically comprehensible existential form. But other relationships may occur, of which I will highlight only one. Below, I will define phobic experience existentially as a disproportion of intersubjectivity that overvalues the other (see Sect. 3.2). This incomplete definition is given here merely to enable the presentation of this example. From this description, we might make a nosological diagnosis of a person as having a phobic personality. In this case, we would be saying that the essential characteristics of phobic disproportion tinge their personality, constituting itself in the state of anthropological proportions that guides their existential development. In other words, that their personality is marked by the hypervaluation of the other-pole to the detriment of the self-pole. In this case, the essence of the phobic experience imposes itself tenuously but continuously on their personality. In the same way, we could say that phobic disproportion may invade existence acutely, manifesting itself as phobic anxiety or panic attack. In this case, the nosological psychopathological entity would be defined as an acute and dramatic invasion of the same anthropological disproportion that defines the phobic personality. However, they are two different, autonomous and fully fledged nosological psychopathological entities based on the same anthropological disproportion, the same phenomenological diagnosis.

The development of psychiatric nosology and nosographies based on a work of phenomenological psychopathology would require a whole additional analysis that falls outside the scope of this work (Rovaletti 2001). Nonetheless, it must be stressed that no psychiatric nosology can do without its foundation in phenomenological diagnostics. A lack of attention to this principle turns nosography into a terrain of working opinions that are merely the result of consensus about what a mental disorder is understood as being, leading to a state of conceptual chaos, in which psychopathological entities multiply without their ontological value being properly elucidated (Zachar and Jablensky 2015).

Part II
Psychopathology and Substance Misuse

Chapter 3
Anthropological Disproportions (Anthropopathologies)

The first stratum at which existential alterations are manifested is the *anthropological level*. At this level, disturbed experiences are essentially anthropological disproportions, or simply anthropopathologies. Anthropopathological experiences are essentially expressions of hindrances to the free and pliable dialectic movement of the conditions of possibility of existence, without compromising the fundamental constitution of reality.[1]

The journey of existence involves a perpetual transformation of anthropological proportions. Falling ill, on the other hand, results from a reduction of the capacity for transformation (Messas 2004; Sass 2010). This reduction leads to an existence dominated by one typical form of anthropological disproportion. The continued domination of existence by a specific proportion is what makes an anthropological disproportion an anthropopathology. Let us look, for example, at the experience of grief following the loss of a loved one. At first, the absence of the other appears as a striking presence. The pain of absence reveals the enormous value of this specific intersubjectivity for the whole of existence. From the point of view of anthropological proportions, the domination of existence by otherness, in this case, absent, defines the state. The subjective experience of the bereaved is tainted by pain, apathy or longing owing to the absence of this otherness. The experience of grief is in essence a typical anthropological disproportion, hijacking existence in such a way that the missing otherness dominates all other conditions of possibility. There is nothing pathological about this experience. As we will see, a typical form of anthropological disproportion determines all cases of anthropopathologies. In contrast, every resolution of an anthropological disproportion involves the resumption of dialectics between the conditions of possibility of existence. In this example, a healthy resolution of grief would occur when the bereaved is able to find support for existence in other dimensions rather than an intersubjectivity focussed on an absence.

---

[1] I will refer to this in the next section concerning structural disorders. Anthropological disproportions are essentially analogous to any human experience of suffering that originates in a reduction of the capacity of existence to transform itself over time (Messas 2004).

G. Messas, *The Existential Structure of Substance Misuse*,
https://doi.org/10.1007/978-3-030-62724-9_3

In the context of anthropopathologies, the point of transition between normal and altered experience is determined in a relatively arbitrary manner by observing the relevance an anthropological disproportion takes on in relation to the existential whole. How one anthropological disproportion relates dialectically to the global movement of existence is crucial for making an anthropopathological diagnosis. Thus, between normal and anthropopathological anxiety, there are many points, which, if not clinically similar, overlap. Only by making a detailed examination of the relevance of anxiety to the dialectic capacity of the existential whole can their boundaries be discerned. There are two situations that provide the conditions for diagnosing an anthropopathology. In the first, the anthropological disproportion ossifies the whole of existence to such an extent that the historical self experiences the need to reduce it. The historical self feels that the emerging anthropological disproportion is undermining its purpose and ambitions. In this condition, the subjective experience is ego-dystonic, since it collides with the value sense of existence. In such conditions, the use of psychoactive substances becomes an important instrument for the historical self to self-modulate its own anthropological proportions. I will call this anthropological mechanism *self-management*. Self-management is central to the understanding of substance misuse in the context of a general psychopathology.

Most substance misuse in states of anxiety or depression fits this definition. This perspective also facilitates the understanding of more specific and less severe cases. In these cases, the anthropological disproportion disturbs a specific aspect of existential plans, without, however, putting the whole of existence at risk. An example of this would be the case of a person suffering from aviophobia who gets a new job which involves travelling. Although this has not been a major issue in the individual's daily life up to this point, the new existential conditions mean that the moment at which it emerges – in this case, the evolution of a professional identity – becomes sufficiently uncomfortable to characterise an anthropopathology. The divergence between the existential projects and the anthropological disproportion, which emerges as an obstacle to vital development, is enough to justify the use of a psychoactive substance with the aim of reducing or nullifying the distress.

In the second condition in which an anthropopathology emerges, the anthropological disproportion is so great that it hijacks and becomes completely identified with the whole of existence. Such is the case of so-called personality disorders, often associated with substance misuse (Welch 2007). A severe case of schizotypal personality disorder, for example, fits this interpretation. In this case, it is not so much that existence has been appropriated by one typical disproportion (which will be seen below, Sect. 3.7), but that it is completely defined by the disproportion. The disproportion is experienced by the historical self as its identity and, with this, its own value senses are based on the disproportion. The pathological aspect of these situations often originates from a second-person perspective, insofar as it is the harmful effects on otherness that characterise this kind of disproportion. As a consequence, intersubjective relationships become difficult and unstable. When anthropological disproportion defines existence, self-management through substance use is often an attempt to resist inhabiting a world where intersubjectivity does not constitute a genuine foundation for existence.

In short, I suggest that the emergence of an anthropopathology in an individual existence originates in the disproportionate emphasis given to some condition of possibility. The essence of an anthropopathology is always a pre-reflexive overdependence on some existential component, constituting a harmful imbalance of anthropological proportions, which culminates in a disturbance of the dialectical regime of existential development (Messas et al. 2017b). The harm inherent to this disproportion does not, however, stem primarily from the associated behavioural and experiential changes. The problem is that it prevents the kind of existential flexibility consistent with the values and projects of existence or with viable coexistence in the shared world. Therefore, we cannot say that a *harmony* of anthropological proportions is the perfect existential state of health. Rather, we might say that the best possible structural condition for reaching a plenitude of existential potentialities is a *dialectical balance* between states of proportion and disproportion.

Using psychoactive substances is an attempt to overcome such difficulties by modifying the conditions of possibility of existence. There are two ways to self-manage anthropological disproportions: synergy and antagonism. I will explore these two possibilities in more detail in the section on the psychopathology of substance misuse (part III). At this point, suffice it to say that with synergy, the historical self seeks to maintain or accentuate the kind of anthropological disproportion in which it exists. In contrast, with antagonistic use, the historical self seeks to reduce or even modify the essential characteristics of its disproportion.

Thus far, I have used the dialectics of anthropological proportions to define the emergence of anthropopathological experience. This is not the only dialectical perspective with which we can illuminate these experiences. Every essential anthropopathological manifestation can also be grasped by an ambiguous conception of dialectics (Blankenburg 1981; Messas and Tamelini 2018). In this, the innate ambiguity of each anthropological experience is revealed in a positive and a negative face,[2] which in turn establish a dialectic relationship between themselves. This ambiguity is fundamental to understanding the meanings different experiences take on in the different anthropological disproportions and therefore in the decision-making processes for each one.

Take the example of borderline disproportion, which I will examine later. Its positive aspect comes from the oversubmission of existence to the presence of the other-pole. All the clinical manifestations of borderline disproportion thus derive from this anthropological insufficiency of the self-pole. However, in the negativity of borderline, this fragility of the self-pole reveals a healthy aspect for existential development. The weakening of the self-pole makes it more flexible in relation to the directives of professional roles, promoting an unsaturated identity that permits existential creativity, which we do not see, for example, in melancholic persons

---

[2] I understand "positive" here as "according to the psycho-pathological definition" and "negative" as "opposed to the psycho-pathological definition". This definition does not imply any affirmation of positive or negative psychological value.

(Kraus 1996b). There is a dynamic balance within each anthropological disproportion that reveals the ambiguity of all human experience. This ambiguity is responsible for the immanent force contained in every experience which enables it to be overcome. The ambiguous dialectical interpretation suggests that in every anthropological experience, any loss is offset by some gain. The dynamics of existence thus draw on the possibilities of compensation inherent to each anthropological disproportion. This immanent property of anthropological disproportions is invaluable in a therapeutic setting since it indicates how the evolutionary potential of each clinical case should guide the clinical strategy. Finally, I should mention that each anthropological disproportion studied begins with a short clinical vignette designed to exemplify some of the typical biographical features it presents in daily life.

Every anthropopathology is, as I have suggested, a form of anthropological disproportion. I now wish to present their characteristics. As every presentation is based on some specific classificatory principle, I should begin by stating the basic assumptions of my work. The anthropopathological disproportions presented below are classified around different modes of intersubjectivity. Although I could have used a different category for this classification, especially temporality, I opted for intersubjectivity because it is through this channel that the psychopathologist gains first-hand access to the patient's existence (Messas and Fukuda 2018). I therefore give priority to the evidence that each psychopathologist and clinician has immediate access to as a basis for the organisation of anthropological disproportions in a scientific discourse.

The selection of pathological experiences was not therefore guided by epidemiological prevalence. However, epidemiology did play a key role. I tried to organise the anthropological disproportions, seen from the perspective of intersubjectivity, in such a way as to cover the vast majority of the comorbidities empirically observed between mental disorders and substance misuse (EMCDDA 2016; NIDA 2018). Although the emphasis in this section has been on the indication of a general phenomenological psychopathology, the choice of anthropological disproportions examined presupposes some relationship with substance misuse. As mentioned above, my premise is to understand the role of substance misuse in relation to anthropological disproportions from its existential sense, that is, as self-management.

Based on these principles, I determined four levels of intersubjectivity, organised in decreasing degrees of value given to otherness, although there is a significant degree of overlapping and dynamism between these levels. The values of the self-pole and the other-pole are determined relative to each other in terms of dialectical balance. In some cases, the increase in value of the other-pole originates from the reduced value of the self-pole. In others, however, there is a reciprocal loss (or gain) of the poles' value. In yet others, an increased value of the self-pole accompanies a devaluation of the other-pole. At the first level, otherness has elevated value with emphasis on the figure of the other as an *individual force*. This includes borderline and phobic disproportions. The second level includes a valued otherness, emphasising *collectivity*. This group includes melancholic and hyperthymic disproportion. At the third level, the other-pole loses value as a whole person but gains as a part. This group includes the large group of compulsive disproportions (e.g. sexual compulsion, in which the other only has value as the receiving end of sexual intention), which includes addictions; however, this is only addressed specifically in the next section, on the psychopathology of substance misuse. Here, the relative value of the world's materiality increases, meaning that significant objects (food, physical exercise, shopping, etc.), which can offer pleasurable experiences, are overvalued in detriment to the value of the other-pole. The fourth level is that in which otherness is *devalued*. Schizoid disproportion is present at this level. The feeling of some severely schizoid persons that they are unable to feel love or affection demonstrates how the other-pole can lose its value as its observed presence is attenuated.

The non-specific nature of obsessions makes them difficult to classify in these terms, demonstrating the inherent weakness of all cataloguing efforts. Obsessions may originate from a prevalence of ideas of a phobic nature or from melancholic rumination. The former tends to occur in a fragile self-pole surrounded by frightening and sometimes morally fraught overtones. The latter also tends to hem in a weak self-pole, although in this case it is prone to take on greater responsibility. In other words, the phobic self-pole fears dissolution (e.g. the prevalence of jealousy in phobic temperaments, indicating fear of the end of a meaningful relationship), while the melancholic one feels ultimately responsible for any harm. However, it is not always easy to differentiate them syndromically. I will therefore avoid mentioning the generic aspect of obsessive experiences, presenting them only in their strictly anthropological sense. In this sense, obsessive disproportion can be seen as an existential clash with perfection, in which the value of the other-pole is reduced. It will therefore be examined at the third level, together with compulsive disproportion. Similarly, the concept of depression will be treated as a general human experience (Charbonneau and Legrand 2003; Tatossian and Moreira 2012; Souza and Moreira 2018). At the end of this section, I will indicate its relations with anxiety and melancholia.

Finally, before going into the anthropological disproportions themselves, I would like to make four points concerning the use of categories in the text. In the strictest sense, anthropopathologies are styles of anthropological disproportion. As such, they are typical modes of reciprocal interaction among all the conditions of possibility. Strictly speaking, their names should be indicative of these relationships, in terms of the greater or lesser presence of each of them in the disproportion studied. For example, a disproportion in which the other-pole is undervalued should be called the hypopresence of otherness, and so forth. However, such a denomination would seem too abstract and too distant from psychopathological traditions. I have therefore given each of the anthropological disproportions I will present with a term from the psychopathological tradition. This means that the name may only illuminate one aspect of the complexity of each anthropological disproportion. I have done this because it does not seem to me that any traditional name can account for these complexities. I do however highlight the proportional excesses and lacks that characterise each one anthropologically in the description of each type.

Secondly, in order to help the text flow more easily, I use the adjectives that describe each disproportion interchangeably with their respective nouns. As such, schizoid disproportion and schizoidia, phobic disproportion and phobia, mean the same thing. Only when necessary will I point out some distinction in meaning. Thirdly, as the notion of anthropological disproportion indicates a relationship among conditions of possibility, it may indicate more than one existential situation, irrespective of any clinical significance. For example, when I mention melancholic disproportion, I indicate a certain way of existing that can appear at a specific moment in life or throughout a whole life, as a disorder or just a form of existence. Binswanger inaugurated this approach to examining anthropological proportions, bringing together multiple anthropological conditions, in his study about anthropological disproportions of schizoid disorders and schizophrenia (Binswanger 1992a), yielding exceptional results.

Fourthly, I want to point out the pragmatics of the concepts employed here. Whenever I want to emphasise the totality of experience, I will use the term *existence*. When I want to emphasise the essential core of experiences, the subjectivity "for whom" they come about, I will use the term *historical self*. I will also use this term to emphasise the existential core responsible for making decisions and confronting life's dilemmas. In the passages where I want to emphasise the dialectical relations between the world, otherness and the self, I will use the term self-pole as opposed to world-pole and other-pole. I will use the term "person" in as broad a sense as possible so as to encompass every dimension, active or potential, of an existence (Cusinato 2017). Therefore, when referring to interpersonality, I will address the relationship between whole people, in all their incomplete completeness. I will reserve the term *intersubjectivity* exclusively to indicate the pre-reflexive modes in which the self-pole and the other-pole organise themselves reciprocally, in the most technical sense of the word. I will always use the term *experiences* in an imprecise way, as a generic indication of any experience an existence is capable of having. Finally, in order to keep the text as readable as possible, I will use the term *intoxication* (with its related adjectives and verbs) in a broad sense, meaning any change of consciousness voluntarily produced by the historical self in order to modify its anthropological proportions. As such, the alterations brought about by the use of alcohol, generally referred to as drunkenness, are also subsumed under the umbrella term *intoxication*, except when I wish to indicate some specific effect of alcohol.

First Level

3.1 Borderline Disproportion

Clinical Vignette

Jane is 32 years old. Her mother (Anna) brings her for psychiatric treatment after her third suicide attempt. She is suffering from the break-up of a three-week love affair, based on which she made marriage plans. Her mother reports that the other suicide attempts had a similar motive: frustration at the prospect of separation. Her mother also says that she gets very apprehensive each time her daughter has to face this kind of problem, fearing she will again attempt suicide. At the first consultation, Jane shows a certain hostility and voices disbelief that psychiatric treatment could help her, as she has already seen three other professionals and they have all failed and abandoned her. She highlights all the faults the doctors neglected while caring for her. She says she remembers very little about her most recent suicide attempt because she was "blind with rage" when her boyfriend chose to work overtime instead of spending the evening with her at the appointed time. She had drunk a bottle of vodka, taken a packet of clonazepam and thrown herself from the balcony of the building where she lives with her mother.

Her mother says that Jane was an angry child, difficult to deal with, "crabby" and jealous (towards her brother). During adolescence, mother and daughter had many arguments and clashes, especially when Anna tried to control her irresponsible, risky, impulsive behaviour (drinking too much, unprotected sex and dangerous driving). Anna raised Jane and her younger brother, Harry, single-handed since her husband died in a car accident. Jane was nine at the time. The patient idealises the figure of her father and often compares her mother unfavourably with him. Anna says she fails to understand why Jane is so difficult, even though she has received the same upbringing and attention as Harry. The patient, however, believes that her mother always preferred her brother and that she was very strict with her. She recalls in detail an episode in which her mother forced her to perform well in a sports competition and criticised her for being overweight. Her mother has no recollection of this occasion.

Jane has begun several degrees (architecture, marketing and law) but completed none. She has also tried to work, but failed to sustain anything for long. In most jobs, she quit after clashes with managers or colleagues. Her brother describes her as childish, immature, "all or nothing", short-tempered, spoiled and "tied to her mother's apron strings". He chose to leave home a year earlier after graduating from law school because he could not bear seeing his mother "pandering to Jane's whims", afraid of taking a more assertive attitude. Jane has angry outbursts over tiny things if they frustrate or displease her, breaking objects or lashing out verbally or physically (especially at her mother). Once, Anna invited her friends to lunch at her house, to Jane's annoyance. One of the guests asked the patient a simple question about her plans and work. This enquiry made her feel so angry and affronted that she swore at the guests and punched her mother in the face. After this embarrassment, her mother said it was time for her to take responsibility and get on with her life. This was the catalyst for her second suicide attempt.

Jane reports feeling "hollow" in her chest, a chronic emptiness. She says she feels fulfilled for fleeting moments, especially when she is starting a relationship. However, her insecurity about the actions and intentions of the other is as if she "opened a black hole that tears her up and engulfs her". Alternatively, she uses shopping, alcohol and self-mutilation to promote an artificial filling of this void or to overcome her distress and anxiety. She feels that by cutting herself, the physical injury consolidates the diffuse pain of her soul and reinstates a feeling of self-control. Jane reports that many friends and boyfriends have rejected and abandoned her, which increases her emptiness. But then she corrects herself, saying she no longer needs them and that from now on she will make do with her dog for company, as it is faithful and doesn't ask for anything in return. As for herself, she does not know who she really is or what she wants. She only knows that she is chronically dissatisfied with her body. She has a history of changing her appearance, chameleon-like.

All anthropopathological experience reveals the disproportionate participation of a fundamental thematic existential dimension, which stems from a disproportion at the heart of existential development. Borderline (and hysterical, as developed in Messas et al. 2019a) experiences are moulded in a disproportion of the dialectic of attraction-repulsion. The borderline world is intense, colourful, dramatic, and filled with powerful other-poles that the self-pole needs and on which it continually projects itself. The biggest challenge of a borderline existence is to find an optimal anthropological point in this equilibrium of overwhelming attractions and repulsions, which continually unbalance it. The subjective manifestation that best explains this dialectic is the feeling of passion, which the borderline person experiences to the extreme. In borderline experiences, passion is the expression of a form of intersubjectivity in which a valuable and powerful other-pole must be attracted to the self-pole's intimate sphere so as to offer it anthropological security (Fuchs 2007a). Here, I will examine the anthropological roots of this mode of existence, which is one of the ones most frequently associated with substance misuse (Belcher et al. 2014; Kienast et al. 2014; Balducci et al. 2018).

3.1.1   Intersubjectivity: Relational Hyposufficiency and Heteronomy

A disproportion between the poles of intersubjectivity forms the basis for borderline experiences. In this anthropological imbalance, disproportionate priority is given to the other-pole, to the detriment of the self-pole. The fundamental presupposition of this disproportion is the existence of an extremely powerful, sometimes even omnipotent otherness. The fragility of the self-pole, exposed intolerably to the existential strength of the other-pole, is what invokes the exaggerated expressiveness and intensity of borderline experiences (Stanghellini and Rosfort 2013).

In the experience of the borderline person, the other-pole is overvalued, and is therefore immoveable in its self-sufficiency. The borderline historical self must act to remove the other-pole from indifference and draw it to itself in order to reduce this extreme imbalance. With this movement, the borderline historical self seeks to achieve some balance for its insufficient self-pole. This behaviour prompted Schneider to name this personality the "psychopath in need of esteem" (Schneider 2007).

The other-pole is the gravitational centre of the borderline existence. The very unity and coherence of the borderline historical self depend on the capacity of this articulation between the self-pole and the hypersufficient other-pole. Any loss of contact with the other-pole can lead to experiences of existential discontinuity, which are superficially reminiscent of psychotic episodes. In this situation, substance use serves as a powerful tool for offering a supplementary experience of existential continuity. Intoxication promotes a temporary experience of independence from the other-pole by increasing the intensity with which the historical self experiences pleasure or relief. Intoxicated, the historical self feels that it can keep itself unified and strong without the other-pole, albeit for a limited time. Substance use is a common tool in the self-management of the borderline person, given the frequent fluctuations in their experience.

It is important to stress that these occasional pseudo-psychotic experiences still have the other-pole as the tacit object of their clinical manifestations (Sigmund 1997). As a consequence of this overvaluation of the other-pole, borderline persons are pre-reflexively apt to identify themes, identities and behaviours that are capable of producing movement and attention in the other-pole. The main existential interest of the borderline person is the mobilisation of everything that can remove themselves from the position of hyposufficiency, granting them a position of centrality. This centrality is secondary and reactive to the intersubjective disproportion between the relevance of the other-pole regarding the self-pole. The main existential instruments for centrality are opposition, exaggeration and theatricality (Charbonneau 2007). These are all stimulated by substance use. These attitudes give the other-pole the impression of ingratitude, falsehood and inauthenticity to, casting the borderline person into an endless cycle of feeling despised by the otherness and trying to attract their attention. Usually, the result of this vicious circle is unfavourable to the borderline person, making it propitious for intense depressions (Rogers et al. 1995; Levy et al. 2007), self-mutilation behaviours (Oumaya et al. 2008; Stead et al. 2019) and substance abuse (Tomko et al. 2014; Kienast et al. 2014; Trull et al. 2018). In these situations, the main purpose of substance use is to fictitiously raise the importance of the self-pole to obtain a minimum of existential balance.

The anthropological hyposufficiency of the self-pole means that the way the borderline person engages with the world depends mostly on the meanings and values the other-pole imprints on the world. For the borderline person, the other-pole stands in situation of hypersufficiency. It is this dialectic of hyposufficiency–hypersufficiency that gives rise to the seduction often associated with borderline persons, since to seduce means to seize and to offer, immediately and expressively, that which is valuable to the other-pole. The erotic seduction favoured by intoxication is one of the most effective ways of this exercise in self-management.

Another feature of this anthropological subjugation of the borderline self-pole to the meaning imposed by the other-pole is suggestibility. The hypervaluation of the other-pole also justifies some quasi-psychotic experiences related to borderline persons, which sometimes causes their behaviour to be misunderstood as delusional

(Glaser et al. 2010; Adams and Sanders 2011). One example is fantastic pseudology. In this, an imaginative psychosocial fantasy (like being rich or belonging to an influential family), originally aimed at capturing the attention of the other-pole, is taken to its ultimate consequences. Substance use acts in synergy with the increased participation of this imaginative element in existence. This belief in imagined facts is radically different from, say, schizophrenic delusion, because of the distinct anthropological meanings they have and the existential dimension in which they occur (Charbonneau 2010).

Likewise, paranoid and self-referent experiences, usually transient, are frequent in borderline persons (Oliva et al. 2014). Usually, these self-referential experiences lead to aggressive behaviours. Frequently, the aggressive behaviour that arises from the self-referential experience is directed against an other-pole of extreme biographical value for the borderline historical self. It is not an aggressiveness projected against a diffuse and collective otherness, experienced as a diffuse source of risk because of its strangeness (see schizophrenia (Sect. 4.1. or paranoia in *schizoidia*, Sect. 3.7.2). On the contrary, it is an aggressiveness directed against a special historical other, a specific other of personal significance. For example, the borderline person may experience a delay by the clinician in attending them as some personal statement that they no longer want to see them or despise them. In reaction to this experience, extreme aggressiveness may arise against this clinician, filled with ethical complaints or even physical threats.

Similarly, the impulsive behaviour typical of the borderline person is based on the disproportionate appreciation of the other-pole. The intense pain the borderline person experiences, for example, when breaking up an intimate relationship is an expression of the great relative value this historical other-pole has for the historical self. The hurt and excruciating frustration that mark borderline persons are also indicative of the fragility of their existential condition in the face of the other-pole which they experience as crucial to their minimal existential balance. Substance use is often crucial for the borderline person to achieve this minimum of balance (Lane et al. 2016).

This anthropological disproportion gives rise to intersubjective heteronomy. In this heteronomy, the other-pole is pre-reflexively taken as an exclusive, special, even heroic individual, the personal centre of unique power, be it because for their competences, fame, wealth, influence, intelligence, or whatever. The uniqueness of the heteronomy of the borderline other-pole makes borderline disproportion different from hypomania or hyperthymic disproportion,[3] with which it is sometimes – erroneously – identified (Coulston et al. 2012; Paris and Black 2015; Pieri and Castellana 2016). For the borderline person, the self-pole is extremely impotent in relation to the other-pole; in hypomania or hyperthymic disproportion, there is more symmetry of value between both poles of intersubjectivity, as we will see (Sect. 3.4).

This excessive relevance of the other-pole in borderline disproportion makes it useful to investigate how the borderline person experiences otherness. Normally, the

---

[3] These categories are synonymous for the effects of this study.

excesses of borderline behaviour are matched by a corresponding discomfort in the other-pole, experienced as an invasion of its privacy or abuse of its receptiveness. Due to the extreme value of this personal other-pole, the borderline historical self will often seek to go beyond the limits determined by social conventions in their relations with the other-pole, attracting the other-pole to zones of intimacy and giving rise to embarrassing situations.

From the longitudinal viewpoint, intersubjective hyposufficiency and heteronomy hinders the process of existential maturation of borderline persons. The maturity of the personality is based on the interplay of both subjective poles. This interplay depends on there being some alternating value in the self-pole and the other-pole according to the context. In the case of borderline disproportion, as the historical self-pole fixates on a subaltern condition, it is not competent to carry out the alternation that leads to maturity. As a consequence, borderline disproportion is characterised by immature feelings, often taken as "childish", unpredictable, unreliable, or even unauthentic, false and invasive. This impression is based on the impulsiveness and exaggeration that each affection or feeling contains, precisely because they are oriented to the mobilisation of the other-pole (Rossi Monti and D'Agostino 2019). Also, this state of pre-reflexive insufficiency may cause borderline behaviours to sometimes take on a perverse face. However, perversity per se – the pure desire to nullify the other-pole – is not a feature of borderline behaviours. Rather, the borderline historical self seems just to try to keep the powerful other-pole in a state of availability or prevent itself from experiencing the excruciating pain that interpersonal relations usually inflict on them.

3.1.2 Vulnerable and Unstable Temporality

Temporality in borderline disproportion is dictated by the other-pole, which leads to temporal instability. The dimensions of temporality follow the changing ways the self-pole is influenced by the other-pole. Since what matters is the other-pole, temporality is determined by the ways the other-pole is actualised to the self-pole. Every time there is a change of the presence of the other-person with whom the borderline historical self relates, the entire temporality of its existence is adjusted accordingly, making it vulnerable and unstable. The temporal instability wrought by this overdependence on the other may be behind the substance misuse seen in borderline persons. The substance use may serve either as a protection against a fleeting and volatile instant (Kimura 2005), or as a tool for enhancing the instability of the temporality (Lee et al. 2010; Coffey et al. 2011).

Sometimes, the present is what counts the most, when contact with the powerful other-pole can be enjoyed in its entirety. In these situations, the borderline historical self tends to long for eternity, a time completely filled by the other-pole's presence. Here retention is irrelevant as it bears no part in this present and protention is irrelevant as it is already anticipated by the other person's total presence. The importance that the borderline historical self gives to these experiences of plenitude makes it prone to seek intoxication in order to attain it. However, it is not always possible to maintain this total present, this gift of the whole presence of the other-pole, in borderline disproportion. It is easily lost when the other person is absent or refuses to guide the borderline self-pole. In such situations of deprivation, the borderline historical self quickly takes on other proportions of temporality in their bid to control the speed of these changes through intoxication. In some situations, retention is the only dimension that can alleviate the pain of a present that no longer contains the other person's reassuring presence; in others protention is a reference point for an existence deprived of an autonomous pole of centralisation. The following account of a borderline patient may serve as an example of the difficulties involved in this last temporal condition.

> This thing of always thinking about being someone else in the future tortures me. My instability bothers me. I can't be present. I'm always in the future, wanting to be someone else, to have other friends, things beyond my reality. It's like I think so much about others that I don't know what I want.

Discontinuity of the present in relation to retention is the typical temporality in more severe cases. Describing the alterations she experiences in her visual perception, one patient stated "even the sight of the trees is dissociated [...] they are floating images in space: like unsaved text on a computer". This fragmentation of the present has as a dissociative characteristic. It is a pre-reflexive mechanism that suppresses the experiential continuity of some recent fact of great interpersonal significance. The most typical case of this form of fragmentation is post-traumatic dissociation, in which the precise mnemonic and affective segment connected to painful experiences disappears from consciousness, although the person continues to experience existence in the world as before.

In short, temporality is a constant challenge for borderline existence, because the proportions of the dimensions of temporality can change suddenly and radically. Its variations range from a present that engulfs the other dimensions to the absorption of the present in retention or protention. The degree to which these variations overtake existence compels the borderline historical self to intoxication to obtain a minimum degree of self-control. Its complete instability is due to the vulnerability of the borderline self-pole before the hypersufficient of the other-pole, around which it gravitates. This is how we should understand borderline impulsivity: as the result of the terrible instability that dominates its existence. The borderline person's vulnerability means they are led by a psychologically painful stimulus to take thoughtless acts that are harmful to themselves and to others. This occurs because the reaction to a stimulus suddenly transforms the dialectical relations among the dimensions of temporality, causing the person to abandon their usual kind of reaction. Thus, for example, a marital argument may lead a borderline person to attempt suicide, even if their previous psychological state is apparently stable. The person loses all perspective of protention, in reaction to the possible deprivation of the total presence of the other person, suddenly identifying life as a lack of prospects, loneliness and pain. When faced with this annulment of the possibility of existence, suicide presents itself as an alluring option.

3.1.3   The Spatiality of Extremes

Two dialectics characterise borderline spatial situations in the world:

Centrality-peripherality. Borderline relations always occur when one part of the self-other polar dialectic occupies the centre. This part pushes the other to a peripheral position. At a deeper level of analysis, the other-pole will always be the centre of inter-subjective experience. However, the self-pole of a borderline existence may deceptively appear to occupy the relational centre. This vicarious occupation occurs owing to the intense emotions produced in an interpersonal act. Sometimes the vicarious protagonism of the borderline person takes on the form of anger and aggressiveness against the relevant other-pole, usually revolving around topics of social relevance, which galvanise public opinion in favour of the borderline person. The telltale signs of this behaviour include calling out the errors of powerful other, whether small (e.g. a slight delay in starting a consultation) or big (e.g. parental negligence in childhood). Ironically, the borderline person's accusing protagonism results in the criticised person becoming the protagonist, even if for the wrong reasons, maintaining the centrality-peripherality dialectic as the central element of borderline existential disproportion.

Even imaginary errors of others can contribute to this scenario, in which the borderline historical self becomes the apparent centre of intersubjectivity. For example, shortly after a painful breakup, a patient in our clinic reported that someone had abducted her. As a result, those responsible even called the police to investigate the situation. However, the patient later revealed that she had made up the story in order to make her ex-boyfriend feel sorry for her and help contact the law-enforcement agencies.

Distance-proximity: the paradoxical fusional distance. The basis of borderline experiences is an ambiguous and contradictory mix of primordial distance and fusional proximity, both essentially due to an incapacity for true proximity. With distance, the borderline historical self remains elusive and therefore able to sustain the potent other-pole's attraction (as in the above example of kidnapping). In fusional proximity, on the other hand, the borderline self-pole blends with the other-pole in order to find some ontological stability. The borderline historical self is unable to base its relationships on a fertile interpersonal dialectic, from which sound dual unity between adults may result. On the contrary, the borderline person must simultaneously keep the potent other-pole at bay and in extreme proximity. The borderline historical self guarantees the minimal preservation of its integrity through the impossibility of finding an intermediate spatiality between the two extremes. Under the circumstances of intermediate spatiality, in which the self-pole and other-pole could experience each other more symmetrically, the overwhelming power of the otherness would completely overcome the borderline self-pole. The borderline self-pole needs the other-pole to be so far away or so close that its great power is immobilised. The borderline self-pole can only sustain an interpersonal relationship through this paradoxical – and ultimately unattainable – immobilisation of the other-pole. This creates an evident relational impoverishment, which appears in the tormented and harmful interpersonal relationships that mark borderline existence.

This paradoxical fusional distance is what underlies the strength of the borderline person's anthropological dependency on their potent other. This proximate distance is what gives the borderline style its dramatic and unstable overtones. For this reason, the idealised passion at a distance characteristic of borderline emotions is easily transformed, with close contact, into hostility and even physical aggression against the significant other. Idealised passion occurs in the absence of the beloved object, distanced by time and space (the romanticising of other cultures or societies, in which a heroic person may be found to love). The borderline self-pole allows the other-pole on whom it depends to assimilate it in total proximity, to support this idealisation. As its dependence grows and it feels increasingly hyposufficient, the borderline historical self gradually becomes intolerant of the idealised other-pole, generating a vicious circle for its healthy biographical development. The vicious circle involves substance use, which sometimes creates an experience analogous to existential anaesthesia, leading the self-pole to withdraw from the other-pole, and sometimes an exaltation of euphoria, which facilitates the fusional movement.

3.1.4 Hyponomic Fragmentation: Borderline Identity

Extreme ontological dependence on the other-pole directly influences the formation of the identity of the borderline historical self. As the establishment of identity relies on temporality, its formation is unstable when this is subject to intense and lasting instability. The fact that the anthropological proportions of temporality in borderline existence are constantly changing increases the unpredictability of the way in which experiences are sedimented in the historical self, causing a disproportion of ipseity in relation to identity. The borderline person's identity becomes unstable and unpredictable in the way the historical self develops in its social identities, in much the same way as in temporality. When engaging with a borderline person, one never knows exactly what aspect of their existence one is dealing with or which dimension of their being they are expressing. Here, intoxication fosters or reduces identity multiplication.

From the prism of dialectics between identity and ipseity, borderline disproportion is marked by the difficulty of the historical self to assimilate various partial social identities, remaining at the mercy of a broad, indeterminate ipseity commanded by a hypersufficient otherness. The borderline historical self only adheres superficially and tangentially to social identities. Though it is able to comprehend the social roles at its disposal, they are beyond its grasp, because it finds them too indefinite, impersonal and complicated to follow. I call this anthropological disproportion *hyponomic identity*. In *hyponomic identity*, the exaggerated incorporation of identities provided by other persons is what provides for the sedimentation of the historical self. The existential success of their biography depends on their being lucky enough to meet others who are sufficiently stable or capable of recognising and supporting the fragility of their borderline self-pole.

Borderline hyponymic identity is an existence in which each social identity dominates for a short period, soon to be replaced by another. This is why the borderline person may cry convulsively at one moment and immediately afterwards, look happy and laugh aloud, giving the observer an impression of falsity. The transience and excessive plasticity of emotions give a false impression of dissimulation, as their rapid succession and alteration means they experience each state superficially.

The biographical upshot of borderline personal development is thus the sum of what relevant othernesses permit. The historical self's inability to take on lasting and stable partial identities leads to its frequent emotional distress. As the historical self is constituted by shallow social identities with fragile roots, they are often prone to anxiety and depression (Silk 2010). Borderline anxiety is intense, volatile and rooted in the impossibility of reaching a minimum of self-sufficiency. Frequent depressions and feelings of emptiness result from the self-pole's devaluation in relation to the other. At the limit, the root cause of these emotional disorders is not only the experience of personal insufficiency, but also a disbelief in the possibility of attaining self-sufficiency at any point. Often, they can only reach some transient hope of existential autonomy through intoxication.

Borderline hopelessness does not originate in a devalued life cycle, such as seen in periods of exhaustion of existence; nor in reactive pain at the loss of a beloved relationship, for example. In these two situations, the self-pole loses something with which it was connected, but it does not lose the ability to connect with the world and to hope for some kind of re-establishment of the bond. In general experiences of depression (see below Sects. 3.8 and 3.9), the self-pole remains intact and, to a certain degree, the guiding centre of the biography. Borderline depression is rooted in the annulment of the capacity of the self-pole to engage with the world and others. Not only does the world thus lose value, but above all, the historical self crumbles and loses its capacity to conduct its own existence. In this sense, we must understand borderline depression differently from the way I interpret its impulsivity. In its own way, impulsivity still signifies the ability to value the world through a relevant other-pole; borderline depression, on the other hand, indicates that even this last lifeline with the intersubjective world has been lost, shutting off life's options and potentially leading towards suicidal ideas.

The annulment of the historical self's ability to conduct its own biography also sheds light on the serious self-image disorders typical of borderline existence. In anthropological terms, it cannot be said it is only a self-image disorder – a historical self which, following self-examination, is incapable of having an idea which can be shared with its peers. The severity of the borderline experience goes further, revealing a historical self that is unable to attain sufficient autonomy to even have a self-image. The formation of a self-image is thus totally bound to the image imposed by otherness.

The weakening of the self-pole in the process of managing and generating partial identities is manifested as identity fragmentation (Fuchs 2007a). Negative findings, such as loss of memory or feelings of emptiness, are indicative of identity fragmentation. The excessive presence of the other-pole as the source of existential vitality is also a basis of negative clinical findings – the impossibility to escape from or tolerate the continuous relational hyposufficiency, In certain critical situations in which there is an increase in relational tensions, it becomes so hard to leave or tolerate this continuous relational hyposufficiency that dissociative, conversive patterns, such as quasi-psychotic reactive states, are triggered. Substance misuse comes in as an attempt to reduce this risk.

3.1.5   Embodiment

The instability and fragmentation of the borderline existence has direct consequences on its embodiment. An inability to maintain biographical temporality and an incapacity to develop a more autonomous identity causes the body to lose its purpose as an instrument for the realisation of genuine life plans. The primordial unity of body and existence is divorced, resulting in dissociative experiences. In such experiences, the body renounces its role as co-participant of existence and becomes an agent that is external to the historical self. The basic experience of the dissociative person is that they do not belong in their body or, conversely, that their body does not belong to them.

Embodiment manifests the characteristics of borderline spatiality in three ways. First, as an instrument of distance-proximity ambiguity. Distance is manifested in borderline embodiment through the theatricality of some of its expressions, laden with expressive displays, which serve their quest for value and attention. At the same time, borderline embodiment serves the purpose of a fusional proximity, manifested above all in the hypertrophy of risky sexual behaviour (Frías et al. 2016). The borderline self-pole achieves the closest and most physical way of sharing the other-pole's intimacy through the body and sexuality.

Besides these two categories, embodiment plays a role that may be its most radical and ambiguous function in borderline existence, the quest for the unification of the historical self. The disastrous behaviour of cutting is one expression of this function. In these frequent acts, embodiment becomes the setting in which the weakened borderline historical self is able to exert some power to unify and stabilise its existence. The borderline historical self has few effective weapons against the instability that tortures and the fragmentation that terrifies it (intoxication is one of them). The insuperable unpredictability that floods its existence liquefies its world, turning it into a ship without a compass, surrounded by demons of pain and intersubjective slavery. Faced with this bleak scenario, sometimes the only solution for the borderline historical self is to replace the diffuse dissolution of its life with unification in a single solid, stable point produced by physical pain. Physical pain reduces the range of existential pain constantly surrounding the borderline historical self, concentrating it to a given physical point, usually limbs or abdomen. The borderline person's concentration on the physical surface of their body ambiguously permits them to exercise some power of deliberation and regency over the existential devastation of their own life. Subjugated to intersubjective relations, borderline existence finds some consolation for its excruciating suffering in the material solidity of the body it inhabits. When this fails, only the fiction of substance use can offer some relief.

Thus, in borderline experiences, embodiment generally takes on the same paradoxical and extreme profile observed in other anthropological dimensions. The spectrum of existential functions of embodiment extends from its alienation from the historical self to its use as a strategy for its own life management.

3.1.6 Anthropological Ambiguities of Borderline Persons

Can a constructive existential value be postulated for borderline experiences? Could any existential advantage be gleaned from such radical subordination to the other? I would argue that the observation of the ambiguities of borderline disproportion brings to light two favourable points for the borderline person and their personal relationships.

Borderline persons, by establishing intense and unique interpersonal relationships with people they deem special, may initiate a form of creative disruption of the traditional indulgence of habits naturalised by unreflective repetition. Due to their unique intensity, borderline experiences, serve as a counterpoint to the mediocrity of everyday life. The radicalism of their experience shows that every person is ultimately incomparable and irreplaceable, that there is no-one who is not special in some way. Similarly, the biography of borderline people shows that life can be more intense, unique and complete – even if for brief periods of time. There is a paradisiacal nostalgia in every borderline experience, which is fundamental for the understanding of substance misuse and which I will examine later (part III).

Secondly, the excessive importance of the other-pole in borderline existence puts the theme of interpersonal responsibility at the core of each human act. As the other's every act has a profound impact on the borderline person, this magnifies their ethical mistakes and successes and makes them more evident. In everyday life, with its chores and distractions, each person's responsibility towards others is not always evident. The flow of operations essential to maintaining work, family and social arrangements and thereby rendering community life tolerable dissolves the consequences of the ethical and interpersonal trials and errors of human decisions. By placing emphasis on the value of others' behaviour, borderline people do not allow this spontaneous extinction of the consequence of others' conduct to go unremarked. Borderline consciousness stands out above the stream in which human actions are dissolved and shines a light on the consequences of its abandonment, of the social injustice of which it has been or is a victim, of gender or ethnic iniquity, of the bureaucratic negligence of societies, etc. Paradoxically, because of its intense dependence on others, borderline existence unconsciously attributes supreme value to what others, the family, society and culture are ethically bound to contribute to a human being's dignity.

3.1.7 Dialectics of Proportions and Anthropological Movement in Borderline Disproportion – Clinical Decision-Making

All decision-making derives from a profound understanding of the anthropological proportions that govern an existence, which can be seen to progress as it undergoes successive modifications of these proportions. The clinician must therefore identify how these proportions are modified before they can intervene in these movements of existence and thereby achieve the desired therapeutic effects. A borderline existence gravitates around a powerful and meaningful other-pole. This is propitious for the clinician from the point of view of establishing a therapeutic strategy. Therapeutic success will depend on the clinician's ability to take on the role of the hypersufficient other desired by the borderline existence. Pre-reflexively, the hypersufficient clinician will have unusual power in helping the borderline historical self identify ways for their existence to reach a maximum of creativity with a minimum of harm to their relationships. The clinician should therefore respect the force-lines typical of borderline anthropological disproportion as they identify these paths, always being mindful to maintain the required level of relational intensity. The borderline person can only modify their anthropological proportions if they retain their main point of equilibrium in a hypersufficient other-pole. Thus, the ultimate goal of borderline treatment is not the patient's total autonomy, but the viability of an autonomy where the other will always be the gravitational centre of existence. Passion will always be the driving force of borderline existence, lending the clinician's speech and behaviour unusual power. Since the other is disproportionately powerful, everything the clinician does in the therapeutic relationship will tend to produce great effects. On the plus side, these effects suffuse the pole of the borderline self with intensity and enchantment, both fundamental for therapeutic success; however, they can also induce experiences of anthropological fragmentation. The clinician should carefully manage the existing anthropological disproportion in their favour, above all using their pre-reflexive strength to help stabilise the composition of the borderline person's anthropological proportions. The maintenance of existential stability is crucial for the sedimentation of the borderline historical self's experiences, offering inputs for its maturation. To mature is to proceed from the longitudinal temporality of dawning towards that of maturity (Sect. 2.1.2). To do this it is necessary to reduce the ipseity contained in the historical self's identity. Since the basis of ipseity is hypersufficient otherness, the otherness must mute its own presence to a certain extent so that the historical self can gradually and delicately introduce temporal continuity and spatial unity to its experiences. This is not an easy task, for it contains an internal contradiction. The clinician must take advantage of the passion the patient feels for them in order simultaneously to limit its intensity, with all due care and caution. The capacity to temporalise borderline existence depends on this rapture being reduced. In the ultimate analysis, the great existential theme of borderline existences is the maturation-immaturity dialectic, which is conducted by a continuous anthropological disproportion in which the self-pole will always be inferior to the other-pole.

3.2 Phobic Disproportion

Clinical Vignette

Daniel seeks psychiatric care on referral from his cardiologist. He has been to A&E on numerous occasions thinking that he is having a heart attack or a stroke. For 6 months, he has been experiencing tightness in his chest, palpitations, paraesthesia, sweating and fainting. He reports that the numerous clinical examinations he has undergone have not shown any organic alterations. For about 3 months, he has also avoided leaving home alone for fear of falling ill or fainting and not having anyone to help him.

Daniel reports that during his childhood he was very weak, insecure and fearful. The horror stories his cousins told frightened him, he could not sleep in the dark and had great difficulty in adapting to preschool. He reports believing that his mother would disappear, leaving him alone in the world. He states that at that stage he had consultations with a psychologist, because in addition to all these symptoms he had night-time enuresis. He was always skinny and had frequent asthma attacks requiring hospitalisation. He says that his mother was very understanding, sweet and caring, but his father was strict and authoritarian. He recalls in detail the beatings and scolding he received for "wetting the bed" again. He also says that whenever he heard of a serious environmental tragedy or someone's death, the news would stay on his mind for weeks.

He says that when he was a teenager, he did not know how to deal with his classmates and with girls. He felt awkward, ashamed of the pimples on his face and convinced his walk was ungainly. He thought everyone noticed his deformities and his clumsy way of walking (which a physical examination did not confirm). He often blushed in front of others, even when among his childhood friends. He says his problem with girls was a cause for mockery among his peers. He felt bolder going to parties under the influence of alcohol. The idea of studying engineering was not his choice, but his father's decision. He passed the entrance exam of a prestigious university in São Paulo city, where he now lives, and also one in his hometown in São Paulo state. He preferred to remain close to his family rather than face such a radical change. He reports the anguish and anxiety he experienced when confronting his father to communicate his choice. For this, he needed his mother's reassurance. At university, although he had no difficulty keeping up with the coursework, the presentations and group work were excruciating, as if he were naked in front of his colleagues. He often felt anxious, exposed, embarrassed and afraid of getting bad grades.

After graduating, he started working in a small company, revising maps of pipelines. He could not imagine himself working in a large corporation, managing employees or being responsible for creating projects, even though he had received job offers of this nature. Daniel believes he is incapable and prefers steady, regular, isolated, low-profile work. He only relates well to his boss, who welcomed him when he was still a mere trainee at his work place. He always tries to invent an excuse not to take part in get-togethers to avoid the embarrassment of not knowing what to say or how to talk to his colleagues.

He married a childhood friend who made him feel safe because she was his opposite, confident and determined. He finds it very hard to stand up to his wife for fear that she will no longer want him. For example, although he was not sure whether it was the right time to plan for a child, he gave in to his wife's desire.

Seven months ago, his mother passed away from stomach cancer and his first child is due in 2 weeks' time. He believes he will never get over his mother's death and he will have the same fate as her. He already feels sharp pains in his stomach. This has only exacerbated his existing concern about having a serious illness. He also believes he will not be an ideal father, and now he can no longer count on his mother to deal with this uncertain and challenging moment. As he puts it, "I am afraid to go out when it's raining and when there's a storm, but what if my son gets sick? What will I do?" He feels totally lost.

3.2.1 Phobic Hyperspatiality – Fragmentation and Proximity

Spatial disproportions can lead to phobic experiences. In a phobic person's world, existential movements occur from an amplification of spatiality in relation to the other anthropological dimensions. The core theme of the phobic person, expressed clinically in agoraphobia and its reverse, claustrophobia, is a dialectic between anthropological widening and constriction. Their dilemma resides in how to manage this overly spatialised existence in which the world always appears in varying volumes of consciousness. One patient, who suffers from a phobia that her husband might disappear at any moment, clearly reveals the power of phobic disproportion, which goes beyond mere symptomatology. Treated effectively with fluoxetine, she no longer exhibits explicit phobic symptoms, but has started to fret at her new mental state since her symptoms were brought under control. She says: "the cure for the phobia is frightening because it opens up a spectrum of alternatives in the world. I feel different now. Before, I had an uncontrollable fear that my husband would disappear. Now, I feel like there are so many things and I have to make decisions about more things than I can manage". Controlling the symptoms associated with amplified intersubjective risk (disappearance of her husband) does not bring about a redefinition of her phobic anthropological disproportion. Overspatiality comes back in the form of excessively complex existential possibilities, which are experienced as too broad for the historical self to manage.

There are two main consequences of excess spatiality: a widening of spatiality or its constriction. In the former, risk is associated with increased spatiality. Spatial dimensions may expand to such an extent that the threat of anthropological fragmentation emerges. At this point, it resembles borderline disproportion. Phobic anthropopathology arises when anthropological amplitude widens to such a degree that the tissue of the anthropological layer of existence may be torn. A typical manifestation of this ruptured anthropological unity is the panic attack. Basically, this involves two breaking points. In such cases, the lost unity of the historical self is experienced as depersonalisation and loss of material support, or as derealisation, the most typical of which is "walking on air". In the most common cases, as in agoraphobia, the entire surrounding space seems liable to dissolve. This causes the self-pole to feel it may lose its sense of unity as it is dragged into a mundane space, now transformed into an abyss, which will swallow it up. It is worth remembering that even in the middle of a panic attack, the structural unity of existence remains intact. This makes the experience of panic quite different from that of schizophrenic derealisation or depersonalisation (Colombetti and Ratcliffe 2012; Madeira et al. 2017). The latter affect the structural unity of existence (its constitution), as we will see. It is not always simple to distinguish clinically between these two experiences. One useful way to do so is to observe how the historical self which experiences the alteration of reality interprets its own experience. Immersed in spatial amplitude, the phobic self-pole also experiences the other-pole as magnified, in terms of existential importance. This enables it to feel sufficiently confident to protect itself from potential fragmentation by approaching them. The phobic person experiences the other, pre-reflexively, as enlarged and therefore powerful enough to protect them (although they can also experience them as threatening, as we will see below). The patient often expresses the fear that they will experience phobic symptoms when there is no known person around. The safety offered by the proximity of known persons shows how important the other-pole's presence is in a phobic existence. Only a strong and intact other-pole is able to make the historical self feel safe. The other-pole always figures as an existential last resort. In general, this insecurity does not feature in experiences of schizophrenic depersonalisation or derealisation, in which the constitution of the other-pole is also compromised. In these conditions, the other-pole usually appears as just a shapeless source of threat.

The second threat from excessive spatialisation comes from its constriction. This signifies a hyperproximity of the self-pole with the other-pole and the world-pole. This excessive proximity leads to a magnification of the risk contained in each world experience. Phobic hyperproximity amplifies the way in which threatening or repugnant objects loom into consciousness. Typically, this takes the form of simple phobias – of animals, for example, mainly poisonous ones, such as snakes or spiders, although risk-free creatures, such as cockroaches, can also feature in such experiences (Rovaletti 2007). In haemophobia, for example, the amplification brought about by hyperproximity has a metonymic effect, in which the intensity of a visual perception – the sight of blood – is experienced as total dissolution, death. The excessive proximity between the world-pole and the self-pole in phobic existence means that just one of the meanings associated with blood – its most intense – is interpreted as representing its entirety. The self-pole exists in a state of continuous terror, living in a world marked by imminent threat due to the overwhelming proximity of the objects of the world. An intense, threatening, even phantasmagorical overtone colours each phobic experience like an expressionist film, creating the atmospheric background that is the hallmark of phobic disproportion. The fear a phobic person experiences is not the result of experiences learned by their historical self, but is born of a world where all experiences harass the self-pole. The phobic person lives all the most terrifying and dangerous experiences in the world pre-reflexively. Thus, the beleaguered phobic self-pole distorts the historical self's experiences in a succession of tensions between fear and relief. Substance use becomes a source of immediate and, at least initially, effective relief.

In extreme cases, this anthropological disproportion may jeopardise the development of existence. The excessive spatial proximity experienced by the phobic self-pole may mean that its primordial meaning, the meaning that is inherent to the species (blood as a symbol of life, animals as a threat to life), not the individual (biographically influenced), ends up invading and taking over the whole of personal experience, preventing any personal meaning from being experienced. In this case, the history of the species overrides personal meanings.[4] The hyperspatialised experience of the phobic person can dominate their existence so entirely that the risk-safety dialectic becomes the core motive around which they gravitate. Reactively, the main value sense for the historical self becomes security. As a result, they can become trapped in an oppressive process in which their whole existence revolves around an incessant quest for security. This then opens the door to substance misuse, with the fictitious experience of protection it can induce.

Existential restrictions in the phobic person also lead to an extreme of spatialisation, producing the aforementioned phenomenon of claustrophobia. The over-presence of the world-pole oppresses the self-pole in such a way that phobic existence inhabits a world divided between protected and dangerous zones.

Always retreating to protected spatiality, a phobic person leads an impoverished existence. The family space is identified as a protected area, while all unknown spaces become high-risk zones. Existence becomes a prisoner to everything that is already part of its identity and rejects all unknown spatiality, which overflows into a kind of xenophobia. This existential xenophobia, which often takes on a conservative hue, is, however, anthropologically different from what we see in melancholic disproportion, for the reasons set forth below.

3.2.2 Devouring Temporality

Phobic persons will sometimes express conservative attitudes in their behaviour. A phobic existence completely tainted by fear favours the temporality of sedimentation, of the familiar, of whatever can be incorporated safely in their identity. However, we should not imagine that this preference for retentive temporality, supposedly espousing tradition, has anything to do with the experience of melancholia. In reality, the temporality of phobic existence implies an excessive amplitude, in which every instant of the present seems to be engulfed by the indeterminism of protention. The same hugeness observed in spatial terms reappears here, now in the

---

[4]There are obviously experiences that cannot be interpreted individually, like suffocation caused by lack of oxygen or the approach of a dangerous animal. What I refer to here are experiences that most healthy individuals could have a more personal interpretation of.

form of a disproportionately threatening protention which the historical self cannot manage. The myth of Chronos, the Greek god who devoured his children, gives the most accurate depiction of the phobic person's temporality. The primordial dispro-portion of this existential type is the devouring time of the present, which ravages the phobic historical self. The conservative behaviour it sometimes displays is first and foremost a type of phenomenological compensation it invokes to reduce the disproportion of protention. Unlike in melancholia, this conservatism is tentative, dictated by the threat of dissolution facing the historical self (as seen above). The temporal anthropological reason for the insecurity and fear that assail the phobic person is the very indeterminate nature of the protentive dimension. Adopting con-servative behaviour is the best way this existence finds to put down temporal roots in the face of the indetermination of behaviour in society. By so doing, the phobic historical self invests in its security by enlarging its retentive temporality and reduc-ing the anthropological disproportion of its excessively protentive temporality. The anxiety that plagues the phobic person also has anthropological roots in the deter-mination of its existence by indeterminate aspects of experience. The dialectic of temporality in the phobic existence oscillates between terrifying protention and a retention that offers some relief. The existential temporal function that drives the phobic historical self to substance use constitutes a new dimension for its compre-hension. More than a tool for seeking relief from anxiety (Randall et al. 2001; Virtanen et al. 2019), substance misuse is indicative of a quest to reduce the indeter-minacy of each new experience in a phobic personality. Substance use creates a shield against the temporal disproportion that restricts the phobic person's existence.

3.2.3 Phobic Intersubjectivity – Hypertransparency and Its Corrections

The dimension of intersubjectivity should be employed when observing phobic hyperspatialisation as this gives a broader understanding of any associated sub-stance misuse and a global framework that is more attuned to the psychopatholo-gist's clinical needs. The dialectics of ambiguity mark phobic intersubjectivity in such a way that the psychopathologist's failure to notice it can impair their capacity to direct their patient's care. The dialectic regime between distance and proximity leaves deep scars on phobic intersubjectivity, as I will show in the following.

3.2.4 Social Phobia and Its Phenomenological Counterphobic Compensations

The experience of social phobia describes a relationship with the world in which otherness appears pre-reflexively as a potential threat. The excessive intersubjective proximity inherent to phobic disproportion means the other-pole is so primordially close to the self-pole that it becomes a source of unease. The unease exhibited by phobic persons in their intersubjective relations does not arise from an effective threat to the anthropological or structural integrity of the self-pole, but from an uncomfortable transparency. This excessive pre-reflexive transparency makes the phobic self-pole feel invaded by the other-pole, as if the psychopathologist's eyes, for example, had a magical power to reveal significant intimacies of their biography. We should emphasise that this apparently privileged access of the psychopathologist's gaze into the patient's existential depths does not stem from a historical sedimentation of their repeated encounters; in that case, the psychopathologist's acuity would be the result of the natural maturation of the clinical-patient relationship. Such an intersubjective form should not invoke fear in anyone. The phobic person's discomfort arises from a primary disproportion of intersubjective spatiality, which makes the other-pole seem very close to the self-pole. The power of the other-pole over the self-pole does not stem from the patient's biography, but from a pre-reflexive and pre-biographical anthropological disproportion. That is why the self-pole experiences the other-pole at the very least as an outsider and a nuisance, if not an actual intruder of its intimacy.

This kind of experience is quite common in phobic patient care. Indeed, the psychopathologist's experience of feeling powerful or all-seeing in relation to a patient could be seen as a strong indication that they are dealing with phobic anthropological disproportion. Hypertransparency with regard to otherness is the essential anthropological disproportion of phobic intersubjectivity. An uncomfortable and exhausting dialectic between revelation and concealment marks the phobic person's relationship with an annihilating and investigative other. The primordial intersubjective positional sense of phobic existence is transparency. Hypertransparency, its anthropopathological condition, is the existential foundation of so-called social phobia. Social phobia is of great interest to us, as it is one of the mental disorders most frequently associated with substance misuse. (Randall et al. 2001; Thomas et al. 2008).

The discomfort inherent to this situation leads the phobic historical self to devote a significant portion of their energy to counterphobic phenomenological compensations to mitigate the uncontrollable power of the other-pole's presence. In social phobia, substance misuse serves as a crucial instrument for the management of counterphobic phenomenological compensation by opacifying hypertransparency. The identification of two major counterphobic alternatives is essential for the psychopathologist. I will emphasise this behaviour in its manifestations in the therapeutic relationship, although obviously it can also be observed it in patients' daily lives.

The first of the alternatives is the intensification by the patient of their already intense intersubjective spatial proximity. The patient who experiences the psychopathologist as clairvoyant (and often wise, too), surrenders completely to the relationship, exacerbating their own hypertransparency. In a way, this behaviour serves to reduce the psychopathologist's disproportionate power, liberating them from the need to strive to unravel the intimacies of phobic existence. There is, so to speak, an implicit invitation for the psychopathologist to relax their professional attention, reducing the acuity of their investigative acumen. The consequent reduction in the psychopathologist's power even gives the patient a degree of psychological comfort by decreasing the intersubjective asymmetry in the respective strength of the psychopathologist's and patient's self-pole.

The compensatory intensification of phobic hypertransparency is the ambiguous face of a phobic existence immersed in spatio-temporal complexity. This hypertransparent compensation appears as kindness in interpersonal contact or even extreme care in avoiding any interpersonal friction between patient and clinician. Sometimes, the patient appears to overstate their account of the positive aspects of their treatment, as if they wanted to make the clinician satisfied with the treatment they advocate. The clinical relationship between psychopathologist and patient, characterised by ease, collaboration and trust, allows for the formation of a genuine therapeutic bond. The increased hypertransparency, counteracting the self-pole's exposure to a putatively powerful other-pole, sometimes resembles performance anxiety, from a descriptive psychopathological viewpoint. It is often not appreciated as a cause of discomfort. Indeed, overall, phobic persons are generally interpreted as taking pleasure from making others happy.

The second counterphobic alternative is the more ambiguous of the two. In it, phenomenological compensation is guided by an attempt to achieve intersubjective distancing. In this case, the existence brings about a reduction of its hypertransparency by enveloping its biography in mystery, concealing subject matter or feelings from the psychopathologist. The psychopathologist does not cease to be pre-reflexively overpowerful in their capacity to penetrate the patient's very being. However, this disproportionate power is mitigated by the intersubjective distance tacitly proposed by the patient. This option for distance in the relationship impoverishes the thematic fabric of clinical encounters, limiting personal accounts to the bare minimum. In cases in which pharmacotherapy is a central or important element, compensation by distance may be demonstrated in a patient who only shows interest in the pharmacological aspects of their care. This limitation may even prevent the clinician from speaking about more complex existential aspects of the patient. In more intense situations, this form of compensation may even lead the patient to miss appointments. It is important to keep in mind, however, that we should take care when qualifying all this kind of behaviour as compensatory, to avoid wrongly interpreting trivial aspects of human relations as examples of anthropological disproportion. The disinterest of a patient in the existential dimension of their pathology while suffering a panic attack may merely indicate that they do not need this kind of reflection in order to evolve clinically. It is crucial for the other-pole to retain its hypervalued status before a patient in order to identify any compensatory behaviour. In other words, a patient's behaviour can only be called compensatory if it gravitates around a powerful other-pole, i.e. that of the psychopathologist; if, for example, when an appointment is missed, it is possible, by means of phenomenological comprehension, to interpret this as an attempt to reduce the intersubjective power of the other-pole without, however, attempting to break the bond. In this case, missing an appointment is significant, paradoxically indicating the disproportionate strength of the bond. The phobic patient, in their specific dialectic of ambiguity, can place great value on a therapeutic relationship if they can maintain sufficient distance so as not to feel completely exposed. Spatial distance is what enables them to reinstate an anthropological proportionality that allows them to pursue their existential trajectory safely.

This excessive transparency in relation to otherness characterises all the phobic person's interpersonal relations. Therefore, the phobic person lives in a torment of constant anxiety. Every interpersonal relationship harbours tension, requiring complex manoeuvres to simultaneously reduce the other's value and maintain their importance. The phobic person cannot withdraw sufficiently from the other person to despise them; nor can they approach them in a harmonious and symmetrical manner. Modifying its state of consciousness is a powerful way for the historical self to increase its own relative value, placing itself on an equal footing with such a powerful other-pole. Alternatively, intoxication can serve to annul the value of the other and the world, bringing some relief to the historical self's agony. The number of times that substance misuse is associated with social phobia shows how important this kind of self-management can be for phobic existence, however undesirable it may be.

3.2.5   Tormented Embodiment

The threat of anthropological fragmentation often reaches the dimension of embodiment. This danger appears most clearly in the experience of a panic attack. Here, the solidity of the living body is diminished. The somatic pole of existence expresses this threat through the same autonomic signs that warn of imminent threats to life, such as tachycardia, high blood pressure and excessive sweating. As the autonomous somatic system cannot differentiate between biological existential threats to life and subjective ones, this triggers a general alert reaction. Both intermingle, generating systemic distress, which only goes to amplify the phobic person's harrowing experience of acute crisis.

3.2.6   Phobic Ambiguity and Clinical Decision-Making

The ambiguous oscillation of phobic existence between proximity to and distancing from a powerful otherness is what determines the conditions under which clinical decision-making takes place. Much of the difficulty lies in identifying the patient's principal movement. If the patient opts primarily for distance, the clinician should favour decisions that imply minimal overall existential involvement with them. By doing so, they prevent their over-presence from disturbing the progress of the therapeutic bond. This can only progress if the clinician can prevent their presence from becoming threatening. Thus, they should be parsimonious in their interpretations while offering reassurance and support to the patient. Conversations should revolve around the patient's habitual and family contexts. No abrupt or radical changes in the patient's life should be proposed. If possible, the clinician should formalise a therapeutic plan in terms of a protocol. The formal rigour of a protocol will reduce the relative significance of the patient's uniqueness, diminishing the effects of excessive exposure in which the patient feels trapped. The aim of treatment is to reduce change, while the clinician should be guided by efforts to preserve the retention of the historical self. Only then will they be able to inspire enough confidence in the patient to be able to approach themes from their existence with sufficient security to attempt some significant change. As the phobic person's experience of change is massively augmented, the clinician must prioritise avoiding any increase in spatial anthropological disproportion. This conservative mode of clinical management, although effective in strengthening the therapeutic relationship, is often undesirable in cases involving substance misuse. The effects caused by substance misuse can be so harmful and pressing that the clinician must take incisive action. This may, however, upset the patient and cause them to drop out of treatment.

In cases in which the patient tends to increase their hypertransparency, throwing themselves entirely into the clinician's hands, decision making should give priority to the authenticity of the patient's personal values. The patient's excessive surrender may lead the clinician to make clinical decisions guided by their own values instead of the patient's. Although this may initially seem fruitful because it gives the patient some existential direction, it may subsequently prove harmful, precisely because of the mechanism described above. The patient's total surrender may quickly turn into a sudden impulse to escape. In these cases of surrender, the patient will often ask the clinician for advice on topics that are very central to their existence, as if they could solve them without needing any self-reflection. The clinician's role is to suggest caution and seek to amplify the patient's own awareness of their values. In this way, the clinician also curbs the devouring temporality of the phobic patient, helping their existential decisions to be taken in a pacified temporality, where they can ponder any options for change until the point of maturation. In both situations, the clinician should be aware that a phobic patient may be more committed to treatment than they seem; that their distance may not only be a sign of commitment, but also a precondition for satisfactory evolution. In a way, the clinician, as a person, is always present in the life of a phobic patient.

Second Level

3.3 Melancholic Disproportion

Clinical Vignette
Raphael, 64, was hospitalised for severe melancholia with significant suicidal tendencies. He has a history of recurring melancholia. Raphael feels that he has failed and dishonoured his family and his death is the only possible solution to his condition. According to the patient, he was responsible for the bankruptcy of the family's coffee business, so his brothers have every reason to accuse him of mismanagement. He also says he is guilty of abandoning his employees' families. His children point

out that the patient's perspective of the situation is exaggerated, because many of the factors that led to the bankruptcy were beyond his control (weather, changes in the world export market, national agricultural policy) and that the brothers who accuse him never showed any interest in what was happening to the company. Raphael made enormous efforts to avoid conflict with his brothers.

Raphael is the oldest of seven siblings. Son of a traditional oriental family, from a very early age he took responsibility for carrying on the family name, a commitment he undertook fully. In childhood, he seemed much more grown-up than his years. He was obedient, well behaved, conscientious and easy-going. He took over the family firm and emotional and financial care for his parents naturally and unquestioningly, while his siblings followed other paths. As head of the company, his employees loved and respected him and he never allowed himself to take holidays. In the absence of one of the employees, he would do the job himself. His brothers interpreted his ethical manner, his sense of responsibility and his conciliatory treatment of the employees and suppliers as naivety and weakness.

Raphael is married and has a son and a daughter. His wife considers him a very dedicated partner, who is always attentive to her needs and those of their children. She points out that, even having an excessive work routine, he always finds a way to devote himself to his family. He likes to have his family together at every mealtime and is interested in what everyone has to say about their routine. His children emphasise that he has always done whatever he can to give them the best, but that he is also strict and demands (sometimes excessively) that they must always behave correctly and responsibly. The family says that the patient lives in a state of constant stress, worried about getting into debt or failing to fulfil his duties. He has almost daily migraine attacks and chronic insomnia, worrying about problems he has failed to resolve. At one point, he used alcohol to "get out of his head" and make it easier to sleep.

His first melancholic episode occurred when his son decided to leave home and went to live in Italy to do a postgraduate course in architecture. Raphael knew it was a unique opportunity for his son and that he was happy, but he was acutely aware of that empty place at the meal table. He was also disappointed because his son had chosen not to follow the family tradition for the firstborn. He improved with a selective serotonin receptor inhibitor. The second melancholic episode arose after he suffered an acute heart attack. Impotent in the face of the limitations imposed by this ailment, he thought he had no right to be absent from the company and feared his family would suffer financial hardship (even though his children no longer depend on him financially). At the same time, he blamed himself for his negligence with his own health. He blamed himself for causing his heart attack with alcohol, cigarettes and stress. However, he was unaware of the extent to which he had annulled himself. In all his melancholic episodes, he repeated the lament that he had become a burden, a hindrance to his family.

The basis of the experience of melancholia is the anthropological theme of *socialisation*. All the dilemmas surrounding the melancholic person stem from difficulties in administrating the anthropological proportions of the dialectic between the individual and the collectivity to which they belong and on which they depend to exist. While in the cases of borderline and phobic disproportion, existence is vertically tilted off-balance towards an other-pole endowed with power, what we have here is power distributed horizontally, producing symmetry between the self-pole and the other-pole. The guiding principle of this symmetry is collective normality: the precepts, values and customs of social conduct consolidated in society over time. Collectivity is the overarching Gestalt that organises the patterns of relationships between the self-pole and the other-pole. As a result, both the self-pole and the other-pole are stripped of their power in the face of this superior order, which emanates from everyone, but no-one in particular. Both poles are identical in terms of their anthropological participation in existence. This leads to a world in which there are no powerful individuals, in which power mostly emanates from the impersonality of the collective norm. This is why any solution for a melancholic existence will never come from a redemptive other. Here, the great hope and dread that attracts and terrifies borderline and phobic persons is replaced by the mediocrity of people and behaviours. The melancholic person is guided by an ordinary, mediocre world.[5] They are circumscribed in their lives by the established norms. Their sufferings are secondary to their failures in their attempts to detach themselves from them or to follow them strictly. The following observations are narratives of this dilemma.

3.3.1 Identity – Hypernomic Behaviour

Kraus defines the melancholic personality as an anthropological disproportion between identity and ipseity, which he calls hypernomic behaviour (Kraus 1991a). Generally speaking, the profile of any existence is given by the singularity the individual stamps on some of the norms they learn from their social environment. This attributed singularity results from a dialectic between the roles of a normative collective identity and the creativity of idiosyncratic conduct. In the melancholic person, this dialectic tends strongly towards the collective, so that the entire personal identity revolves round social roles, leaving little space for personal aspirations and imagination. In general, the most important identity role tends to be the one that is responsible for concentrating the identity complex. An example of this is certain mothers who identify so strongly with their maternal role that when their children grow up and no longer need them so much, they feel as if their whole existence is a void and they fall into melancholic depression. This condition clearly appears in the statements of one patient: "I have lost myself in others"; "I don't know how to put myself first"; "I've lost my ability to know what I want"; "I always stay in the middle ground, because of others. I can't pursue a personal project because of my duty to others".

---

[5] This also occurs in hyperthymic disproportion, although while the melancholic person submits to it, the hyperthymic person tries to use it to their best advantage, as I will show further on.

Hypernomic behaviour is marked by a concomitant reduction of the ipseity of existence. A restriction of its identity creativity dominates the whole existence, which becomes vulnerable to changes in partial identities immediately leading to psychopathological situations, often severe. Melancholic depression induced by retirement (Tellenbach 1983) is another example of the risks involved in the anthropological disproportion of hypernomy. Retirement requires existence to seek new identities to sustain the propulsion of biographical development. Hypernomic restriction hinders this necessary renewal of identity, transforming the loss of the professional role into a loss of support for almost the whole existence. It makes little difference whether or not the retiree enjoyed their work. Quite often, they longed for retirement, but paradoxically, reaching it depresses them.

The hypernomic historical self matures serenely and gradually from the sedimentation of experiences that originate pre-reflexively from the assimilation of current norms. Its existential maturation is usually painless, since it does not face existential dilemmas arising from any tension between the aspirations of the self-pole and the demands of the world-pole and otherness. However, the psychopathologist should recognise the ambiguous face of this comparatively easy maturation. The melancholic person has little leeway to transcend ordinary situations because they are accustomed to develop their identity through the sedimentation of norms. They have difficulty in assimilating anything non-normal, which is why they have trouble adjusting to existential transitions. In general, they lack the creative ipseity necessary for the transition between life periods of longitudinal temporality. It is easier to understand the melancholic person's difficulty in transcending their immediate, middling experience if we examine it from the perspective of spatiality, as I will do next. First, however, we must point out an anthropological ambiguity inherent to hypernomy. The melancholic person performs social roles with consummate skill and integrity, precisely because their identity fits snugly to the collective identity. They are by nature the epitome of interpersonal reliability and personal dignity. The very anthropological disproportion that reduces their existential creativity is what maximises their value as a pillar of the collectivity and of human relations. As one patient expresses it, "my melancholia is good for my [professional] persona, but it's tough on me". Effectively, it is duty towards others that moves the melancholic person rather than passion or personal ambition. Their basic feelings are satisfaction or sadness. Their anxiety stems not from fear of the future but from unfulfilled duties. Their main dialectic is between commitment and the exhaustion of daily life. Their maximum value for themselves and the society to which they belong derives from the sedimentation of these experiences in their historical self. The basis for melancholic substance misuse can therefore be understood as a quest for an exogenous power of resistance in a world of duty and routine that offers a dearth of creativity and transformation. Intoxication offers the melancholic person, incarcerated in the world of their peers, a way of transforming this prison into something remotely tolerable.

3.3.2 Spatial Hyperintegrity

The prism of spatiality contributes to a further understanding of hypernomic identity. The spatiality of melancholic existence is marked by a disproportionately high participation of pre-reflexive integrity, with a corresponding reduction of fragmentation (making it the opposite of borderline spatiality). Hyperintegrity determines that compactness and inflexibility mark the melancholic person's lived experiences. The natural function of this spatiality is to reduce the dialectical fragmentation of experience. Compact spatiality hinders the emergence of contradictory or irreconcilable contents of consciousness. Melancholic existence, marked by spatial hyperintegrity, inhabits a world of experiences that are saturated, full, refractory to the multiplicity of perspectives. A melancholic person has a particular psychological integrity, which is granted by the cohesive and comprehensive way in which experiences dominate their consciousness. In a certain sense, the melancholic historical self already has, in advance, the coordinates to navigate the world. Unlike borderline or phobic persons, the melancholic person gives pre-reflexive preference to unifying their field of consciousness. Their experiences are lived in a clear and defined way, governed by principles of continuity and internal coherence. An example of this state is the difficulty that some melancholic patients have in receiving any suggestion about their life or interpretation about their behaviour that does not adhere strictly to what they are accustomed to and what people expect of them. They do not seem to understand the meaning of a suggestion, for example, that they modify some exhausting activity, such as caring for a chronically ill parent alone. It does not seem to cross their mind that there are alternatives to alleviate the situation. The spatial hyperintegrity of melancholic existence excludes from its field of consciousness all experiences that are disorderly or contradictory to its whole identity. The melancholic person's existence therefore develops by incrementally adding experiential elements that are coherent with their integrity, which means their process is gradually shaped by a sum of repetitive experiences, with little affective or sentimental variation (although they are usually quite profound). Regularity and reliability sustain the melancholic person's biography. The integrity of anthropological spatiality itself prevents the experiences that are most contradictory or inconsistent with its central line of development from penetrating consciousness. There is a kind of existential blindness to ambiguous and uncertain elements. Nonetheless, the melancholic person does not live in a world of certainties. Rather, the melancholic historical self occupies a spatiality permeated by a dialectic between right and wrong actions or between the necessary and the superfluous, always choosing the former. Nor is the typical melancholic historical self affected by corrosive doubts. Above all, its dilemmas arise from its ability, or not, to carry out its tasks. Its main dialectic concerns its performance in the face of failure. As such, one fundamental dimension of substance misuse in this case is its synergy with performance, either to enhance it or to render it tolerable.

The saturation of the melancholic existence's personal identities by hyper-integrity makes it especially vulnerable to situations in which existential ambiguity cannot be escaped (Kraus 1996a; Ambrosini et al. 2011). This intolerance to ambiguity induces a pre-reflexive simplification of the world that leads to mediocre behaviour and personal ambitions. A kind of rigid belt around the self-pole, the other-pole and the world-pole limits their expansion and restricts their capacity to modify and amplify each experience. It is as if every melancholic experience took on a solid, sculptural form, while the fragmented experiences of borderline persons are fluid and pliable. In short, melancholic existence exists in a narrow, rigid spatiality.

In more severe situations, the hyperintegrity of spatiality is transformed into existential shrinking. This shrinking is an important transition point for us to recognise the difference between a melancholic personality and a melancholic anthropopathology. The recognition of this shrinking is fundamental for understanding the most serious melancholic anthropopathologies (as it is for structural melancholic pathologies; Sect. 4.2). When this occurs, spatiality becomes so restricted that it distances existence even from its underlying intersubjectivity, and crushing it into a self-pole that is practically isolated and browbeaten in its solitary task of bearing all the world's responsibilities.[6] The name of this condition is solitary hypernomy. Melancholic guilt is the usual sentiment of solitary hypernomy: a guilt deriving not from some individual conduct but from the opacification of the world. This guilt does not sprout from the consequences of the decisions of a free historical self, but from the fact that this historical self is no longer capable of freedom (Blankenburg 1978). The Greek myth of Atlas is the pictorial representation of solitary hypernomy in the form of a gigantic self condemned to carry the world on its back. We should not misunderstand this enlargement of the self-pole: it does not result from an expansion of the self-pole's participation in existence as a whole, but from a shrinking of existence towards the self-pole. In this anthropological disproportion there is an intense harrassment of the self-pole. This phenomenon should also be observed from the perspective of embodiment in order to better gauge its magnitude.

3.3.3   Embodiment: Embodied Feelings and Inflexibility

The shrinkage of existence towards the self-pole also transforms the anthropological proportions of its material support, embodiment. In melancholic disproportion, exacerbated constriction transforms feelings into bodily sensations. Feelings can only be felt if the self-pole interacts with the world-pole. They are like an expansion of the self towards the world. For example, the feeling of anger is a way of relating

---

[6] It is not, therefore, a spatiality of distancing, as is seen in phobic disproportion, where the self-pole essentially continues to gravitate around a powerful other. Here, the self-pole tends to isolate itself from connection with the other-pole, constituting a deformity from which no liberation is possible.

to an other-pole when it appears important for bad reasons. When the severely melancholic person loses connection with the world, their feelings take on a totally isolated form, focusing only on the solitary historical self. This affective concentration on the isolated historical self means that all experiences take place in the body, the final refuge of the historical self. The result is an excessive embodiment of feelings. The clearest example of this is the precordial anguish seen in the most severe melancholic states. These patients have such intense psychosomatic feelings that in practice it is hard to distinguish them from somatic heart diseases (Buchmann et al. 2019).

Spatial shrinkage also reduces the body's capacity for the full exercise of existential cyclical movements. Body rhythms change, resulting in an indifferentiation between the poles of biological cycles. Examples of this are changes in the sleep-wake and hunger-satiety cycles.

3.3.4 Conservative Temporality

A low tolerance to ambiguity, as presented above, fills the melancholic historical self with mediocre experiences in terms of creativity and excitement. The paucity of these elements is transmitted to temporality. Thus, melancholic temporality is an anodyne temporality, marked by a disproportionate participation of retention in relation to existential protention. The density of this retention overwhelms the present, so that even individual projections of the future tend to be restricted to a vision of continuity. As one young melancholic patient said, in the course of an anthropopathological state of moderate severity, "I centralise my concerns on what has happened, and what will happen". Her choice of words precisely describes the situation in which she lives, as it implies a paradox. The patient uses a verb that indicates concentration of action at one point to the detriment of others. After all, when something is centralised, it must have a nucleus. Yet when she explains the object of her centralisation, she refers to the whole extension of temporality! She is quite simply concerned about everything, both the centre and the periphery. This temporalisation results from the integrity of melancholic experience, now extended to temporality. Everything is the object of her concern, and protention is already contained in a retention that permeates her present consciousness of suffering and restriction. Saturated temporality reduces the capacity of protention to protect existential creativity.

We can also see the prominence of temporal conservation in the melancholic person's preference for occupations that already exist in the family. As retention is disproportionately relevant, it can go back to the transgenerational dimension of an individual existence, inducing the melancholic person to continue family traditions, which, by dint of their roots in this relevant past, can even override any individual ambitions they may have.

In melancholic disproportion, therefore, there is no easy way to find solutions for indeterminate situations. The main symbolic reference for melancholic existence, the dialectic between individual and society, is quietly resolved through the annulment of the self-pole. The melancholic person's temporality settles for the collection of facts experienced modestly, but regularly. Their excessively unified spatiality offers great capacity for the accomplishment of necessary tasks for the community, family or company, because the sef-pole identifies with its professional identity. However, their retention-oriented temporality reveals its frailty when times of indeterminacy and emptiness have to be faced. In such cases, a melancholic existence may not have the flexibility to multiply its partial identities, lapsing into conditions that are often marked by nostalgia and total hopelessness with regard to the future. This is the point at which substance misuse comes in. The associated alteration of consciousness serves to recover feelings, memories and desires of a past time to which the melancholic person can retreat, making the ambiguity they face tolerable. Above all, it provides a kind of synergy for their temporal disproportion.

3.3.5   Clinical Decision-Making in Melancholia – The Incarcerated Clinician

The typical dilemmas of melancholic existence reduce the dimension of ipseity of the self-pole and the other-pole. As we have seen, both are determined by the higher force of the collective. This is what dictates the clinician's role in the melancholic patient's life. If, when treating patients with borderline and phobic disproportions, the clinician can become a beacon to show the way, in melancholic we have a totally different state of affairs. The clinician enters the patient's life as an agent of clinical normality. This makes the clinician's decision-making somewhat less complex. The patient will expect the clinician to perform a role as established in impersonal scientific therapeutic protocols. Their main demand will be to reduce distressing and unpleasant subjective experiences. There is little space available for existential interpretation. During treatment, the clinician will figure more as a technician than as a whole person. Their decisions involving their patients must be guided by the values of the maximum conservation of daily routine. The main existential sense that a treatment takes on is to expand the restricted spatiality in which the self-pole is incarcerated. Usually, the clinician is unable to obtain major re-proportions of intersubjective relevance. Mirroring the patient, the clinician will also be entirely incarcerated in their partial identity as a doctor or psychologist.

Take, for example, this statement from a young patient treated for mild melancholia, which 60 milligrams of fluoxetine can easily control: "I don't like psychotherapy because I don't like to open up. Here, there's nothing improvised in our consultation. I prepare myself first. I don't like to arrive with nothing to talk about". Her sincere statement reveals how she restricts intersubjective space for existential creativity. Melancholic persons prepare themselves in advance with pre-determined roles that are limited in their potential. The interpersonal relationship is restricted to a therapeutic relationship and any possible silence during the consultation constitutes failure, a lack of investment in the social duty prescribed by the role of the patient in relation to his/her doctor. All indefinition is expunged from the interpersonal relationship beforehand, thereby limiting it to repeated reiterations of the same experiences and an overall restriction of creative ipseity.

3.4 Hyperthymic Disproportion

Clinical Vignette

Andrew, 22 years old, seeks psychiatric care because he considers that his limited attention span and insomnia are obstacles for his plans to achieve career success. He is contradictory as regards his insomnia because he knows that lack of sleep makes him irritable and slows his thinking, but he cannot refrain from using every available moment of his day. He is a fourth-year economics student and is convinced he will become a renowned financial market professional.

He reports that he was an active, extroverted, sociable child. Often, his teachers would call in his mother for a meeting because he would never stay quietly at his desk, would approach his classmates during classroom activities, would quickly lose interest in his tasks and was inattentive. Andrew did not present cognitive difficulties; on the contrary, his intellectual performance was above average. During school time, he was always responsible for leading his classmates, who regularly elected him class representative. He also engaged in student council activities, represented the school enthusiastically in basketball competitions and was the singer in a rock band. At university, he has followed a similar course. The Academic Centre elected him president, he manages the students' consulting company, never misses college matches, even if he is injured, and is a volunteer teacher for disadvantaged teenagers preparing for university entrance exams. He is resourceful and generous both in dialogues with university authorities on behalf of the student body and with his disadvantaged students. However, Andrew recognises that his peers consider some of his actions and attitudes to be grand and superficial. He tries to be agreeable to everyone while also being open to criticism. However, lately, he has started feeling more intolerant and annoyed with his mediocre and slow-witted peers.

Andrew has an athletic build, is always well groomed, with hair and beard neatly trimmed, and dresses impeccably in designer clothes. The technological devices he uses are all state-of-the-art. He speaks with pride and a certain vanity of the attention he attracts when he goes to parties. He has no stable love relationship at present and emphasises the importance of enjoying himself. He fears a love affair might interfere with his plan to study at the prestigious Stanford University after finishing his degree. He emphasises that he intends to make his first million before turning 28.

Andrew complains of feeling impatient during classes. He has been unable to choose what to focus on. He says there are unnecessary classes about subjects he will never need to achieve his goals. He also complains that the teachers themselves are not interested in improving the classes. During these classes, he either stays at home sleeping (to compensate for insomnia) or goes and reads books on other subjects. He says that especially during exam times, he has been using methylphenidate to feel more productive and be able to cover the content of the whole semester in a single day. He is unaware that his use of the stimulant has increased over the last year and spread from the intellectual to the recreational sphere. He has been using methylphenidate with energy drinks for going out, because he feels more alive and enjoys the moment more. Even sleeping is a waste of time for Andrew.

The first sensation that the hyperthymic person evokes is that of enthusiasm and energy towards life. This preliminary perception gains depth when associated with an understanding of these characteristics in relation to the existential theme that underlies them. Hyperthymic disproportion gravitates around socialisation, just as melancholic disproportion does. Melancholic and hyperthymic disproportions, however, reveal two distinct existential solutions to the same dialectic of the horizontal tension between self-pole and other-pole, in terms of reciprocal importance. I will now consider the anatomy and dynamics of this high-energy enthusiasm.

3.4.1   Hyperthymic Intersubjectivity – Endoxia and the Collective Other-pole

Fame is the byword of hyperthymic existence. An etymological examination of the meaning of the ancient Greek word for famous, *endoxos*, offers the best explanation for this typical form of experience. Let us separate the prefix from the root, examining the meaning of each part. "En", like the English word "in", has the function of adnominal adjunct of place, indicating the idea of *inside*, the place in which something occurs. *Doxa* indicates public opinion (esteem). Together, the particle and the root indicate the occurrence of something "within public opinion". I propose the neologism endoxia, in the context of existence, to convey the idea of public opinion within a spatial perimeter. Having identified this structure of anthropological proportions, two perspectives can be taken to observe it: spatiality and intersubjectivity. Let us begin with the latter. A pre-reflexive relationship of equality between the self-pole and the other-pole determines both hyperthymic and melancholic existence. As I suggested above, the identity roles offered by society at a given historical time fully capture both. The hyperthymic person also devotes their existence to the reproduction and improvement of ambitions and attitudes regulated by social roles – restricting temporal protention – taking these pre-established social values to the extreme and exploiting projects and themes from a particular cultural moment to the ultimate degree. In this sense, both are hypernomic.

However, this typical anthropological disproportion takes on a specific configuration in the hyperthymic person. The indication of this particularity lies in the way the other-pole participates in the totality of existence. The hyperthymic self-pole maximises its visibility to the other-pole to actualise its need for complete identification with a social identity (hypernomy). It does this by approaching the other-pole as a collective other. This closeness then creates a tight bond between the self-pole and the other-pole, both as representatives of the collectivity. This bond gives hyperthymic existence a sense of solidity. For this reason, hyperthymic disproportion has even less ipseity than melancholic disproportion. The latter, with a self-observant historical self to verify the rectitude or error of its social actions, is to some extent more independent from social rules that determine its and others' roles. Hyperthymic disproportion involves an overvaluation of intersubjectivity, in which the powerful presence of the other-pole, always as a proxy for collective roles, continuously endorses the identities of the self-pole. The legitimation and justification of stable social rules is the focus of a reciprocal dialectic between the two poles. The collective other-pole is an indispensable concrete element in hyperthymic experience for the self-pole's performance of the required social identity. The extreme proximity of the two poles raises the social determination of the hyperthymic person's identity, making it hypersocial.

The behavioural result of this dynamic of anthropological proportions is the quest for fame, popularity, for the endless proximity of the other-pole to the self-pole as a vehicle for sociability. In the hyperthymic person, everything is social. Thus, the socialisation offered by intoxication is the first prism through which to understand hyperthymic or hypomanic persons' frequent substance misuse.[7] The hyperthymic historical self seeks consciousness modification to enable a strong tie with the social world, creating a broad attunement in which the identities of the self-pole and the other-pole adhere strictly to the norms (e.g. co-working).

Nonetheless, we should not mistake this hyperthymic existential form for the compensatory result of some insufficiency on the part of the self-pole. The hyperthymic historical self does not need fame, in the sense of someone seeking to elevate their self-esteem. What we are looking at here is a different anthropological situation. The hyperthymic historical self seeks fame because this is the language in which the collective's rules and values appear with greatest clarity and prominence. For the hyperthymic person, existence means fame or nothing. As one hyperthymic patient put it at the beginning of her care, "I came here to become famous". Although her initial desire was to cope with an anxiety disorder, her statement could not be clearer for understanding the anthropological basis of hyperthymic anxieties.

The feelings that express eudoxia reveal a basic existential state in which there is a pact between the historical self and the opinion of the other, always as a proxy for the collective. Two paradoxical feelings emerge from this: generosity and impatience. Generosity stems from the fact that any movement of the hyperthymic historical self encounters the other as its first and most important object; the hyperthymic person directs everything they produce towards the other and shows a unique capacity to fulfil the needs of the other, in that this other represents collectivity. Yet, they can have a very diminished perception of the other as a specific person. In terms of the dialectic between collectivity and singularity, we can say that the hyperthymic existence has a disproportionate bias towards the collectivity over singularity. This imbalance between the collective and the singular other causes the hyperthymic person's impatience and frequent irritability in relation to the other or even

---

[7] See note 3.

behaviour with cruel pseudopsychopathic overtones. The effects of substance misuse may magnify the latter. The hyperthymic historical self has low tolerance for
others' failures to conform to the dictates of social expectations, getting annoyed
with them and often acting with contempt. Rather than a whole person deserving of
respect, the other becomes an obstacle to hyperthymic hypersociability. For example, the hyperthymic person may be intolerant with a bad driver in traffic or with the
weaknesses or idiosyncrasies of a colleague who fails to observe their employer's
productivity goals. Hyperthymic hypersociability also requires the most objective
possible metrics to measure existence. As a result, the dialectic between social success and failure is another thematic pair that dominates hyperthymic eudoxia. Both
are clear, unquestionable expressions of the social results of an existence.
Hyperthymic disproportion does not enjoy subjective evaluations regarding the
results of life. This overinterest in objective results gives an understanding of possible hyperthymic pseudopsychopathic behaviours, such as validating a lifestyle in
which the ends justify the means.

3.4.2   Temporality of Conquest – The Paradox of Linear Hyperprotention

The characteristics of hyperthymic intersubjectivity are particularly illuminating of
hyperthymic temporality, which is particularly paradoxical. The hyperthymic person is, above all, someone who follows the rules of social identities, which means
their existence develops by circulating between predefined roles. The hyperthymic
person particularly projects their ambitions on the actualisation of identity projects
that already exist, making their temporality similar to the saturation and density of
melancholic persons. However, the hyperthymic person is future-oriented, always
investing energy and enthusiasm towards what they can achieve in the world. The
temporal preference of hyperthymic disproportion is for what is new, meaning
whatever has not yet been incorporated into their personal identity. However, this
significant openness to the future is designed to conquer objects and social positions
with pre-established value in their cultural context. The hyperthymic historical self
does not seek to determine itself by an existential leap into the unknown, but rather
by the conquest of new territories which are already occupied. From an anthropological point of view, we must not allow the frequent exploratory experiences of
hyperthymic persons to confuse us. Their subsequent progression to unusual places
or positions will in fact be generally successful. However, the hyperthymic person's
apparently indomitable spirit is rooted in the search for an expansion of familiar
areas of identity. For example, we can look at the biography of Alexander the Great,
who apparently had several manic experiences and who said that whenever he
looked at the horizon he always wanted to conquer it (Gregory 2013). The existential structure for understanding his achievements is not the renewal of existence

itself, but rather the expansion of the social attributes of a general. The hyperthymic person is more of a conqueror than a trailblazer. Therefore, their substance misuse functions in the sense of increasing the power with which the historical self surrenders itself to the world and others.

All this means that, paradoxically, there is both expansion and contraction in hyperthymic temporality. The protentive temporal dimension may be the most prominent, emphasising expansionist projection and conquest, yet this hyper-dimensioning of protention is restricted to a linear temporality of increases and transitions that are pre-programmed by social identities. In hyperthymic existences there is continuity in the maturation of the personality. As we observe the course of their life, we see that each step is the logical consequence of a previous one, so the progress of a hyperthymic existence can be predicted with a degree of regularity.

3.4.3 Hyperthymic Spatiality – Horizontality and Clarity

Horizontality is the spatiality of human coexistence, a preference for the shared to the individual, the plural to the singular. In this space of sharing, existential advances are based on clarity and regularity. We have seen how hyperthymic existence launches itself in the world through a succession of conquests occurring in an arena predetermined by social clarity, both of objects to be conquered and social identities. The predominant movement of the self-pole in this clear, horizontal space is shaped by its proximity to the other-pole and the world-pole. This in turn elevates the relative importance of worldly objects to the self-pole. In its intense relationship with the world, hyperthymic existence generally interacts with it in two specific ways.

The first consequence of this overvaluation of worldly objects is distraction. As the world contains a multitude of valuable objects homogeneously distributed in space, the interest of the hyperthymic historical self flits between them, sometimes unable to fix itself on any one of them. For the hyperthymic person, the face value of objects eclipses their deeper meaning, making it hard for them to choose which object to enjoy first. If everything is interesting, nothing deserves a more profound and detailed examination. The hyperthymic historical self can get lost in the superficiality of an excessively clear and horizontal world. The second consequence of this overvaluation is irritability. In a spatiality packed with a vast array of enticing objects, the hyperthymic historical self is keen to try them all out, but ends up being trapped in its haste to jump from one to another (Binswanger 2000). This haste tends to prompt an emotional state of continual irritation and impatience. Substance use has an important self-management function here in enabling the hyperthymic person to actually enjoy the world.

3.4.4 Hyperthymic Identity – Hypersymmetry

The hyperthymic historical self dwells in a fascinating and colourful world. It is extremely close both to the world and to those who live there. This proximity gives it easy access to the world and its appreciation of the world makes the objects that compose it inherently interesting. This combination of proximity and interest is what gives rise to the central experience of hyperthymic identity: manageability. The dialectic between the self-pole and the world- and other-pole stems from the capacity of the hyperthymic person to manage this world. The hyperthymic person's identity is defined by their ability to move the world or the other in favour of the temporal movements they propose. A hyperthymic person's identity is completely filled by actions in the world, which ends up saturating it (in the same way as the melancholic person), leaving no room for any dialectic relationship that serves no measurable functional purpose in terms of practicality, clarity or productivity. The relationships of the hyperthymic person are relations in which action is the metric, often leading to experiences of vanity. However, hyperthymic vanity should not be understood as an overvaluation of the self-pole over the other-pole. Paradoxically, the hyperthymic person's vanity derives from a historical self whose identity is filled with the values and gazes supplied and confirmed by the collective other. In this paradox, although it may appear narcissistic, the vanity in this behaviour is far from being so. In genuine narcissism, the historical self demonstrates blatant disregard for the other-pole, which serves as an instrumental object of domination. In hyperthymic vanity, the self-pole and the other-pole are locked together in constant combat, forever compared to one another without either pole ever coming out on top for long. We call this state of anthropological proportions *hypersymmetry*.

In the hypersymmetrical identity of hyperthymia, the historical self engages the other in a battle for hegemony. The ultimate goal of this battle – seldom apparent to the patient themselves – is to rid themselves of the excessive symmetry of value which imprisons them. This dialectic leads to an alternation of experiences of submission and supremacy. The self-pole quickly gains value in relation to that of the other; but conversely, it soon experiences the other-pole as more valuable. The hyperthymic historical self alternates on a scale of temporary triumph or transitory contempt, or one of obedience and subservience; between imposition and submission.[8] The euphoria of success and the humiliation of failure are habitual characteristics of the hyperthymic person. The enormous contribution that the hyperthymic person often brings to society results from this ambiguity. The hyperthymic person's eternal connection to society includes the simultaneous desire to stand out. They therefore direct much frenetic activity – often eased by substance misuse – to the development and offer of products that are valued and useful to the groups to which they belong. The hyperthymic person's existential pain thus comes precisely from the excessive value they place on this all-consuming collective otherness

---

[8] Some phobic people may superficially reproduce this pattern of domination and submission. However, their capacity to shake off this pattern grows as they mature existentially.

which shapes much of their individual conduct. In hyperthymic disproportion, the projects of the historical self tend to merge with the identities of the collective.

3.4.5 Iconic Hyperactivity – Embodiment in Hyperthymia

The horizontality of spatiality determines that the gaze of collective otherness galvanises hyperthymic experience. In the bodily dimension, this condition takes on the form of emphasising modes of social appearance. The hyperthymic body thus becomes an icon of collective visibility. The hyperthymic person expresses eudoxia by always standing out, a body adorned with symbols of social success. Fashion is the best way to that goal. The prominence given to brands, labels and cosmetic beauty is typical of this embodiment. Hyperthymic embodiment is public and its aesthetic display therefore presents and represents the preferences of the society in which this life develops.

Hyperthymic embodiment is also a primary instrument for the horizontal occupation of social space. The hyperthymic person directs all their energies to the realm of their equals, their peers, where they engage in activities designed to transform the world. This primordial giving to the world makes motricity the second capital element for understanding hyperthymic embodiment. Frequently, this motor hyperactivity reaches such a disproportion that it prevents the historical self from focusing on one thing. From an anthropological point of view, much of the behaviour semiologically referred to as attention deficit and hyperactivity disorder (ADHD) has roots in the disproportional participation of horizontality in motor behaviour and is therefore of hyperthymic origin.

3.4.6 Hyperthymic Ambiguity and Clinical Decision-Making

Intersubjective hypersymmetry endows hyperthymic experiences with ambiguity. On the one hand, very close and continuous contact with the other causes frequent annoyance and tiredness; on the other hand, this same condition is the source of existential success. Thus, the ambiguous demand that the hyperthymic person makes on the clinician is to help bring them closer to others without this exhausting them (very often, their substance misuse serves the same purpose). The task is not easy from a pharmacological point of view, because any pharmacological treatment of irritability will tend to induce an experience of detachment from the world, which is felt as an undesirable imbalance rather than a healthy balance of anthropological proportions.

Generally, the hyperthymic person will rarely tolerate (or only temporarily tolerate) any modification of the spatiality of their experiences. They prefer occasional bouts of relaxation or distension which are not so intense or time-consuming as to diminish their enormous energy and vitality. They experience any reduction in vitality as an undesirable loss of identity. From a psychotherapeutic point of view, the intersubjective ambiguity of the hyperthymic person means that the clinician has little room for manoeuvre, since the patient experiences any more incisive interference in their life as an annoying attempt to subdue them. The clinician should prepare to take on the role of a neutral spectator, supporting the conquests of hyperthymic existence and commiserating with their occasional failures. Their interventions should be short-lived and focused and should rarely aim at crucial aspects of the patient's life. The clinician should not employ existential counselling as their main conduct. A hyperthymic person generally carries out their own decision making, with little help from the clinician.

However, the clinician should not interpret this type of intersubjective relationship as unimportant. The basic symmetry that constitutes the intersubjectivity of the hyperthymic person often makes them an excellent partner in therapy. Hyperthymic persons can develop great loyalty to their therapy and friendliness to the clinician if the clinician takes the abovementioned approach. Often, the clinician feels as if they cannot clearly apprehend the life plans of a hyperthymic person. They do not feel competent to help them existentially. This stems from the fact, indicated above, that their projects are so assimilated by social identities that they do not seem authentic or even seem to exist. However, given the very nature of hyperthymic identity, these plural projects are the most genuine in their existences. The clinician should therefore keep in mind the perception that their main function will be to adjust the hyperthymic existence to previously adopted social identities. This work is sometimes more akin to social skills training or merely the dispensation of pharmacological or psychological aid to help them withstand tiredness and irritation. This is the profound therapeutic approach for a hyperthymic existence.

Third Level

3.5   Compulsive Disproportion

Clinical Vignette
Isabel's husband, José, takes her for psychiatric evaluation because she has been increasing her consumption of alcohol and cocaine, which has caused marital and work-related issues. Her husband feels she does not seem to care or worry about what happens. As he puts it, "she promises to stop, but ends up relapsing...lying... she's not afraid that she's killing herself, doctor".

As a teenager, Isabel took part in a gymnastics team. She was very hard-working but her technical performance was average. She functioned well in the hierarchical structure governing the group and was unaware that she often took a submissive position. She absorbed criticism passively. When she was 14, she was not selected for the competition squad. From that period on, she changed her eating habits and experienced massive weight gain (reaching 110 kg). Isabel would lock herself in her room and eat, especially sweet things, in large quantities, even when she was not hungry.

She could not explain exactly what kind of situation would trigger this behaviour or what she felt while she was eating. As her condition worsened, she no longer enjoyed the act of eating, did not savour the tastes and textures of the food and could not break the cycle until she felt sick. She told a nutritionist she could not understand why her weight was increasing. She tried several slimming programmes and managed to lose 10 kg with Weight Watchers, but she did not sustain the loss. At the age of 20, the patient underwent bariatric surgery and reduced her weight to 75 kg.

At 22, the patient left her job as a receptionist to devote her time exclusively to the care of her mother, who had been diagnosed with colon cancer. After 8 months of her life revolving round her mother's illness, she felt bewildered by her death. During this process (her mother's illness and death), the patient started to use alcohol and cocaine. Isabel had already tried cocaine and amphetamines at the age of 19 to lose weight, but not habitually. She reported that cocaine was the only way to bring a little excitement into her life. She could not feel pleasure in anything else. Nothing else interested her. She was doing six to nine lines of cocaine a day. In her own words, "cocaine fills me up, because I can't eat any more" (because of the dietary restriction and side effects of the bariatric surgery). Isabel tried to get back into the job market, but lost her job for showing up intoxicated and flirting with a client. This inappropriate behaviour is just one example of how the patient lost the overall ability to interpret the context of situations and personal relationships.

The patient has been married to José since she was 25. They married 5 weeks after their first date. It was the solution she encountered to have a home, since at this time she was facing eviction for non-payment of rent. Isabel acknowledges that José is very patient and understanding. She says, "I really don't know how he can stand it ... if it were me, I'd have left ... I only have him". She says she has had sex outside her marriage, but has felt guilty and regretful afterwards. José says he is tired of the same old excuses: "it was just a sexual urge, no emotions attached", "it won't happen again". He says he really does not see any malice in Isabel's attitudes, since she is always open and sincere. He appreciates her life story and tries to encourage her to resume her studies or think of some business venture they could do together, but nothing flourishes ("she's stuck"). Isabel sees no sense in her husband's suggestions.

Currently, Isabel has followed the psychiatric and the multidisciplinary teams' guidelines to the letter, especially those related to short-term behavioural control (one day at a time). Her husband has acted strictly and inflexibly in his control of medications and in the fulfilment of the therapeutic project. Isabel is also showing surprising commitment to Alcoholics Anonymous, with which she feels identification.

One of the principal founding dialectics of human existence is the relationship between the parts and the whole. The classical concept of the hermeneutic circle, embraced by Jaspers in the early days of psychopathology, highlights the importance of the relationship between existential unity and its constituent elements. The dialectic-proportional model focuses on these dialectics, as is seen in the presentation of spatiality as divided between integrity and fragmentation (Sect. 2.2.3). Ambiguity is also a feature of the objective relations between the self-pole and the other- and world-poles. As such, every time the other- and world-poles become evident to the self-pole, a dialectical tension springs up between the part and the whole. For example, sexual desire for another is a yearning to access the other partially (as a sexual object), while nonetheless experiencing them as a complete person (not merely a receptacle of this desire) and therefore equal in their entirety to the self-pole. The relations between self-pole, other- and world-pole are dialectic relations between the partial and the general. The condition I will now examine presents the problems that occur when there is an overwhelming presence of a specific part of the world and the other, bringing forth a corresponding part in the self-pole. I call this existential condition *hypermeria*[9] for reasons that will be made clear in the following exposition. Here, the part is dialectically more important than the whole. This distorts the experience of the world and the other as wholeness. This is not a fragmentary occurrence, undermining integrity, but a distorted overpresence of the part in the whole (a condensation of totality), without the part–whole dialectic being lost, as I will explain below. We will now look at the inherent characteristics and risks.

3.5.1 Spatial Compression of the Compulsive Person and Hypermeric Embodiment

Of all the anthropological disorders, it is in compulsive experiences that we observe the greatest spatial proximity between the self-pole and the other- and world-poles. The compulsive person's spatial disproportion creates a tendency for adherence between the self-pole and the other- and world-poles, resulting in an existence compressed around one point in the objective world. It is therefore a variant of excessive horizontal alteration, this time marked by extreme compression. It is a dysmetry of horizontality: a loss of a healthy spatial measure in relation to the objects of the world- and other-poles. In healthy individuals, the self-pole and the world-pole are protected from each other by a minimum of distance, allowing objects to appear as part of a wider context. This pre-reflexive distance is what enables the world to be apprehended as endowed with relationships between parts and whole. Let us consider the spatial perspective. Perspective permits us to know that a tree is part of a forest, or that we should divide our personal budget between expenditure for pleasure and for daily maintenance, or that satiety limits the act of eating. In the compulsive person, however, a hypoperspectivity occurs. Faced with a reduced existential spatial perspective, objects appear to the compulsive self-pole as unique and complete, as if they did not belong to a significant whole. For example, the act of eating becomes binge eating: food is devoured in bulk and experienced only as a

---

[9] Hypermeria is a neologism, based on the association of one of the meanings of the prefix *hyper* in Ancient Greek, above measure (Liddell et al. 1940), with the noun *meros*, meaning part, portion. Hypermeria is literally "the condition in which the parts are more than they should be", which results in an undesirable state. An identical use can be encountered in the term hypermetria – meaning "passing all measure".

mass to be incorporated, rather than being enjoyed as a complex interaction of flavours, textures and colours, gradually leading to satiety. The same applies, mutatis mutandis, to compulsive sex and pathological gambling. In these, the object relating to the self-pole (the personal other or an object to be manipulated, respectively) floods existential spatiality, dominating consciousness in a tyrannical manner.[10] The object takes over the consciousness of the one who experiences it, leaving no room for limits. Consciousness is overcome. Thus, the satiety that should follow the hunger, the person behind the sexual impulse, or the whole budget behind the urge to win when gambling all vanish. In the same way, the personal pleasure obtained in substance use disappears, giving way to a state of total intoxication, in which the self-pole and the other- and world-poles take on a *fusional relationship* (Pringuey 2005; Kimura 2005). The historical self then disregards the existential spaces of its historical development and merges with the pleasure-giving pole, constituting a dense, cohesive nucleus that is impervious to complexity and dialectics. (This theme will be further explored in the part III) In this fusional experience, the self-pole is frozen in a single subjective state produced by the force of exogenous intoxication. Addiction, from the point of view of compulsive disproportion, entails a fusional dereliction of the personal history (Binder 1979; Zutt 1963b).

As a result, the compulsive historical self perceives the world-pole as filled with massive, dense objects. This aspect of objects attached to the self-pole heightens the world's materiality, magnifying its bodily aspect (Messas et al. 2016). (It is worth remembering that the body is always present.) The compulsive person abdicates their capacity for freedom in their surrender to material aspects of the real world. Their existence involves a compressive surrender to food, sex, shopping or substance abuse, in a radical adherence to the materiality of the world, which essentially enslaves them. We will explore the consequences of this materialisation of the world in the section on the psychopathology of substance misuse (part III).

In compulsive experiences, spatial compression also has the effect of emphasising specific aspects of embodiment. The body's interactions with the world are overconcentrated on a specific point, which becomes the focal point for the signification of the whole of existence. An example of this condition is the focus on the erogenous zone as the principal representative of all bodily desires.

3.5.2 Homogeneous Temporality

The rhythm of healthy life can be seen most clearly in the phenomenon of fruition. Three articulated, heterogeneous moments can be detected here. Initially, the self-pole detects an object that fulfils one of its current needs. For example, feeling hungry induces the historical self to seek food. We can use this principle to understand abstract notions: a beautiful object may attract the consciousness of someone who desires to possess it. Following the initial moment, the self-pole approaches the

---

[10]Although, as we will see below, the ability to experience whole-part dialectics is not lost.

object, seeking to assimilate it, acquire it, or just spend time in its presence. This functions as existential fulfilment. The distinctive characteristic of fruition is precisely the passage from this second stage to a third, in which consciousness reduces the physical presence of the object. Someone who enjoys something, once they have attained their object, experiences a mitigation of the temporal movement leading to the object. Once this happens, the end of the cycle is reached, and the dimensions of temporality are accordingly made available for other experiences. The importance of the present, when the self-pole and its object come into contact with each other, is reduced to allow a greater proportional participation of protention. Thus, the rhythm of existence demands a dialectic relationship between lack, fulfilment and end, corresponding to an alternation between the value of the present and the value of protention.

The compulsive person's temporality eliminates the third stage, at which protention reorients existence. The present dimension, where assimilation or contact with the object occurs, is so hypertrophied that it stops experiences of fruition passing to retention or giving rise to a new opening for protention. Homogenised, the compulsive person's temporality requires continuous stimulation to enshrine a hypertrophied present. The historical self resorts to substance misuse precisely to maintain this stimulation. Nothing is more powerful than intoxication to sustain the unique form of the present, as the endless stimulus of an existence where the present is homogeneous. This overwhelming, indissoluble present distorts the threefold form of temporality itself, damaging the longitudinal processes of existential maturation.

From a longitudinal point of view, this all-encompassing present makes it difficult to learn from experience, which is the bedrock of existential maturation. Learning depends on submitting both positive experiences (to be enjoyed) and negative ones (to be forgotten) to a figure-ground dialectic, through which everything experienced at some time with the force of the present is modified in its temporal meaning. It is necessary to transform experiences from the present instance into an attenuated form, provided by retention, in order to incorporate them into the process of existential maturation. Only thus is it possible to incorporate experiences into existence and use them as a guide in the quest and appreciation of new adventures. A continually present experience cannot serve as a guide for existential development, as it lacks the capacity for historicisation. In a temporality where there is no end, there is also no beginning. The compulsive person's homogenisation of temporality, when taken to the extreme, acts in the opposite direction to biographical development, leading to subjective and behavioural alterations which have to be examined through the dimension of identity, as I will do now.

3.5.3   Identity in Compulsion – Adhesive Condensation and Subidentities

The essence of compulsive disproportion is the *adhesive attachment to partial aspects* of otherness or the world, limiting the value of interpersonal relationships. This limitation, as we have seen, does not stem from the person's incapacity to perceive the significant totality of the world and otherness, but from an excessive proximity of a partial aspect of the self-pole over a partial aspect of the other- and world-poles. An anthropological distortion occurs, characterised by adhesive condensation of identity at some point in reality. I reiterate: adhesive condensation does not affect the historical self's capacity to apprehend the whole meaning of its surroundings. The condensed relationship between the self-pole and its object of compulsion (e.g. the other as an object of sexual desire or the continued use of a psycho-stimulant) coexists with the totality of which it is part (e.g. the individual other or the need for moderation in substance use). This coexistence of modes of relationships between the self-pole and the other-pole and world-pole lends the personal dialectics of identity-otherness a particular overtone. Adhesive condensation causes partial segments of identity to direct behaviour disproportionately. For example, the erotic partiality of a person with a compulsive sexual desire unbalances consciousness as regards the social identities available in the class or social group to which they belong, or beyond what the historical self recognises as appropriate within its value structure. A subidentity originating from excessive existential condensation conducts the relationship with the world from the partial aspect of its own identity. This subidentity acts out of tune with the person's value senses taken as a whole, even though their value system remains intact. Every compulsive act of identity entails a dialectic tension. While refusing reduction to that role, the person's adherence to it completely dominates their existence. This dialectical tension gives some insight into two frequently interlinked observations in compulsive disproportion. The first is antisocial behaviour, often linked to compulsive actions. A partial aspect of identity that contradicts the historical personal identity will be manifested in lies about substance use (even in the face of evidence) or uncontrolled and irresponsible sexual behaviour (of which the historical self is usually ashamed). The compulsive person who lies about their behaviour knows they are lying and feels ashamed of doing so; however, they often mention that an inner force compels them to this undesirable behaviour. Compulsive subidentities are the shadow that terrorises compulsive existence, a kind of Mr. Jekyll which, while never totally incorporated into the identity, lurks as a threat that distorts anthropological proportions. This experience differs, for example, from potentially antisocial behaviour in schizoid persons (which we will see below), since this is based on an inability to perceive the other as a whole. In antisocial schizoid behaviour, evil or disrespectful actions emerge from an inability to attune to the other as a person. Conversely, the self-pole suffering from compulsive adhesive condensation does perceive the other pre-reflexively as a whole; however, only one of its subidentities is capable of taking an interest in some partial aspect of the other-pole. Feelings of guilt often follow compulsive acts. Indeed, guilt is the second most common finding in compulsive experiences (Dearing et al. 2005; Matthews et al. 2017). It indicates that the individual's set of values remains intact behind the partial actions. The compulsive action, while it lasts, obscures values that guide the habitual conduct of the historical identity. However, immediately after the compulsive act, the historical self regains awareness of its values as a whole. This return to its own values forces the historical self to compare its compulsive act to conduct it deems correct. A compulsive person's ambiguous, sometimes heart-breaking, behaviour, condemns it to an anguished and shameful state of concupiscence and guilt. Typical examples of this situation are guilty feelings (and forced vomiting) following binge-eating episodes, or profound depression after abusive substance use.

3.5.4 Subidentity Condensation and Phenomenological Compensation

As we have just seen, subidentity condensation may be primary – constitutive of the typical anthropological disproportion of a singular existence – or secondary. In this case, it functions as a compensatory mechanism for the historical self's unsustainable dialectic tension. We may consider the following case: a patient, highly successful in his career and family life, quite often hazards his reputation with risky sexual behaviour. On these occasions, he strips himself of his identity as a very successful professional in his field and becomes a ferocious sexual predator. He begins to forfeit his reputation in his social context because of this behaviour. Despite these initial losses, he continues his risky sexual behaviour, always stimulated by substance misuse. He considers the risks he is taking are unreasonable. He even fears there will be substantial losses in his life if this goes on. However, he says it is difficult for him to give it up because, in his words, it "releases me from my professional self. It's very important to me, because I can't bear the burden [of the professional self] any longer". The longitudinal perspective of temporality helps us to understand this subidentity disproportion and its related compensation. The exhausting professional role – despite having reached social maturity – leads to a temporal imbalance, without any prospect of protention. The social identity dominates the whole identity and its exhaustion means that no temporal alternative appears to give the historical self some hope. However, an alternative to temporal closure arises in the form of a subidentity. This subidentity provides some temporal perspective for existence to continue, despite its limited capacity for temporalising existence. The sexual compulsion emerges precisely because of the patient's inflexibility in dealing with the depletion of the value of his professional role. Rather than engaging in a renewal of his whole identity, the whole complexity of his identity is condensed towards a single subidentity, producing compulsive behaviour. This compulsive behaviour induces a kind of existential intoxication reverberating in an existence whose temporality is numbed.

3.5.5 Relationship with the Object – Hypermeria and Paradoxical Transvaluation

A horizontal compression of spatiality generates compulsive experiences. The adhesive condensation of parts of the self-pole makes objects and experiences offer themselves to consciousness in the hypermeric form. This manifests itself both in relation to objects and in interpersonal relationships. It takes on specific character-istics in each case. Let us first examine how these relations operate in the case of the polarity of the self with non-personal objects.

The self-pole's dysmmetrical approach to the world, in compulsive disproportion, relies on exaggerating the value of an object or state of consciousness that possesses an intrinsic value for existence, such as food, aesthetic pleasure in shopping or subjective pleasure obtained through psychoactive substance use. Dysmmetry distorts the appearance of objects by simultaneously overvaluing and reducing the object's value. The object is worth so much that it ends up losing its value for existence as a whole. I call this phenomenon *paradoxical transvaluation*. The object or experience has such relevance that the self-pole apprehends it in a distorted manner. The *trans* prefix indicates that the accentuated value granted to an object surpasses the intrinsic context of its existential meaning. The most obvious case of paradoxical transvaluation is addiction, where the incarceration of existence in an altered state of consciousness appropriates the initial pleasure of altering consciousness. There are other examples linked to daily routines. We value food both for nourishing the organism and for sensory pleasure. We can increase this intrinsic value in a healthy way. For example, gourmets may devote a great deal of time to improving the appreciation of fine food, without it becoming compulsive. The dividing line between the gourmet and the compulsive person is how valuable food is to dimensions of existence that even the historical self deems inappropriate. Thus, extending the valuation of the act of eating to anxiety reduction or simply satisfying some diffuse voracity are examples in which an inflated value exceeds reasonable boundaries, distorting the value of food as an object. Another frontier of normality are historical profiles of temporality. Someone who gambles for so many hours that he cannot work the next day distorts biographical temporality, reducing the future in favour of a homogeneous present. This also applies to exogenous pleasure obtained from psychoactive substances. In both situations, the increase in value occupies a paradoxical, transvaluational terrain. Transvaluation is a change generated by the ambiguity contained in an overvalued experience, which itself reduces the value. Paradoxical transvaluation is when a value takes on an excessively high position in the world, without ceasing to be a value in itself, and without ceasing to be part of a significant whole. For this reason, relinquishing a compulsion does not generally mean discontinuing the existential value of one's original experience. Herein lies the paradox and difficulty of overcoming compulsions: they refer to the genuine value framework of an existence. The addict who quits using substances or the pathological gambler who quits gambling does not relinquish their sense of pleasure; instead, they try to restrict it to a healthy existential form.

To identify a compulsive disproportion correctly, it is important to emphasise that the existential meaning given to the object of compulsion must be identical to its meaning in non-compulsive experience. Thus, a compulsion for food has a nutritional function at its original existential core, while a transvaluation of nutrition defines compulsion. The fruition of nutrition is the significant whole that defines the compulsive partiality. This knowledge is important for establishing differential diagnoses. We can consider the difference between binge eating episodes and pica.

In binge eating, the total meaning of eating, as a source of pleasure and nutrition, is never lost. However, in pica, the eating of ice or bricks does not indicate an exaggeration of the original value of nutritional enjoyment, but an exotic appetite which the historical self identifies as strange. In the same way, in compulsive shopping, we must differentiate the person who buys dysmmetrically for the excessive pleasure of owning aesthetic objects from the one who, for example, buys several items because they are from the same collection. In the first case, there is a paradoxical transvaluation; in the second, there is an obsessive desire for symmetry (see below, Sect. 3.6).

In short, someone who intoxicates themselves, eats, or shops compulsively never ceases to believe that there is a pleasurable and familiar aspect to their behaviour, but that they have taken it to unacceptable extremes. Intrinsic values that they could respect but do not are what guide the existence of the compulsive person. It is in relation to these values that we should understand how otherness manifests itself in compulsive dissymmetry.

3.5.6   Hyperequal Guardianship – Intersubjective Ambiguity of the Compulsive Person

In a compulsive experience, excessive proximity of the self-pole to the other-pole, as the example we have just seen, establishes an intersubjective ambiguity: although the self-pole only focuses on part of the other-pole (as a sexual object, for example), this partiality does not prevent it from having contact with the whole person. On the contrary, there is an exaltation of the presence of the other as a historical person. The other person appears to the compulsive historical self in two simultaneous and paradoxical dimensions, which we will see below.

In the first form, as seen in sexual compulsion for example, which perforce requires another, there is a metonymisation of relations between the self-pole and the other-pole. The paradoxical transvaluation makes the other appear as a part representing a whole, in the manner of metonymic transvaluation. The other-as-sexual-object results from a condensation of the values of this other, in which the erotic part becomes a synthesis of the whole personality. This other-pole appears to the self-pole as a category of world object, just like food or other consumer goods. Evidently, this metonymisation of the other-pole reduces its total value. The manner in which compulsive patients can neglect their closest personal relationships or abandon them in favour of their compulsive urges demonstrates this reduction clearly. The high dropout percentage of these patients is evidence of this in the therapeutic relationship (Jensen et al. 2014). The compulsive historical self's tendency to abruptly give up a therapeutic strategy or even a personal relationship seems to be deeply entrenched in their intersubjective possibilities.

On the other hand, there is a second way, which interests us more, for its clinical consequences. This presentation of the other derives exactly from the extreme proximity between the self-pole and the other-pole. Subsequently, they become so close that they are equal in terms of identity. This is a phenomenon that I call *hyperequality*. Hyperequality is a form of identity saturation in which the experiences of the self-pole tend to merge with those of the other-pole. It is a typical experience of collective intersubjectivity.[11] Hyperequality is very visible in the ease with which compulsive people organise themselves – in a productive and healthy way – into mutual help groups, to apply self-control to their behaviour. This facility shows that the groups' participants are able to share their problems easily. There is thus great homogeneity in the experience of compulsive behaviour, which means each individual experience is much less unique. This homogeneity can be harnessed effectively in mutual help groups, especially in cases of substance misuse (Parkman et al. 2015). To explain this notion better, I propose to contrast this with a totally opposite situation, involving the groups of schizophrenic patients. In these, although there is effectively a reciprocal empathy between the patients in terms of suffering from a mental disorder, we cannot say that their experiences are homogeneous. In fact, they are extremely diverse, and the one thing they share – suffering from a severe pathological condition – is what actually isolates them from each other. On the other hand, in groups involving the hyperequal intersubjectivity of the compulsive individual, the experiences are similar precisely because they all derive from the similarity between the identities (or subidentities, in the case of pseudo antisocial behaviour associated to compulsion). The compulsive person's other can thus comprehend their subjective experience with clarity and immediacy, for it is fused with them. This capacity of the compulsive person to fuse their experiences in a group relationship makes the hyperequal other's presence essential for the progression of compulsive people's lives.

Intersubjective hyperequality transforms the other into the guardian of the biographical integrity and the personal values of the patient's historical self. The other will be responsible for reminding the historical self of its life's value senses, or in other words, adjusting it to the anthropological proportions that allow its personal values to be lived as such, and not as transvalues. The other is an external element who imposes limits on the historical self's spatiality. This allows, for example, the binge-eater to recover the meaning of food or the obsessive shopper to derive pleasure from the object consumed when shopping, and it liberates sexual activity from the lust that depersonalises the other. Ultimately, it enables the person consumed by addiction to find a genuine path of life development.

As fusion with its object distorts the selfpole, the hyperequal other-pole must act in the opposite direction, recalling the historical self to its usual identity forms. The hyperequal other will lead to a demetonynisation of intersubjective relations. In compulsive intersubjectivity, it is up to the other to recall the historical self to its most valuable and cherished anthropological proportions. In precise terms, the hyperequal other serves to re-value compulsive experience. Re-valuing does not mean here the reconstruction of a shattered value (as seen in schizophrenic psychoses or in overwhelming existential situations), but simply the decondensation of an

---

[11] This is a stronger form of hyperthymic hypersymmetry.

existence previously endowed with a value sense, which has lost its positional sense. Existence distorted by compulsive dysmetry does not encounter anthropological proportions that fully allow it to access and live its own set of values, and needs the other to dismantle the disproportion.

The compulsive person's intersubjective ambiguity springs from the very nature of hyperequality. Being equal to the historical self, the other can be invaluable, because only they can lead compulsive existence back to its familiar paths. For exactly the same reason, the other is worth nothing, because they and the self-pole have already lost themselves, due to their inability to be guided by the values in which they believe. Compulsive existence shifts between equals and its good biographical development relies on the peculiarities of this dialectic between homogeneous identities. This last sentence already leads us to think about how the clinician may approach the compulsive person.

3.5.7   The Compulsive Person's Cohesive Otherness and Clinical Decision-Making

The role of great importance the compulsive person endows other with puts a lot of responsibility on their shoulders. In compulsive disproportion, the other must figure as cohesive, decided, utterly capable of acting in accordance with their own value senses and as a guardian of the patient's biography. The other will protect the biographical cohesion of the patient's life. When dealing with a compulsive person, clinicians themselves must offer clarity and resolution to their patient. Given its anthropological proportions, the compulsive historical self is comfortable accepting the presence of strong resolute others, who act to organise its life. The compulsive person usually permits strong interference by the clinician or the peers in their life. The firmness of the clinician's and peers' action guarantees the patient's continued ability to guide its historical self by its own values. Strictness and firmness are therefore routine components of the clinical management of compulsive people. They do not indicate any intention to subjugate the other over the compulsive historical self, as might appear in a hasty analysis. On the contrary, they act in the interests of the historical self's aspirations, in what it needs most profoundly for the restoration of its personal integrity. Previous knowledge of the patient's values and personality are very important for clinical decisions in compulsions, because the aim of the treatment is to reorient existence to these pre-consolidated values. Compulsion therapy is not, therefore, a technique of creative construction of meanings, but a reorientation towards solidly established meanings. The opinion of relatives or peers who share the patient's cultural environment is very important in clinical decisions. From the point of view of identity, the primary purpose of clinical strategy is to decompress identity, dismantling the subidentities that so hinder the biographical progression of compulsive patients, and reorient their lives to the values of the historical self's identity. The treatment's aim, from a spatial point of view, is to promote a detachment of the self-pole from the other-pole and the world-pole.

The compulsive person's anthropological disproportion, from a relational point of view, allows two clear alternatives for the clinician: negligence or firmness. As the compulsive patient's value senses are very clear, the clinician has little margin for reflections of an existential nature. Either they engage in energetically controlling the compulsive person's behaviour or the patient will construe them as indifferent to their problem and will abandon them. This limited flexibility in clinical decisions concerning the treatment of compulsions makes the clinician's work both easy and complex. Treatment can be easy because the patient makes few interpretative demands; they require the mechanical control of their behaviour, not comprehension. However, the demand for immediate, resolute action without reflection can isolate the clinician. Often, they feel confined, having a clear strategy in hand, but unable to implement it in the reality of the case because the patient resists discussion of the difficulties they face. Sometimes, the clinician feels that only they are interested in the treatment. The greatest ambiguity in the clinical management of compulsions lies in the fact that therapeutic strategies are simple, but their execution is rarely so.

3.6 Obsessive Disproportion

Clinical Vignette

Lucas reports that he needs help, as he has been unable to get organised and keep up with a course he has started. He says that he "may be losing his grip". Lucas works as an infectologist and started his PhD project a year ago. He says he has been making copies of his patients' prescriptions so that if any doubts arise about what he prescribed, he can show them as confirmation. He adds that he is unduly worried that he may have made a mistake reading an exam and communicating the diagnosis to the patient. He leaves work with a pile of prescription copies, and spends a long time mentally reviewing the cases he has dealt with during the day. Although he finds this activity excruciating, the verification process brings him relief. He keeps the copies in his car, to avoid having to explain this accumulation of papers to his wife. Regarding his PhD, he says he missed the deadline for submitting his first draft because he had trouble managing his lab work and writing the paper at the same time. He says he has wasted time on experiments, because he redoes them almost infinitely even with no concrete reason to justify the repetition. As for the text, he reads voraciously, but lacks the power of synthesis. This has earned him criticism from his academic advisor, who accuses him of wasting laboratory resources and missing an important deadline. Lucas was upset by his supervisor's verdict. He believes he is diligent and careful. He has the same meticulous relationship with his finances, which cause him great concern, as he wants to guarantee provision for his old age and any unforeseen circumstances.

Lucas had no problems during his development. He always did well at school and got on well with his classmates. He was considered a bright and conscientious child. He took a long time to get into university, taking the entrance exam four years running, insisting on his first choice and oblivious to external pressure to try other courses. During medical school, he maintained a high level of performance, distinguished by his organisational capacity and dedication. His colleagues coveted his abstracts, and he had a reputation for being very meticulous, with strict critical standards. During group work and internships, he was considered stubborn and annoying for wanting to impose his own productivity standards and ethical principles. He prefers not to request help at work, even when he gets in trouble or behind, because no one can do exactly what he asks. Sometimes, when gets annoyed with others' delay, he takes over their tasks. He is known to be extremely meticulous in his actions and verbose in the clinical reports on medical files.

Lucas reports that his marriage is also going through a rocky patch. Rosana, his wife, says she has been feeling abandoned. As she puts it, "When someone wants to be in a relationship, they find time and make themselves available, don't they, doctor? He never makes a plan for us to have holidays together. He shows up late for our dates. He never gives me a treat or brings me a surprise, saying presents are unnecessary expenses. He's stingy. He rarely joins me at dinner with friends. If he goes, he's awkward, frowning and insists we leave early. He never spontaneously says he likes me. It just seems that for him our relationship isn't a priority". On the other hand, Rosana points out that, as he is reasonable and thoughtful, the patient grants her stability and confidence.

Lucas used to jog as a hobby, but ended up quitting. He says he chose running because it only depended on him. He had an obsessive commitment, waking up every day at 4.30 am to train. If he had to miss it one day, he would double the distance the next day. He loved the feeling of mastering the mechanics of his own body. He would get frustrated if he fell short of his idealised performance. He had an obsessive desire to break his personal record every time he ran a marathon. A stress fracture in his tibia forced him to give up this exhausting routine.

The patient tried using cannabis as an alternative way of alleviating his distress and nervousness when he was overcome by his worries and the need to stay on track in his daily tasks. He described the experience: "It was very bad...it did relax me, but then I completely lost control ... I got totally stoned ... and then I was distraught". He also says that he uses cocaine sporadically, because it makes him feel more clear-sighted and focused to deal with all the details of his work. However, he stresses that he is terrified of losing "balance" and becoming dependent on it.

The anthropological basis for obsessions is perfection. One of the underlying themes of human existence is the implicit idea of an arrangement of reality, which needs nothing added and nothing removed. The idea of perfection is designed to represent a state of supreme equilibrium in the components of reality, where all their dimensions are organised in such a way as to appear simultaneously and definitively. The idea of symmetry is inherent to perfection. Symmetry implies a kind of democratic principle, by means of which each component of a complex form receives the same prominence as the others. In symmetry, all the parts are equally represented in the composition of the whole. This equivalence is also what gives the arrangement its definitive nature: if all the parts have an equivalent value in the whole, there is no pressure for them to move. Immobility is therefore also contained in the idea of perfection.

The idea of order is also often part of an implicit notion of perfection. The perfect form is one in which each component organises its relations with the others based on a rationally justified principle. Thus, a row of children would be perfect if all the participants followed an order of increasing height, for example. The crystal clear logic behind the organisation of the row propitiates the sense of relief that perfection can bring. Symmetry and order are part of the spirit of perfection.[12]

Perfection, however, is a costly human dream, because the dialectic dynamics of reality act to prevent achieving perfection or, maintaining it, once achieved. Ultimately, every notion of perfection is an unattainable ideal (Mallinger 2009). It is more a yearning to embrace the complexities of reality than a possible end in itself. The impossibility of finding the ideal experience of perfection in daily existential reality is precisely what leads to obsessive experiences, as we will see now.

3.6.1 The Present Perfect of Obsessive Existence

In theory, the concept of perfection in temporality is a contradiction in terms. It is impossible, because to be perfect means having found a definitive form, which by definition would have to be unaffected by time. The temporality of the obsessive person is therefore extremely distressing. The obsessive historical self does not experience protention as a gateway to possibilities, nor as a melodic theme by which existence runs its course. The dimension of protention represents imperfection, a rupture in the sequence of perfections that should organise life. For this reason, the very course of existence is experienced as consisting of undesirable and tormenting deviations from the order essential for them to be at ease in the world. The trinary nature of temporality torments the obsessive historical self because of its implicit imperfection. The obsessive person's temporality focuses on the form of the present, since the present is the temporal dimension in which all reality can be examined in toto, as the obsessive historical self prefers. The future is virtual and so cannot be examined, only predicted; the past has already elapsed and so its entirety is not available to the scrutinising consciousness of the obsessive person. The present, on

---

[12] It is important for the progress of this book to distinguish the concept of perfection from that of plenitude (Sect. 7.2). In plenitude, there is a suppression of the dialectics of the constituent parts of experience, an option for the supremacy of the whole over the parts. The goal of plenitude is the absolute. On the other hand, in order to experience perfection, it is fundamental for the parts that compose a whole to appear simultaneously in this structural arrangement. Perfection is an arrangement in which all the parts appear and so the notion of dialectics is not only maintained, but is accentuated. The conflict of the obsessive person is precisely the difficulty of maintaining a perfection that is constantly vanishing. Whereas the notion of perfection is an aspect of complexity, plenitude, is one of simplification, as I will explain further on.

the other hand, allows all details of reality to be placed side by side and articulated in a coherent and unifying order. It is the dimension closest to the perfection to which the obsessive historical self pre-reflexively aspires. By enclosing itself in a present that does not flow smoothly towards protention, the obsessive temporal experience mutates into a *present perfect*. The obsessive historical self devotes itself to the details of this hypertrophic present in order to dwell in perfection, the only zone of existence in which it can actually exist. The present perfect never runs out, nor does it spill out to retention or protention because it always contains a new element which deserves the attention of the obsessive historical self in its quest for order. That is why one severely obsessive patient, for example, begins to relate some fact of her life, but immediately interrupts the account to restart the sentence from the beginning because of some grammatical error. For the same reason, another patient, when reading a book, goes back to the beginning of each line after she finishes it to make sure she has read and understood it correctly. Both examples show a kind of experience for which the flow of the present toward protention is not important. On the contrary, the present revolves around itself to achieve a perfection which is closed, circular, and directed towards filling itself with all possible meanings there may be in a given period of time (Rovaletti 2005). Normally, for existence to flow naturally in its temporality, we have to discard part of the multiple meanings contained in each experience. For example, we know tacitly that we do not need a detailed understanding of all the ideas contained in a text explaining how to get somewhere to grasp its overall meaning. How to get there is the focus of our reading of the text. The future result is worth more than the means to achieve it. In the temporality of the obsessive person, on the other hand, as the present closes in on itself, the self-pole's gaze takes in all the complexities contained in that perfect temporal instant, removing the examination of these details from its practical dimension and its articulation with other dimensions of temporality. In obsessive disproportion, the examination of the details contained in the present is worthwhile in its own right and leads to nothing.

Similarly, retention receives no special attention in obsessive experience. Unlike melancholic people, with whom they may often be confused, obsessive people do not retain a remote past of values and habits to underpin their lives existentially. Rather, their retention is curtailed, immediate, contrived as an appendix to the immediate present. It is a retention which belongs directly to the perfect temporality of the present. Thus, the perfect temporal experience gives preference to short memories of purely operational value, to the detriment of retention of existential value. A classic example of this is the obsessive checking seen in some patients. A patient cannot leave home because they have to repeatedly check they locked all the doors and windows. This inspection is grounded in a hypertrophy of the circular present of perfection; retention serves here only as short-term memory, just enough to remind them that they have not yet achieved the desired perfection. In obsessive checking, retention does nothing to inform existence about the reasons for leaving home, for which locking doors and windows is needed. In more severe cases, the patient's experience may even be of a disconnect between the present and retention. This is how a patient tormented by an obsession for cleaning complains about her suffering (relating her need to wash the glasses countless times after a meal): "It's as if I forgot everything, forgot I just washed up and had to wash up all over again".

3.6.2 Order and Chaos – The Rigid Dialectics of Obsessive Spatiality

Perfection is, above all, a bestowal of spatiality. Spatiality is the ultimate expression of the complexity of how reality is organised. This is because spatiality permits simultaneity. Simultaneity is the state of the world in which all objects emerge at the same time and can therefore be examined in detail. This is why the ultimate expression of obsessive experiences is to be found in perfect forms of organisation of spatiality, symmetry and order. The immobility inherent to the experience of perfection is what makes them the favourite spatial form of obsessive persons. Patients who suffer from obsessive experiences fuss about everything that is not symmetrical; their attention is riveted on objects that are not aligned with perfection, intent on correcting them, aiming at perfect order. For example, they must keep their shoes in the same order, their shower must follow the same ritual, and they must shave exactly the same way. The force with which symmetry and order guide obsessive spatiality is, dialectically, what determines the importance of its reverse. We might say, reflectively, that the opposite of symmetry and order also guides obsessive experiences. There is a double thread governing obsessive existence. This duality guides its behaviour dialectically both in the quest for symmetrical order and the urge to escape whatever cannot be organised through perfection. We must therefore investigate the spatiality of the dialectics of order and its reverse if we want to understand the suffering of obsessive people (Morin 1982).

The reverse of orderly symmetry is chaos, an indeterminate space which can only be defined as negative. Chaos is whatever cannot be bound to any order, whatever lies outside the outlines of the forms of objects in reality. Chaos is thus anti-form (or anti-eidos, as von Gebsattel (1966a) characterised the core of obsessive experiences in the classical period of phenomenological psychopathology). The obsessive person focused on perfection draws clear boundaries between what is perfect and what is not, dividing reality into two rigid and incommunicable expressions: perfection or chaos. To a certain extent, the absence of perfection represents death for them (as seen frequently in their fears of contamination and illness). This lack of intermediate elements between perfection and nothing afflicts obsessive existence in its everyday activities, because it leaves it suspended between the total consolation of perfection and the affective experience induced by the absence of form.

Strictly speaking, it cannot be said that chaos is affectively terrifying, as it is unfathomable. Nonetheless, it cannot be said that a lack of form has no impact affectively on such a form-oriented existence as that of the obsessive person. The way they experience formlessness, first and foremost, is as degeneration and decomposition (Straus 1938; Bürgy 2005; Dörr-Zegers 2018). The main feeling that an experience of a decomposing world provokes is repugnance and disgust. All that is imperfect repulses, terrifies and disgusts the obsessive person, both in the world's physical material sphere and in its abstract senses, such as morality. Examples of the former are obsessions with dirt or the risk of contamination by some disease; examples of more abstract feelings appear in the constant fear of committing some moral misdemeanour or in obsessive sinful thoughts, which so infest obsessive consciousness. The division of spatiality into perfection and chaos permits them to divide reality between a space of purity and a space of impurity. Another form of obsessive dialectics is the profanation of sacred space by the space of impurity. That is why obsessions may go beyond the realm of personal morality to enter the realm of religion. A religious patient suffering from a very serious obsessive condition complained painfully of an imagetic obsession in which she saw herself having oral sex with Jesus Christ!

In anthropological terms, the disgust and upset experienced by obsessive persons must be seen in a specific way. It is not exactly fear or anxiety in the face of a terrifying situation. Nor is it a deviation from the general values that shape their personal morality. In a way, the anthropological basis of obsession is more impersonal in nature. Obsessive experiences result from the human impossibility to inhabit a world of perfection and orderly simultaneity. It is therefore a general situation, specific to the human condition. What happens to certain people is that the dialectic tension between perfection and repulsive deformity attains levels that impede effective existential development.[13] With these observations in mind, we can say that substance use in obsessive persons serves to offer some relief from continual tension. Its function in obsessive disproportions is mainly to counteract the obsessive person's excessive need to inhabit a perfect, orderly world. To a certain extent, intoxication gives the historical self licence to experience some pleasure in the chaos and disarray of real life.

3.6.3   The Apollonian Formalism of Obsessive Intersubjectivity

Surrender to a life dominated by the dialectic of form-chaos is the hallmark of the intersubjectivity of obsessive experiences. In the eyes of the obsessive self-pole, the other-pole should always exhibit perfection. This perfection is expressed primarily through the ability – even the need – to apprehend the other in their entirety. Therein lies the main asset of the intersubjective style of obsessive disproportion, which engenders a respectful way of building personal relationships. The obsessive person is impelled to accept the other in all their complexity, due to their total and simultaneous appreciation of all dimensions of reality. The obsessive historical self

---

[13] It is important to indicate here that this analysis considers obsession in its strictest sense. As indicated above, there are obsessive experiences that refer mainly to personal morality, which are based pre-reflexively on personal retention. That is not what I am talking about here.

perceives the other as a complex, ambiguous unit full of paradoxes. Indeed, for the obsessive person, the other may appear as a fully-fledged individual in all their dimensions. Similarly, the obsessive person faces the other in all their complexity and proposes a relationship in which even the slightest of contradictions in the relationship should be respected and articulated. Nothing can be hidden in the obsessive person's intersubjective relationships. The net existential result of this kind of intersubjectivity and its emotional result are opposites, as we will see below.

Existentially, all facets of the intersubjective relationship deserve the obsessive historical self's attention. That is why, when obsessive persons express an opinion to their interlocutor, they often take care to take into consideration any of the interlocutor's different views, even before they express any opinion on the subject. Obsessive persons act as if they should contemplate all interpretative possibilities contained in each statement, sentence or attitude for the conversation to occur normally. It is common for obsessive persons to express their opinion before immediately retreating and offering another perspective on that same opinion, or reveal voluntary indecision, as if leaving room for potential future objections. This whole process leaves no room for the natural flow of a dialogue. The whole dynamic of statements and retractions makes any dialogue stilted, even in the most every day of circumstances. As there is inevitably a multiplicity of possible opinions on any given topic, even the most banal, this difference – even without it causing conflict – is enough to fill the obsessive person's life with hesitations, changing views, uncertainties and the quest for other opinions, all in a bid to grasp the totality contained virtually in every interpersonal act. Obsessive intersubjectivity therefore bears a burden of bitter contradiction. On the one hand, it allows all the complexity of human relationships to arise in each interpersonal contact: nothing escapes the intersubjective relationship of the obsessive person. But on the other, it prevents naturalness in any relationship. All intersubjective ease presupposes some partial exclusion of the other. When we say something about politics, for example, we implicitly recognise that the other who is listening to us may have a different opinion to ours. This does not mean we despise their opinion or their person, but that we are taking a first step towards a conversation that may lead to a productive exchange. This affirmative step in which there is a partial and temporary exclusion of the other is taken by the obsessive person as a sign of imperfection and should therefore be shunned. The obsessive historical self's actions to amend this flaw have effects on the emotional dimension of its intersubjectivity.

The baseline emotional state of obsessive consciousness is one of restlessness, which causes considerable discomfort in contact with their fellow men. This restlessness stems from the difficulty of attaining relational perfection, which is the only form of interaction acceptable to the obsessive person. However, this excessive care with others' feelings results in a degree of formality that has precisely the opposite effect from what is intended, erecting a barrier in their intersubjective relations and making them appear stiff, inauthentic and, above all, uptight. It is this that sometimes calls for the relaxing action of some psychoactive substance.

The main anthropological disproportion of obsessive intersubjectivity thus involves submitting the bonds between two people to the necessities of the dialectics of form-chaos. This governing of existence by the dictates of formal perfection causes something of a reduction in the value of both the self-pole and the other-pole. Both become a kind of impersonal instrument in the Apollonian search for the perfect form. It is precisely this taste for Apollonian impersonality that makes the obsessive experience the opposite of the compulsive person's experience. If the latter gets lost in a sub-personality attracted by the quasi-fusional material aspect of reality, the former subsumes their personality in a superior world in which rational forms can be worth more than the people who give rise to them. The positive value of obsessive existences stems, dialectically, from this voluntary submission to the formal dimension of reality, expressed as respect for others, politeness and openness to the contradictory and complexity inherent to every human exchange. The obsessive person's sense of justice and abnegation can elevate human relationships to an extraordinary level rarely achieved in other styles of anthropological disproportion. Unlike the melancholic person, for example, who may exercise a sense of justice in the name of their cultural tradition, which provides the boundaries for their ethical action (and the feelings associated with it), obsessive existences can rise above their own needs (and traditional feelings) in the name of a greater truth, based on an act of perfect reason. Obsessive experiences are the rational apology for complexity and ambiguity.

3.6.4   The Obsessive Person's Servile Motricity

The pursuit of the perfect anthropological form absorbs all the attention of an obsessive historical self. It is afflicted by all the contradictions and tensions implicit in the rationality that guides its conduct. Obsessive embodiment is equally a field in which the tensions inherent to the quest for perfection are played out and the most powerful instrument for obtaining some relief from them. The embodied expression of the quest for perfection can be seen in the need for bodily purity, the care the obsessive historical self takes to maintain a perfect state of physical and biological integrity, and its obsessions with disease and hygiene. One obsessive patient, for example, suffered immensely from the obsession that there was pubic hair wherever he went. As he himself had pubic hair, inhabiting his own body became intolerable to him because it could never reach the required level of purity. Apollonian purity can also be detected in obsessive people's intercorporeality. They maintain only a minimum of physical contact with others, since they also perceive the other's body as a source of contamination and virtual death.

But it is in the compulsive acts secondary to obsessions that we can see the main existential function of obsessive embodiment. It serves as a concrete instrument to reduce the tension contained in impurity and chaos. The obsessive person experiences their body as the main agent responsible for the production of perfection and reduction of the experience of chaos. For this reason, the obsessive historical self investigates every corner of reality to find out where it is wanting in terms of symmetry or purity. Every time it identifies a sign of disorder, it employs its embodiment to reduce it, either by cleaning a supposedly contaminated surface or by arranging objects symmetrically or by checking for the risk of some unnoticed inaccuracy.

The principal form of expression of this embodiment is motricity. This is simply because it is easier for the historical self to manage. For example, as long as I have no neurological or orthopaedic disease to impede my movement, my power over my right hand's motricity is greater than my ability to induce joyful or relaxing sensations in myself. It is true that simple acts of representation may be as manageable as motricity. For instance, we can easily imagine a dog by our own volition. However, this ability to produce a simple image has little impact on the emotional ability to reduce basic obsessive tension. On the other hand, if we are worried we may have left our house unlocked today, the easiest way to alleviate that concern is to go home and check it. The motricity that leads us to our home is thus more effective in relieving tension than simply conjuring up a mental image of our locked house. Motricity is embodiment's most obedient dimension and it is therefore this that is hypertrophied in the obsessive person's slavish embodiment.

Continuous surveillance and remediation of the immediate environment are the hallmarks of the obsessive person's movements. Their embodiment is subjugated to the Apollonian dimension of reality and is therefore instrumentalised in a somewhat impersonal way. Motor vigilance of immediate reality is the essential function of obsessive embodiment, making it constricted and disconnected from the main purposes of existence. Obsessive embodiment is slavish, meagre, a manifestation of the present perfect and the rigid spatiality of the existential condition in which it occurs.

3.6.5 Rationality and Hyperrationality in the Obsessive Identity

Understanding the penetration and duration of obsessive experiences in an individual existence is key to understanding how they affect the historical self. The historical self's identity may undergo different consequences depending on how it is influenced by the anthropological disproportions of its obsession. The temporality of the present perfect is propitious for the slow and gradual maturation of its personality, oriented by the principles of precision and balanced consideration of all reality's possibilities. One healthy outcome of this, as it were, programmed slowness is depth of personality. As every experience is minutely elaborated, both emotionally and rationally, it has deep existential roots, reflecting its complex incorporation into personal identity. This incorporation takes place after evaluating and comparing various facets of an experience in a psychologically tense appraisal of the ambiguities of reality. The way various perspectives of reality are valued is especially unique to each individual and so the way the whole of an obsessive experience is psychopathologically comprehended will be strongly marked by the personal perspective. The obsessive person experiences all reality's dimensions in a bid to achieve a unique personal synthesis.[14] For example, they may hesitate for a long time about how to act professionally as a teacher. Sometimes they will think that they should offer their students clearer explanations to help them understand; then they will immediately worry that by acting this way they will compromise the depth of their explanations and make the learning superficial and incomplete. Similarly, when preparing an exam, they will waver between setting simpler or more complex questions. They are afflicted by not knowing whether to be friendlier or more formal with their students. If they are friendlier, they may be better liked, but lose credibility; if they invest in credibility with a more serious identity role, this may affect how their role is perceived by their students, making them less receptive to the knowledge imparted. Obsessive teachers torment themselves with this dilemma, attenuating the maturation of their identity, toing and froing in repeated attempts to strike a perfect balance between the possibilities offered by their role until they finally find the best way to adjust this identity to their existential style. As the form, it finally takes stems from a long, painful personal process, it is well rooted in their personality, making for a solid and thus dense and reliable identity. Often, the obsessive person is proud of their career when they see it matured.

The pre-reflexive search for absolute truth therefore has the power to grant the obsessive identity originality, truthfulness and devotion to reality. As we have seen, Apollonian rationality is responsible for a process which results in preference being given to the complexity of reality. This protagonism of complexity, can, however, mutate into *hyperrationality*. Understanding this illuminates one aspect of substance misuse in obsessive person.

To understand hyperrationality, we must first emphasise the function of reason in the dialectic regime of obsessive experience. The rational manner in which the obsessive historical self struggles with reality can also be seen as an anthropological disproportion. Rationality is the obsessive historical self's preferred route for connecting with the world, to the detriment of feelings. With its broad effectiveness in imposing order on the complexity of reality, reason allows the obsessive historical self to articulate opposing tendencies. Reason examines and compares, collates and contrasts contradictory aspects, and finally tests them to draw a conclusion. Meanwhile, the way feelings are endowed for the historical self is more diffuse and does not allow them to be synthesised rationally or conclusively. Feelings reveal a world in its raw state to the historical self, where pre-reflexive decisions regarding objects are taken without the input and control of reason, making it impossible for perfection to be attained. The reality they endow us with is one-sided: we like or dislike a film even before we have the chance to wonder why. This gives the obsessive historical self an underlying sense of uneasiness, which they can only mitigate by appealing to reason. Reason enables obsessive experiences to be incorporated healthily because it can organise complexity. So, it is that in obsessive existences, reason is hypertrophied to the detriment of emotional experience. One of the main functions of substance misuse in obsessive persons is to enable an emotional and

---

[14] There is some resemblance to the schizoid person in this spirit of originality, as we will see.

imperfect experience of the world. Intoxication gives the obsessive historical self a sense of relief in the world that it cannot obtain through its own rationality. It offers, so to speak, a hierarchy of values that obsessive disproportion alone cannot offer. This feeling-enhancement of existence through intoxication may even help the obsessive historical self to make certain decisions that are causing them difficulty. For example, a patient with severe obsessive traits would take a dose of zolpidem before making any important decision. He felt that this had the effect of dispelling the doubts that afflicted him and enabled him to accomplish what he wanted. The diminishment of consciousness induced by zolpidem temporarily mitigated his hyperrationality and allowed him to tolerate and dwell in an imperfect world.

However, there are situations in which the obsessive experience is so great that the salutary organisational function of rationality is distorted. Here, the power of rationality spreads into areas where rationality is inappropriate. It is in this existential terrain that superstition paradoxically emerges. For example, although one obsessive person knows rationally that going round a chair three times will not reduce their chances of falling ill, they feel compelled to do so because if they do not, something imponderable may happen. Although another obsessive person is well versed in the logic that determines probabilities of aviation accidents, they cannot refrain from mentally counting the first 60 seconds after take-off because otherwise the plane may crash. At first glance, it appears completely contradictory that an obsessive person so guided by reason and so committed to the complexity of reality would employ superstitions to confront that same reality. Apparently, superstition is a renunciation of the primacy of reason. However, it is misleading to think that obsessive superstition stems from a loss of reason. On the contrary, it is rooted in a hypertrophic expansion of the attributes of rationality, particularly logic, leading to hyperrationality. Hyperrationality extends the logical canons of rationality to the major threats in the world. Although the historical self knows superstition makes no different, it cannot break away from the idea that every experience of reality must be addressed logically.

Superstition (and often the magical thinking seen in more severe cases of obsession) is reason taken to its ultimate consequences. Instead of leading an existence forged in gradual maturation and depth based on coexistence with the dilemmas of reality, the obsessive historical self throws itself into constructing a translucent existence in which everyone and everything are connected in logical, rationally comprehensible ways. The superstitious obsessive existence forges its maturation in the sedimentation of perfection and reason, resulting in an impersonal world oriented by cold and mysterious movements. Personal identity thus becomes, paradoxically, an identity whose biographical coherence is shaky, unstable, as if the historical self were the plaything of a hypercomplex world dominated by supernatural forces. The obsessive person's hyperreason degenerates into the detached, cosmetic superficiality of reason within a world whose complexity is warped into the supernatural. Meanwhile, existence exhausts itself in empty passing matters of minimal existential significance, becoming cold and little inclined to form intimate bonds with the people and values of its society. Intolerance of or irritability with others for the most trivial of reasons, like the way they look or how they park their car in the garage or silly mistakes they make can dominate the hyperrational person's existence, making them grumpy and morose.

3.6.6 Clinical Decision-Making in Obsessive Complexity

The complexity that dominates obsessive existence requires the clinician to deal with two basic situations: to help their patient in the clinical decisions involving the control of their anthropopathological condition, which is usually obsessive-compulsive, or, in less severe obsessive conditions, to help them make decisions of an existential nature. In the case of decisions related to anthropopathological obsessions and compulsions, the clinician does not face a dilemma. The patient's suffering calls for positive action to be taken to reduce the obsessions. Clinician and patient act in synergy envisaging the same goal, which is to mitigate the anguish of the patient's experiences. Indeed, in this case, it could even be said that they are matched in their quest for a new perfection, this time in clinical care. There are no real existential dilemmas involved, simply joint action against an unhealthy condition. Anthropologically speaking, the function of clinical care is to help get the patient's existence to flow again. Resumption of flow is brought about by enhancing the capacity for protention, which means increasing temporal existential asymmetry, which ultimately means producing imperfection. This elevation of temporalisation inevitably also brings a degree of spatial disorder. This makes the patient very uneasy, prompting experiences of spatial asymmetry, anxiety, dirt or risk of death, and calls for great patience on the clinician's part.

There is one particularly interesting facet of the anthropological significance of clinical care in cases of obsessive-compulsive disproportions. The patient's improvement is brought about by temporal amplification; however, this does not necessarily lead to a resumption of personal projects. Clinical cases are usually so severe that this level of re-protention is seldom achieved. In everyday cases, one feasible therapeutic goal in terms of anthropological proportions is to create an asymmetry or imbalance in the obsessive person's present perfect by electing one theme as more valuable than the others. In the present perfect, all objects of consciousness must be in simultaneous symmetry and order. In a normal state, human consciousness distinguishes one object from others. When we are hungry, food supersedes, say, the day's news. The treatment of the obsession endeavours to re-establish this prominence, producing a preference for at least one thing in the patient's present. This prominent object in the present then becomes the magnet to pull the patient's existence forward. In one case, for example, a very severe obsessive-compulsive patient could no longer leave home, despite using all the available therapeutic procedures. All he did was revolve around his obsessions of symmetry and impurity. However, he began to succeed in going out, albeit rarely, to see football matches when his favourite team was playing. Those games were the only times in the week when the intensity of his obsessions and compulsions decreased. Although, sadly, this did not improve the evolution of his case, it shows how producing a focus in the world by introducing some asymmetry that makes some objects or situations worth more than others can be a way of mitigating obsessions. The highly prevalent link between substance misuse and obsessive-compulsive disorder (Ferreira et al. 2020) suggests that this exogenous instrument of productive disarrangement of world order may have a greater existential significance than can be appreciated by the concept of comorbidity. Intoxication does not so much reduce anxiety as actually reconfigure the obsessive existence's positional sense, giving them a temporary perspective on the ways in which existence gains colour and meaning.

In situations where the obsessive historical self has to deal with primarily existential themes, complexity arises in the clinical relationship, making decision-making processes exhausting and slow. To decide means to exclude, to divide up the whole so one part of it can proceed, to abandon symmetry and order and instil some disorder, even if only in the short term. When we decide to move to another country, for example, we have to leave behind the one in which we live. This process begins with a detailed investigation of the advantages and disadvantages of each country and losses and gains implied in such a transition. The obsessive patient carries out this process very well. However, the second part of change depends on the capacity to abandon symmetry and rule out some option. Ultimately, every decision is an act of imperfection that can never be hedged completely. There is an element of chance in every biographical progression. As deciding means opting for doubt, an obsessive patient has great difficulty in doing so, often inadvertently inviting the clinician to decide for them. The clinician often faces a bitter dilemma: to take the lead in deciding for the patient – thereby potentially not doing what is in the patient's best interests – or stepping back, and thus matching the patient in terms of existential inefficacy and indecision. The ethics and emotional state governing each decision are the clinician's inescapable priorities when dealing with the obsessive person's existential themes. A deep knowledge of the patient's positional sense, that is, the way they experience the world, is ultimately the only compass to guide the clinician in any decisions they may propose to the patient.

Fourth Level

3.7 Schizoid Disproportion

Frank has sought psychological assistance on the suggestion of his wife, who said to him, "if you go on like this, you'll lose your son". Frank does not seem to understand very well what his wife means by these words, but he expresses a desire to try to improve the relationship. Another of his wife's requests is to keep an eye on his excessive use of cannabis.

Frank is a 50-year-old geologist. He works as a consultant for large contractors working in infrastructure development. He usually spends the whole week away from home, working on site, sometimes in other states. He returns home at weekends. He is the second of three children. He has been married to Marina for about

25 years and has a 22-year-old son, Robert. Frank has used cannabis regularly since he was a teenager. He cannot explain exactly what effect the substance has on him, nor if it helps him in particular situations. "I just use it without thinking about it, doctor", he says. This is all the information obtained in the first consultation, because the patient is taciturn and reports on his life out of chronological order.

According to his wife, Marina, Frank has always been quite independent and self-sufficient. She says he rarely shares either good news (such as getting a new family car) or bad (such as failing to win some promising contract), and she is often caught by surprise. Marina says Frank's return home makes everyone tense because nobody knows how to respond to his unpredictability. They cannot figure him out. She says: "I don't get it. When does he get angry? When is he in a good mood? When is he stoned on marijuana? When is he flirting with me?" When he is away on business, the atmosphere at home improves. Marina feels emotionally closer to Frank when he is traveling, as he calls to find out how they are. When he is at home, there is a lack of dialogue. He stays glued to the TV or the computer. He also refuses to go to the cinema with her and seemed uncaring and indifferent to her after she had an operation. Marina says Frank's indifference to her became more noticeable when Robert grew up and no longer needed to be the focus of her attention. Several times she has tried to speak to him about the indifference with which he treats her, but it is impossible to discuss their relationship, because it always turns into a monologue that goes nowhere. In her words: "he's immune to criticism and praise". All this led Marina to wonder whether he was having an affair, but she has no evidence of this. There is always a question mark in the air. Something else Marina cannot understand is how Frank manages to keep up with his club acquaintances or colleagues who share his passion for vintage cars, since he acts so differently at home. As she says, "he behaves like someone else...I don't recognize him...two different people". At the same time, she admires and envies his nonchalance, because Frank does not get upset by missed deadlines, lost contracts, criticisms or fines.

Until his son's 15th birthday, Robert's maternal grandfather was responsible for his upbringing, without any great objection from Frank. He accepted the interference passively. Until then, all he shared with his son were topics related to old cars and motorcycles. When his father-in-law died, Frank had to take on the role of father. Initially, difficulties between father and son were not so evident, because the mother managed to mediate their relationship. In a way, she acted as an interpreter. However, this role was untenable in the long term. Frank seems to have difficulty understanding that his son has cultivated interests other than cars and motorcycles and cannot analyse his own feelings of frustration, anger or disappointment. The expression of any kind of dissatisfaction always appears as a bad mood. Robert says he is tired of trying to talk or argue with his father, because he does not understand formal nuances and is inevitably stubborn, intransigent and self-centred. The son says that no matter what he does, Frank only sees him as a spendthrift or a wastrel.

Frank was an introverted, isolated and distracted child. During his childhood, he was even suspected of being on the autism spectrum. He did not interact much even with his brothers. Currently, he only maintains sporadic contact with his younger brother. He does not explain why he cut off his relationship with the other brother and not even his wife knows what happened. He is very fond and considerate of his mother, but even she seeks Marina if she needs to communicate something to Frank.

I shall now deal with an anthropological disproportion which has no consistent terminology to refer to it. I will use the term "schizoid" to refer to every phenomenon which would be officially classified as belonging to the group of schizoid personality disorders or light cases of schizophrenia spectrum disorders. However, this denomination is too narrow for the phenomenological tradition of psychopathology. In this tradition, the term schizoid has always been used to describe a way of relating to the world that is marked by sensitivity and introversion (Kretschmer 2007; Bleuler 1950, 2011; Minkowski 2000; Kapfhammer 2017). Phenomenological psychopathology has always identified the term with a psychic constitution (a temperament, in current terms) that is complex and underpins distinct, empirically observable experiences (Helman 1980)). Therefore, the definition describes a less severe and more comprehensive condition than a disorder. This existential style has been given different names throughout the development of the discipline, each aiming to encapsulate the most central aspects of this temperament. From schizoid, this temperament came to be called schizorational and finally rational (Minkowski 1999a). Although I recognise that the term "rational temperament" is less stigmatising than "schizoid", I use the latter, which is closer to a concept of mental disorder because it is capable of picking up the fragmentary nature which I consider to be a core element of these experiences. The notion is based on the root "schi", indicative of splitting. As we will see below, however, fragmentation is not the only distinctive element of this anthropological disproportion (as seen above, borderline disproportion is also marked by fragmentation). Ultimately, the term is so established that it does not justify the creation of any new concept to describe these existences.[15]

The anthropological phenomenon that underlies schizoid experiences is autonomy. All existence inevitably derives from the dialectics between one form of organisation of existence that emanates from itself and may be called autonomous, and another, derived from the demands of otherness and the world, which is called heteronomous. All existence is ultimately balanced in the dialectical interplay between autonomy and heteronomy.[16] From the perspective of its existential constitution, autonomy consists in a reflexive attitude of identity. Any notion of self-governance depends on the constitution of this self. As all that is self stems from dialectics with otherness, autonomy is actually just one of the forms of self-pole-other-pole dialectics (Stephensen and Henriksen 2017) – a form in which a historical self already constituted by the other is capable of reflexively governing itself. That is to say, under normal conditions. In the situation I now examine, there is an anthropological disproportion that allows a dangerous supremacy of autonomy in its relations with the collectivity. As it is in dialogue with the collectivity that the biography progresses, any weakening of dialogue detaches the schizoid historical

---

[15] Similarly, I would argue that the notion of rationality is too nonspecific to capture what I see as central to this form of anthropological disproportion.

[16] We have seen above, for example, how melancholic disproportion is born from a heteronomic imbalance.

self in an ethereal and sometimes sterile solitude. Schizoid disproportion reveals a world in which the self-pole is disproportionately turned in on itself. The rampant autonomy that results from this (which is therefore the opposite of genuine autonomy, born of a more friendly relationship between the self-pole and the other- and the world-pole) is the foundation of schizoid experience, which I examine below.

3.7.1 Schizoid Verticality

In one of the best-known classics from the science of psychopathology – in which the notion of anthropological disproportion was used for the first time in phenomenological psychopathology as a foundation of mental disorders – Binswanger immortalised the concept of verticality (Binswanger 1992a). According to this concept, existence takes place in two basic anthropological directions (Depraz et al. 2011; Chamond 2005), which are bound together by a dialectic dynamic. The horizontal direction describes the movement through which existence relates to the demands of the world, of others, of shared values, actions directed towards the collective, everyday demands – in short, all dialogue with the other experienced as an equal. The vertical direction, on the other hand, describes how existence rises up, raising the value of its self-pole above the space shared with its fellow beings. In verticality, the historical self observes from afar and from on high the scenario in which existence is played out, as if it were on a mountain top which, precisely for being removed from the heat of the contact and friction with peers, offers it a broader, more distanced, rational and strategic view of its own position in social coexistence. The verticality of schizoid existence means it is primarily concerned with personal matters to the detriment of collective ones, independent and disinterested imagination to the detriment of practical and consequential imagination, idiosyncratic feelings to the detriment of shared ones, abstract concepts to the detriment of more practical ones. Verticality is therefore a mode of the spatiality of distance. Sometimes, this verticality causes schizoid existences to devote great effort to confronting the world intellectually or spiritually, leading totally intellectual lives or lives moved by more abstract aspects of reality, such as reason or faith. One net result of this spatiality is sometimes reduced communicability, making schizoid existences virtually incomprehensible or even enigmatic to most people. It is this ascent towards a uniqueness in which there is little that can be shared and little emotional warmth that makes the basic existential climate of schizoid experience reminiscent of the detachment and isolation of a mountain: rarefied, cold and introspective. Substance use in schizoid persons must be understood from their relations with verticality. There are two central uses of intoxication by the schizoid historical self. If synergy is sought, the self-pole's experience of self-sufficiency is stimulated, causing the schizoid person to become ever more enclosed in their world of dreams and ideas, in which otherness hardly participates. This reinforcement of self-isolation explains, for example, the abuse of cannabis in schizotypic personalities or even in schizophrenia (Davis et al. 2013), as it represents the option to withdraw from the world. To understand these people, it is important to keep in mind that withdrawing from the world is sometimes their natural tendency, and is merely accentuated by substance use. There is no conflict with the world, only a primordial impression that surrendering to the world is no better than closing in on oneself. At the opposite pole to synergy, intoxication can also be used to bring the self-pole closer to the world. In cases like this, the historical self normally realises that vertical isolation actually jeopardises the very structure of its existence, and so voluntarily seeks some exogenous support to bring it closer to other people and objects. The use of stimulants and alcohol is how this horizontalisation of existence is normally brought about.

3.7.2 Peninsular Intersubjectivity of the Schizoid Existence – Aloofness and Independence

In schizoid disproportion, intersubjectivity is marked by scarcity. As the self-pole is vertically detached from the world, a distortion occurs in the naturalness and the extent to which the self-pole and the other-pole are synchronised and engaged in the co-constitution of the world. Unlike melancholic or hyperthymic existences, for example (which we may here call syntonic, as they are innately attuned with the world), the schizoid existence bases its intersubjectivity on fragments of shared experience. That is why we are able to pre-reflexively tune in to the schizoid person's ways of feeling and acting only up to a point, after which we can no longer appreciate how they feel. From this point on, we can only access them through an act of comprehension; i.e. the hermeneutic reconstruction of their experience. For example, one schizoid patient reported that he could not feel any joy even when very important positive events occurred in his life. He listed some of them: his wedding, the birth of his son, the signing of an important deal, a professional achievement. He knows rationally that he should be happy on these occasions and recognises their immensely positive and desirable features, but he cannot make his existence react emotionally to them. He says that all he feels is a great emptiness, which, he adds, he knows will fill with joy as the days go by, as if it took time for the feelings to germinate in his consciousness. Initially, then, what he feels cannot be shared with those around him. A schizoid person has an isolated experience of the things they know intellectually to be valuable to themselves and others. In this case, they can only partially share the emotional reaction. Only someone who knows their peculiar values and characteristics can rationally understand their typical style of existence. It is only through an act of interpersonal comprehension that we can get through to them in their values and feelings, not through our intersubjective spontaneity, or at least not at first.

In the intersubjectivity of the schizoid existence, the other-pole thus remains only partially bound to the self-pole, forming a peninsular style of intersubjectivity. By peninsular intersubjectivity, I mean that like a peninsula, where only a narrow strip of land forms a link to the mainland to which it belongs, the schizoid person's self-pole remains integrated with intersubjectively constituted reality (after all, it is not psychotic) through restricted shared experiences. It is important to emphasise that this narrowness does not necessarily imply superficiality. On the contrary, the intersubjective areas where sharing occurs tend to be profound, dense and stable.

As so much – or even most – of their way of experiencing the world cannot be shared pre-reflexively, they often give others the impression they are exotic, extravagant, indifferent, odd, bizarre, hostile, arrogant or intransigent. As this is a two-way street, it may also be said that schizoid persons themselves often have a distorted perception of others. This impaired or distorted capacity to apprehend others in their entirety, and therefore their intentions and positional sense, is what gives rise to their experience of paranoia, often in association with substance misuse (Verheul 2001). Paranoia originates from the impossibility of experiencing the intersubjective relevance of a relationship or social situation. It is not an experience that is entirely impossible to empathise with. If we imagine ourselves alone in a foreign country whose values and habits we barely know and whose language we do not speak, we can appreciate the schizoid experience of paranoia. Paranoia is not exactly the result of a hostile world, but stems from a person's incapacity to recognise and protect themselves against some hostility. That is why it is so important to distinguish transient schizoid paranoid experiences from borderline ones. In the latter, the self-reference stems from the fact that the self-pole depends ontologically on an excessively powerful otherness. The other's excessive power is at the root of their paranoid unease. For the schizoid person, the cause is the fact that the other is not revealed entirely as another, but is experienced as a spectre lurking in the self-pole's intimacy. Although semiologically the two experiences may resemble each other, anthropologically they are brought about by disproportions of quite different natures. This is why it makes sense for an experience of substance use that propitiates detachment from the world, such as cannabis-induced intoxication, to lead to the emergence of paranoid experiences. The excessive distance from the other-pole renders it indecipherable and mysterious, and therefore a bearer of imminent risk to the self-pole.

In the most disproportionate situations, the other-pole is so far distanced from the self-pole that it cannot be understood pre-reflexively as a whole person. The fragmentation of schizoid experiences also fragments the constitution of the other's personal unity.[17] These are the anthropological mechanics behind much severely anti-social behaviour, based on impassiveness and an inability to empathise. Existential peninsularity in fact imposes limits on feelings of a purely intersubjective nature, such as empathy for the pain of others. A severely schizoid person's interpersonal conduct may be driven by an outlandish, idiosyncratic idea, with their being quite unable to appreciate its consequences on others. A case of a serial killer from many years back clearly shows how this anthropological disproportion can

---

[17] Note how different this fragmentation is from that of borderline experiences. In them, the self-pole is fragmented due to its weakness in the face of a hypersufficient otherness. Here, we have a relatively hypersufficient self-pole, for whom the other-pole appears smaller (although the self-pole also fragments, as we will see below).

give rise to criminal behaviour. The serial killer would kill young boys in the name of saving them for eternity. In anthropological terms, an idea of salvation emerged in the vertical, peninsular consciousness of the criminal in such a disproportionate manner and so misaligned with horizontal intersubjectivity that it failed to include the other as the person to be saved. The result was cold, inhuman, unilateral salvation. The idea of the other's salvation completely occluded the other as a person, and emerged as disconnected from the reality in which humans live and share their existences.

However, there is an ambiguous aspect to schizoid intersubjective peninsularity. The fact that the self-pole is relatively distant and isolated from the world-pole may be propitious for two of humanity's most sublime experiences: independence and commitment to the truth. A schizoid existence that manages, in its proportional orientation towards intersubjectivity and the horizontality of the world, to constitute a rich intersubjectivity is able to protect itself from excessive mundane pressures and develop as a free subject guided by its own convictions. This is the bright side of schizoid conviction. It gradually germinates – since it dispenses with the rhythms of the world – and slowly and profoundly permeates through existence (in a similar way to mild cases of obsessive existence), enabling the schizoid historical self to identify clear, solid, and above all authentic values on which to build its life. The formation of this conviction is painful and uncertain, but if it is fruitful, it permits the most independent and authentic of all possible human existences.

Schizoid existences harbour both great risk and great existential opportunity. As the self-pole is detached in its vertical peninsula, it manages something the world cannot decipher until it is ready. The product of this solitary and oblique process may be extreme. It may result in an existence guided entirely by solid, unshakable abstract values, since it is conceived in the most authentic and dogged search for existential truth; or it may lead to nothing, to barren emptiness in an uninhabited intersubjective peninsula. In this case, abstract values are often quite beyond the schizoid existence, which turns to substance misuse as its last resort to obtain some value for its existence. The ambiguous existential dilemma of the schizoid person is between either enlightened ascension to the most civilized heights of human existence or crude descent to the most barbaric of depths, in which base instincts guide an existence incapable of identifying any value sense for itself.

3.7.3 The Threatened and Unpredictable Temporality of the Schizoid Person

The temporality of schizoid persons is consistent with the type of disproportion seen in this form of existence. Here, the dialectics are between the time of the self-pole and the time of the world-pole. Here, too, schizoid existence struggles to find a balance that permits it to achieve the autonomy that is its vocation. The time of the world-pole is an assurance of existential harmony with one's peers, achieved by interlocking safely and smoothly with its whirring cogs. However, the peninsular interior of the schizoid self-pole is able to lock into this clockwork only to a certain extent. Above all, it obeys its own temporality, oscillating between independence and personal creativity. And even when the ripples of world time lap over the temporality of schizoid disproportion, they may be unwelcome, seen as an undesirable intrusion into an autonomous temporal process of diminished empathic comprehensibility. Intoxication acts in synergy with this rejection of the world, because it enables a state of complete consciousness, in which it is possible to live without leaving the confines of the self-pole's citadel.

It is no accident that in this conflict between two temporalities, schizoid existences have trouble adjusting to the cycles dominated by the time of the world and its circadian rhythms. Clinical experience shows that personalities with schizoid characteristics (or on the autistic spectrum) often switch day and night, as if they were unable to keep in step with the metronome of their peers (Ruiter et al. 2012).

Part of the schizoid person's temporal suffering stems from their need to build a future based on criteria spawned by the historical self with limited input from others or the world. A young and quite productive schizoid patient who suffers from various psychiatric symptoms puts it in the following terms: "I don't know what the future's like; I don't know what I have to build. So I demand too much from myself, do everything, fill any gap". Attempting to build a future based on socially established criteria offers no relief for the schizoid existence; they do not feel the future is a topic that can be shared. Their future only concerns them, and even if they do not know how to fill it – which is typical of the slow personality maturation of schizoid person – they agonise over the void that is quite simply the risk of the complete annulment of their existence.

In response, they do something, anything, to fill it, to counteract the intolerable emergence of nothingness that is always lurking in their existence. The restlessness that is so common in the face of this existential void is quite simply caused by the act of filling present time while waiting to construct a meaningful future. The price schizoid existence pays for subordinating the world's temporality to its own-pole's is the risk of finding itself cut off from any and all temporality. Schizoid temporality is a temporality harassed, a temporality under the constant threat of extinction. Fear of temporal discontinuity and interruption is often seen in the accounts of patients characterised by schizoid disproportions, demanding the immediate relief of intoxication. One of the main functions of intoxication by the schizoid historical self is to manage temporality, counteracting the imminent threat of its fragmentation.

However, the self-pole's independence from the world lends schizoid temporality another characteristic, specifically in its longitudinal dimension. This phenomenon is characterised by an original arrangement of the progress of time in each existence, making it impossible to predict its biographical evolution. If, in hyperthymic disproportion, the line of biographical evolution is overly linear, here, the opposite occurs. It is impossible to describe or predict the schizoid person's longitudinal temporality in terms of any equation. Its design is atypical, irregular, extra-Euclidean. Let us look at this statement from a patient with pronounced schizoid traits: "My life hasn't been a continuum, neither up nor down; it's been different steps with different paths, different contexts. I look at people around me and realise

I don't share their references, their clubs, their problems". She feels as if there could be nothing more idiosyncratic than her biography. The way she sees it, hers is definitely not the same as everyone else's. This is not only in terms of having followed very different paths from her peers in the same society (as she did, mainly because of her schizoid disorder), but in a more radical sense. Not only does she not share the social references of her counterparts, but she also does not share the notion of the course of time. She has no sense of continuity; her paradoxical advances are "neither up nor down", they do not even answer to the same rules of the anthropological directions that govern others. Her trajectory is unique, peculiar, irreproducible, typical only of herself.

This unpredictability is precisely what spawns existential hopes and concerns in those who help direct schizoid existences. When you get to know the patient well, it becomes easier to understand and protect their original, idiosyncratic ways of being and to recognise and admire all their intrinsic creativity and uniqueness. Despite their peninsular intersubjectivity, these people can develop deep and original relationships. However, the restriction of their intersubjectivity frequently causes schizoid persons to exclude the people who help them from their life, without them even knowing the reasons. The occasional inconstancy and incomprehensibility of schizoid temporality is the source of a great many difficulties in forming intimate and lasting bonds. Loneliness is a spectre that inevitably haunts schizoid existences.

3.7.4 Hyperipseity and Multifaceted Identity: The Agony of Schizoid Existence

We have seen how schizoid existence seeks to find some balance for an excruciating dialectic: on one side, a self-pole that is hypervalued in its isolation, far from the world-pole and majestically perched in an ivory tower of existential verticality; on the other, a world that does not cease to exist and make demands on the schizoid historical self. The schizoid person knows that if they move too far from the world, life loses its colour and materiality, making the field of emotions an empty and harsh abyss peopled by an imagination that can lose its connection with the figures of the collectivity. The schizoid historical self knows it must let itself approach the world. In the words of one patient: "I need to feel things more; I know feeling is important, but I can't". However, the vertical and glacial schizoid self-pole often finds the world-pole's proximity painful. Schizoid identity moulds itself on an invincible ambiguity. Being distant, the self-pole is cold, rational and isolated. It therefore becomes over-sensitive to any friction with everyday intersubjective dealings, as if the self-pole had a fine-tuned radar to detect any approach to the borders of its isolated land. The horizontality of the world hurts the schizoid self-pole. This happens even if the other's approach is perfectly benign: it is the very emergence of some intersubjective topic, whatever it may be, that causes discomfort simply by heralding the approach of otherness. This sensitivity of schizoid existences can also be called hyperreflexivity (Sass 2014b). Often, such awkward aloofness is understood as shyness, although in reality, shyness is an anthropological phenomenon based on the world's magnitude and the excessive importance of others. It is therefore a phenomenon of phobic disproportion, as we saw in Sect. 3.2. Although sometimes it is difficult to distinguish the two feelings clinically, the anthropological basis of the schizoid malaise is a sensation of the invasion of privacy, making it a phenomenon derived from difficulties related to isolation from the world, whose basic anthropological disproportion is the reduced importance of the interpersonal world.

The feelings that stem from this ambiguity of the schizoid identity already appear in classical works since Kretschmer described binary hyperesthesia-anaesthesia as indicative of this temperament (2007). The schizoid historical self is at the same time sensitive to its fellow men to the point of not being able to live with them, and impervious to them as if it did not share their world (Bowlby 1940; Parnas et al. 2005).

This dialectical regime of extreme ambiguity combines with an anthropological disproportion in the identity sphere. Schizoid experiences display great imbalance of the identity-ipseity relationship, favouring the latter. I call this phenomenon *schizoid hyperipseity.* Every schizoid experience arises from a very high degree of identity indeterminacy. It could be said that the whole of schizoid existence always lies far beyond the boundaries of each social identity (again, at the opposite pole of melancholic and hyperthymic disproportions). This indeterminacy is what spawns the idiosyncrasy of the schizoid person's experiences. Given that the unsaturated dimension of each experience is greater than its saturated dimension, identity can have a very varied range of possibilities from numbness to hypersensitivity. The social roles formed by this hyperipseity oscillate between the particular forms enriched by each individual's talent or personal flair (an exotic artist, for example) and the rough, crude, coarse, irritable and cantankerous forms forged in solitude in intersubjective peninsularity (a hermit, for example). The risk contained in the exuberance of existential creativity is its absence. Every schizoid experience is thus, anthropologically speaking, extremely uncertain and broad in its potential. That is why the way in which schizoid persons act out their social roles is often so personal and original – for both good and evil. It is because of the ease with which their identity takes on new forms that the schizoid person falls prey to substance misuse. Consciousness modification becomes attractive to the schizoid historical self because of how great an impact self-management can have on such an existence. Their excessive plasticity means each act of intoxication can be more than just a trivial shift of anthropological proportions to reach the point of actually re-creating the world. Addiction in schizoid persons represents the historical self's dissolution in the very world it created.

Clearly, this hyperipseity influences the historical self's integrity. This self, repository of all experiences, also becomes indeterminate and therefore unstable. At this point, I should explain this indeterminism better. It is not like the indeterminism we saw in borderline disproportion, in which the self-pole is weak in the face of a hyperpowerful otherness and therefore loses its integrity on the anthropological layer, generating dissociative symptoms. When it comes to its constitution, the schizoid historical self is integral and firm. However, because it emerges in an atmosphere of high ipseity, it is capable of taking different identity forms – as in the aforementioned sensitivity and numbness, or the coexistence of great maturity in some partial identities and great immaturity in others – and it may respond emotionally in different ways to each situation, sometimes giving the impression that the personality is split or even shattered. There are several clinical examples of schizoid persons that change their behaviour with such intensity or in such a short space of time that they seem to dissociate their personality, when in fact they draw on their elevated capacity to fragment it. This mechanism, unlike borderline, is more of an asset than a weakness. I call this characteristic multifaceted identity; it takes shape as a complex centre of experience that is endowed with pre-reflexive creativity, making it enigmatic to others. The schizoid person's historical self has to manage this multifaceted identity because it is co-constituted only minimally by intersubjectivity and it owes more to autonomy than any influence of otherness. In this respect, it also counteracts the fragmentary nature of the borderline historical self, which is strongly intersubjective.

The basic emotional relationship between the self-pole and the world-pole in schizoid disproportion is the dialectic of tension-relief, fuelled by an atmosphere of mutual incomprehension and pre-reflexive friction, giving rise to the overriding feeling of schizoid existence: agony. Agony stems from the tension of an existence that oscillates between finding its own authenticity, usually as personal values of truth or faith, and losing itself in a world in which it does not even find a positional sense for others and the world. The schizoid person balances on the central binary arc between genuine value and absence of value.

However, the schizoid person's frequent agony is also brought about by the mere presence of the minimum of intersubjectivity necessary for it to maintain some intersubjective reference. The presence of this barely comprehensible other-pole also induces agony, because the self-pole tries to harmonise with it in some way. For example, a schizoid person may suffer greatly at being unable to play the professional role requested by their boss. Their difficulty derives less from not understanding the content than from an inability to adapt to the company's rhythms, like meeting deadlines, and the associated social rituals, like justifying a delay. All these intersubjective processes, derived from the protocols of human relations, are largely beyond the pre-reflexive grasp of the schizoid person and therefore agonising. The term agony seems to me the most appropriate to describe this experience as its origin in ancient Greek brings up the idea of a conflict between contenders whose outcome is uncertain.[18] Reducing agony through substance use is an important element for understanding substance misuse in this anthropological disproportion.

The experiences of an existence too detached from the world and too close to the self-pole also reflect the potential for rupture contained in this dialectic. They are experiences of laceration, tearing, breaking, fracture; their themes are terrifying and overwhelming. For the schizoid person, the world brings a continuous threat of

---

[18] This yearning for definition also justifies another typical behaviour in schizoid people, mainly suffering from eating disorders: self-mutilation. Self-hurt is a way to put an end to the indetermination of agonising conflict.

rupture. As an intelligent, severely schizoid patient who had achieved considerable professional success described himself, "I can't get depressed, nor can I stay calm or be happy. My feelings are only agony and relief; I'm always afraid of a loss, of my job, my friends, my work. For me, life is about defending myself from losses that may happen at any moment. It seems that my inevitable destiny is loneliness. That's what stalks my life on all sides. I know it's not rational, because all my life's evidence proves the contrary, but that's how I am. It's as if everything will end from one moment to the next". Schizoid experiences share little of the sorrows and joys that plague their existential opposites, melancholic and hyperthymic existences. For these feelings to occur, the schizoid person needs preconditions that are lacking. The sorrows and joys of everyday depressions to which the patient refers arise from pressures the historical self suffers from a world pressing in on it from all sides. They are experiences of constriction and anguish rare in a world as distant and extensive as that inhabited by the schizoid person.

This specific difficulty of schizoid existence in finding an anthropological proportion that harmonises the dialectics between self and the world leads to multiple existential crises. What is at stake is existence's capacity to identify a value sense for its life. In existential crises, the schizoid person experiences an extreme fear of rupture, of loss of the experience of belonging to reality or of incapacity to maintain their life plans or even, in more serious cases, to possess a life project. Dread of shattering is the state that describes this existential state. It is this substantial weakening of life that gives rise to the high suicide risk observed in antisocial personalities.[19] At the same time that they are unable to experience the other as close to themselves, they also find it difficult to experience themselves as close, making existence pure detachment and nullification.

3.7.5   The Dysautonomy of Schizoid Embodiment

The incompatibility between the verticality in which the schizoid historical self dwells and the horizontality required by the world introduces a constant dialectic tension into the core of schizoid existence, with its quest for autonomy. However, as this autonomy is often excessive or detached from the articulated meaning of existence with its environmental context, it mutates into dysautonomy. This loss of articulation affects embodiment too, producing embodied dysautonomy. Schizoid corporal de-autonomy happens when autonomy is no longer directed by the centre of the historical self, and ultimately revolves around itself in short circuit. Embodiment is the sphere in which most schizoid dysautonomy is observed. Embodiment is the last refuge of the being: when it is at risk of annihilation, the body is the last instrument existence can turn to stay in touch with reality. It is

---

[19] I am of the view that antisocial behaviours are the most visible external manifestation of a variety of anthropological experiences produced in different contexts (Englebert 2019). However, I maintain that at their core, these behaviours generally have some schizoid root.

mobilised as an expression of the most agonising schizoid experiences, such as the aimless, directionless, painful psychomotor agitation that certain schizoid patients exhibit as a catastrophic reaction to some unknown stimulus. These severe cases include the automatic repetitive motor behaviours of autistic people. These movements evoke and raise to the umpteenth power the non-existence of any positional sense. They are essentially the automatic filling of an eroded existence, for which only the void remains. The melody of total void is the mannerisms, automatisms and hand-flapping of severely autistic patients. In the same way, tics can emerge in schizoid terrain. Tics are partial motor expressions devoid of global existential meaning and, as such, are experienced as disturbing by those who suffer from them.

There is also another way in which embodiment participates in schizoid agony. The distance between the self-pole and the other- and world-pole brings, as we have seen, a tense unease, reciprocal incomprehension and numbed hypersensitivity. The body is one of the most explicit vectors for this version of opposition between the self and the world, in which the very existence of the latter renders it hostile. The schizoid body is experienced as pure exposure, an object vulnerable to others' gaze. The schizoid person perceives these gazes, indefinite and disturbing by their very presence, as partially comprehensible, partially mysterious. The schizoid historical self knows that its body expresses its vertical eccentricity and thus exposes it painfully to the sight of others as if it were a gigantic tower in the middle of a plain. The gaze turned to the schizoid patient's body causes them so much discomfort that they will go to great lengths to rid themselves of their bodies, which they feel make them overly exposed to others and a consequent invasion of their autonomy. Anorexia nervosa is the clearest case of schizoid situations where the body is the central arena of anthropological distortions. In it, the centre of vertical incomprehensibility is the body itself. It becomes the absolute symbol of the disproportions suffered by the schizoid person. These patients normally aim to achieve a thinness that annihilates the body's forms – a goal that others cannot empathise with, since they cannot see the excess weight, which the patients experience as a symbol of material exposure. The schizoid historical self's rejection of nutrition functions as a rejection of their own embodiment, in the sense that it permits another to access its interior. Many anorexic patients highlight this aspect in their desire to disappear. In short, the disappearance of the body as a locus of meaning or the disappearance of the body as an object visible to others is the crux of schizoid embodiment (Binswanger 1957, case Ellen West).

3.7.6 Management of Schizoid Verticality and Clinical Decision-Making

Approaching schizoid patients for clinical decision-making first involves identifying their value sense. There are basically two possible conditions. In the first, there is a failure of the patient's value sense, in which case the clinician's decision-making apparatus is quite restricted, being limited to accepting the inability of the patient's existence to derive some sense from their life. The literature shows how the correction of negative symptoms is one of psychiatry's most arduous tasks, precisely because this emptying of meaning is based on the intersubjective peninsularity of schizoid experiences. Isolated "outside" the schizoid self-pole, the clinician has very little means to mobilise its existence. Or when they do, it is more likely to hurt the patient's sensitivity than offer anything substantial. In such cases, the best clinical approach is to opt for conservative decisions that preserve the uniqueness of the patient's temporality and to very gradually guide them towards some horizontalisation of their lives. In these cases, substance misuse is usually severe and intense, since intoxication functions to maintain the patient's existential unity.

However, the individual forms of schizoid experience are often very rich and complex, making the clinician's therapeutic decisions more complex, too. The clinician must initially recognise the values that guide these existences. The singularity of the personal values of schizoid existences can never be overemphasised. Their own anthropological disproportion means these patients need to be guided by their own values much more than the other forms of anthropological disproportion I have examined. In general, the other modes of life manage to incorporate values already given in their surroundings, which means clinical decision-making can easily be guided by gaining familiarity with the values that guide these existences.

This does not apply to the schizoid person, because for them, life either is their personal values or it is nothing. Identifying what value sense governs their life is therefore the first decision that should guide a clinician in relation to a person with these characteristics, (more important, for example, than trying to reduce their symptoms or the use of some psychoactive substance). Once they have identified these values, the clinician faces new tasks of increasing complexity. The first of these is to discuss with their patient whether these values, vertical in nature, should retain their verticality or should be tilted towards the world's horizontality. This is usually a very difficult moment in a schizoid person's treatment and can cause the therapeutic bond to break. The patient is not always sure the time has come, for example, to publish that book they have been working on meticulously for many years, or that series of songs they have dedicated the best years of their life to. Often, the products of schizoid imagination, born from quality criteria dictated by their autonomy, need many changes if the world is to recognise their value. Whenever a schizoid person feels it is time to show their work to the world, they are overcome by extreme agony. It is usually at this time that they seek mental health treatment because of the difficulties they face in developing their products for consumption by others. It is common for them to hesitate, to feel that they should not alter anything in their work at risk of misrepresenting it; or to feel that the world will never be able to identify the value of their creative individuality. In these situations, the clinician should, together with their patient, decide whether the course of existence should continue to be vertical or move towards the needs of the world (often the need for money makes this decision an issue for the schizoid person). The decision-making at this time must be slow and patient, because any haste will hurt the schizoid person's sensitivity, leading them to take decisions based not on autonomy, but on wounded pride. The schizoid person's entry into horizontality is always gradual and reiterative.

Every clinical decision in the treatment of schizoid patients is about management from a distance. Typical schizoid peninsularity keeps the clinician at a distance that they should not perceive as undesirable. If we remember that intersubjective proximity disturbs the schizoid person, we must be mindful that clinical care for such patients should be distant. That is why a clinician often participates deeply in the treatment of a patient without knowing exactly what role they play in their life. However, it is often exactly this distance that allows the schizoid person to rely on the clinician for their existential decisions and to have them as a bastion for their life. Ultimately, these are situations in which we cannot expect to establish a therapeutic relationship in which the patient will be accessible in all their intimate details.

From the perspective of technical management, breaking down temporality is worth considering when putting together a therapeutic strategy for a schizoid person, especially when some operational result is sought for daily life, such as helping them manage their work activities. Breaking time down means offering the patient a clear division of their activities throughout the day. In such a situation, the patient should do neither more nor less than agreed. This prevents them from experiencing the scourge of unlimited activity that often plagues them, feeling like they have to do a whole year's work in a single day. As the schizoid person is always hounded by a feeling of annihilation, they may easily feel like their work will be annihilated if they do not do it all in one go. Fortunately, these patients are generally aware of the problem and they accept the proposal of breaking it down.

3.8 Depression and Anxiety

All existence flows and therefore modifies its temporal anchorage points over the course of time. Sometimes, our existence rests on retention, being guided by everything we have accumulated in life so far; at other times, it is the living and sensory force of the present that keeps our life vibrant; and at others only the hope born of protention, expressed as an idea or desire, can provide the imaginary steps for our journey. This dialectic movement can be lost in many ways, as we have just seen. The commonest way to lose it is depression (Lim et al. 2018). Depression is a universal human experience, which participates in the dialectics of all the anthropological disproportions we have seen, as well as in the structural pathologies we will examine next. It is the great and diffuse anthropopathology, in which the biography's experiences of meaning are at stake. For the same reasons, it is also an anthropological condition often associated with substance misuse (Virtanen et al. 2019; Hunt et al. 2020).

From an existential point of view, depression is every anthropological condition characterised by *the attenuation of parts of the positional senses* of an existence. It is the subjective manifestation of an existence in which the value of a project, a taste, a habit, belonging to a collective or the meaning of an interpersonal relationship is reduced. In the general concept that I use here, it indicates a reduction of existence's commitment to a prevailing positional sense, without the capacity to experience positional senses being altered.[20] The word depression already indicates this meaning, because it indicates the pressure to separate or deviate in such a way as to take existence away from its usual course. When, for example, we take a diversion during a journey along a road, the road itself does not disappear; we know that it is us who have left it. Similarly, when we become depressed, we know that things, the world and others have value, yet we are no longer able, pre-reflexively, to bestow them with the value we previously attributed to them.[21] For example, we may experience depression because we no longer like our job; however, we know pre-reflexively that work must be based on giving existence some meaning, even if it is just the meaning of subsistence.

Because it is a generalised anthropological experience, depression actually forms a heterogeneous set of experiences. The anthropopathology of depression is part of the wealth of possibilities of all anthropological disproportion, without itself being a specific anthropological disproportion. Rather, it is the existential result of the intensity or duration of a disproportion. Therefore, it is important from a psychopathological point of view for the identification of a depression to coincide with the identification of the anthropological disproportion from which the attenuation of the positional sense characteristic of depression derives. Substance misuse in depression therefore takes on the same functions in terms of managing anthropological proportions as it takes on in each disproportion.

Depression can arise from the depletion of the self-pole's value ("my life is worthless"), for which intoxication serves as an antidote. It can also arise from the loss of value of otherness. In this case, intoxication means falsely recreating value for the other ("I drink to make others interesting"). The internal dynamics of each anthropological disproportion determine the existential origin of each depression. Every phobic amplitude can transform existence into a chasm that engulfs the historical self. Every borderline attraction can die out, its dramatic intensity giving way to bland tragedy. Every compulsive behaviour can impoverish the course of existence by repetition, imprisoning it within invisible walls. Every melancholic and hyperthymic standardisation can become intolerable; every schizoid autonomy can turn into empty solitude and every yearning for perfection can freeze the expansive heat of life.

The same goes for the concept of anxiety, also strongly correlated with substance misuse (Pasche 2012). Anxiety is a generic experience that signifies subjective

---

[20]Although in a somewhat distinct understanding of depression, this position is shared by Ratcliffe (2015).

[21]This definition is important in order not to confuse depression with the existential emptying of schizophrenic people. In it, even the capacity to make some positional sense is lost (at least in areas fractured by the disease). Depression must also be differentiated from the experience of grief. In this, there is not exactly a loss of positional sense, but the presence of an absence. As Ratcliffe points out, in grief, "the retention of an intense second-person connection" is maintained. (2015, p.199).

malaise. It is seen in all anthropopathologies, but especially in the ones in which the historical self feels diminished (phobic disproportion) or too close to the world (which becomes overly interesting and therefore an inexhaustible centre of attention, as in compulsive disproportion). Finally, it is also seen in the obsessive quest for perfection, in both the difficulty of attaining it and the ease with which it escapes.

3.9 Depression and Melancholia

I would like to conclude this section with a few words about the difference in meaning between the heterogeneous group of depressions and melancholia. Although these concepts have merged over the decades of evolution of semiological (i.e. non-phenomenological) psychopathology, nowadays, the difference between melancholia and depression is again being upheld, with the assertion that melancholia is an autonomous psychopathological unit (Carroll 2012; Taylor and Fink 2008). Conceived without distinction, the concepts of melancholia and depression may have no psychological validity (Ratcliffe 2015). The indiscriminate and indeterminate use of the two categories also has a major impact on phenomenological psychopathology. The extensive literature on phenomenological psychopathology does not clearly indicate the experience it studies, often mixing the two categories. Although, from a phenomenological perspective, the term that designates an experience matters little, the random use of categories can leave the misleading impression that depression has been widely studied. In fact, as Charbonneau (2010) correctly points out, the conclusions regarding depression in phenomenological psychopathology have almost all derived from melancholia. The author also tries to fill this gap by exploring new categories for depressions, such as paradepressions. Another weakness caused by the assimilation of one term by another which is even more important than the first in anthropopathological terms, is blindness to the different anthropological levels at which depressive or melancholic experiences take place. Ratcliffe (2015) attempts to overcome this insensitivity to levels by coining the term "existential depressions" and endeavouring to separate them from other depressive experiences through empirical study with self-reports of depression. However, he does not make any distinction between melancholia and depression. I advocate a clear distinction between the notion of melancholia, as a typical anthropological disproportion (or structural pathology, as we will see in Sect. 4.2), and the general experience of loss of value of segments of existence, to which we give the non-specific name of depression.

Chapter 4
Structural Pathologies

The second stratum in which psychopathological experiences take place is the structural level, where the conditions of possibility of existence are integrated and unified, making existence itself possible. It is at the structural level that the conditions of possibility actually become a structure, that is, their unitary form becomes more important than their constituent parts. Metaphorically, we could say that existence is a single organism composed of united and interdependent parts, which are its conditions of possibility. Existence is more than the sum of the conditions of possibility, just as a square is more than the sum of its sides. It is in this dimension of existence (see Sect. 2.6) that the self-pole, the other-pole and the world-pole are constituted. What I understand by *constitution* here is the process by which experiences become possible in existence, just as existence itself becomes possible. The structural integrity of existence must be intact for the self-pole, other-pole and world-pole to have the capacity to organise themselves in terms of anthropological proportions. The structure of existence has a transcendental constitution, which means that it depends on factors other than subjectivity itself.[1]

The pathologies at this level are brought about whenever the unity of the structure of existence is fractured and thus seriously modified. Since the possibility of a primordial attunement between self-pole and other-pole is the primary constituent of the structure of existence, I would argue that existence is primarily *co-constituted*, insofar as the first pre-reflexive process that makes reality viable is when it is shared intersubjectively. Consistently with this, structural disorders are based, first and foremost, on *a ruptured capacity for the intersubjective grounding of experiences*. This pre-reflexive intersubjectivity is behind what Blankenburg calls *natural evidence* (2012). Natural evidence is the obviousness of reality that we experience

---

[1] These factors external to consciousness and responsible for its delimitation and final form are not the object of this book, since they ultimately refer to philosophy. The transcendentality behind the constitution of the structure of existence should not be confused with the neurological mechanisms upon which consciousness depends. These are only its physiological basis. I would refer those interested in the subject to Fuchs' work (2018).

© Springer Nature Switzerland AG 2021
G. Messas, *The Existential Structure of Substance Misuse*,
https://doi.org/10.1007/978-3-030-62724-9_4

directly in our everyday life. It is constituted by the fact that the self and the other authorise one another.

However, this primordial fracture extends to other dimensions of existence. Any loss of the intersubjective constitution of existence and reality may be accompanied by modifications of other conditions of possibility of existence, lending the forms in which these pathologies appear in individual existences their specific hues. These modifications range from a paralysis of temporality, as occurs in monothematic schizophrenic delusions (I will return to this Sect. 4.1.4), to an inability to attune to the surrounding cosmic world, as can be seen when sleep and the other cycles of the organism are altered, as seen in severe melancholia.

The typical forms that structural fractures produce can be divided between schizophrenic and melancholic/manic pathologies. Both experiences result from a fracture in the co-constitution of the existential structure. The fundamental difference between the two lies in the way this fracture impinges on the constitution of the structure of existence and the way existence reacts, pre-reflexively, to this fracture. Both stem from a break in the original link that unites us, as persons, to the experiences of our patients. Our difficulty in understanding schizophrenic psychosis or manic–melancholic empathetically is essentially because we are alienated from co-participating in the world in which our patients live. In schizophrenia, this can be seen in the tedium commonly felt by psychopathologists when dealing with chronic schizophrenic patients (who are no longer agitated, but are in a state of relative clinical stability) or the impotence they experience when attempting to persuade a psychotic melancholic patient of the unreasonableness of their statements.

On the other hand, the modes in which structural pathologies emerge in an individual biography can vary greatly: a persecutory delusion can cause personal life to revolve around a single theme; a negative schizophrenic experience can lead to a complete emptying out of existence and detachment from one's fellow man, or even the production of an imagination that loses its focus on the world to become fabulation. A radical melancholic experience is demonstrative of the subjugation of existence to feelings of guilt or ruin. All these psychopathological phenomena are reducible, in essence, to a fracture in the primordial co-constitution of the structure of existence. Although certain psychotic acts may seem more adjusted to the world in the productivity of their execution (a patient with persecutory delusions who, for example, attacks someone in the street), we cannot allow ourselves to be misled by the surface appearance of the behaviour. A psychotic action that needs cognitive planning and is successfully enacted cannot be anything but pathological, because the consequence, that is, the temporal connection to the context in which it occurs, is lost.

An individual existence progresses longitudinally according to its personal style of organising and reorganising its anthropological proportions. This personal mode of structuring historicity is based on the intersubjective co-constitution of the world. In structural pathologies this co-constitution is fractured, hampering the establishment of a personal way of articulating anthropological proportions. The simultaneous modification of the other conditions of possibility hinders or prevents existence

from being constituted in its personal biographical form and, in situations of psychosis, impedes the dialectic movements that are the hallmark of a biography. In this
case, normal variations in anthropological proportions cease to exist. Therefore, it
can be said that structural pathologies occur on an infra-biographical level, and as
such cannot be understood in terms of a single existential temporality (Tamelini
2012). Faced with this infra-biographical invasion of structural pathologies, there
are two main ways in which substance misuse can be understood: firstly, as an
attempt by the historical self to manage the infra-biographical alterations invading
existence – both synergically and antagonistically; secondly, as indicative of specific needs arising from the very form of the structural alterations. (We will see
examples of these two senses below.) The fact that structural pathologies are not
biographical does not mean they cannot be motivated by important biographical
events, nor does it mean they do not take individual forms in each suffering person.
However, I advocate that all personal forms can be subsumed under one of the two
typical pathological forms we will see below. A schizophrenic pathology may, for
example, begin after a breakup, but this is no reason not to still regard it as a serious
pathology that takes a typical form, irrespective of the original trigger.

Although structural pathologies are not always easily distinguishable in the
uniqueness of a clinical case (or may possibly intermingle), they are sufficiently
distinguishable to be addressed as independent pathological units (Sass and Pienkos
2015; Stanghellini and Raballo 2015). I would argue that schizophrenia and
melancholia/mania are existentially distinct modes of structural fracture.[2]

4.1 Schizophrenia

The prototypical disorder involving a fracture in the co-constitution of existence is
schizophrenia. As a result of this fracture, a deep existential alteration occurs. The
experience of the world and otherness changes, making schizophrenic patients'
experiences qualitatively different from those of patients with anthropopathologies.
The fracture in the co-constitution of the structure of existence may occur at several
different points, determining a variety of schizophrenic experiences. Let us remember that in the original formulation of the concept, coined by Bleuler in 1911
(Bleuler 1950), it was referred to as the "group of schizophrenias", emphasising the
plural nature of the condition. This original intuition of plurality within unity is still
valid today, although hidden by the singularisation of the name.

In order to better understand the set of schizophrenic experiences, I must return
to what I said earlier about its infra-biographical nature. Schizophrenia occurs when

---

[2] The most typical clinical manifestation of this melancholia-mania polarity is bipolar affective
disorder. However, the phenomenological diagnosis is interested in the way this polarity comes
about existentially, so it should not be mistaken for the study of the semiological disorder. In order
to speak, in semiological terms, of bipolar affective disorder, the structural alterations described
here would have to occur for a certain time or be recurrent.

there is a fracture in the possibility of integration and unification of existence, which is a prerequisite for the possibility of a biography (Tamelini 2008). This means we cannot think of the totality of schizophrenic existence in terms of an evolving personal unity that alternates between moments of balance and imbalance of anthropological proportions. Everything that is biographical has to do with proportion, so the impairment of the ability to fully develop a biography is consistent with the impossibility of initially comprehending schizophrenia in terms of anthropological proportions. However, we can comprehend a schizophrenic existence secondarily in terms of proportions, since there are some zones of existence which continue to be constituted as normal (as we will see below (Sect. 4.1.7) along with the zones of discontinuity. The relationships between the normally constituted zones and the ones that are fractured may be comprehended as proportions of normality and alterations in a biography. At its core, schizophrenic pathology is shaped by how these zones of discontinuity determine the whole of existence.

4.1.1 The Primary Structural Fragmentation of Schizophrenia

As mentioned above, schizophrenia is, first and foremost, the loss of the intersubjective constitution of existence and consequently the protentive dimension of temporality (Fuchs 2007b). These losses, however, never occur in isolation; they also occur in other existential dimensions (Messas 2014b). Schizophrenia can therefore be understood as a rupture of intersubjectivity (Ballerini and Di Petta 2015) which results in the *structural fragmentation* of the other conditions of possibility. By structural fragmentation I mean the reciprocal relationships in which the sum of the fragments does not constitute an existential whole. Schizophrenic existence is therefore a structurally fragmented existence. This fragmentation is the primary spatial precondition for this pathology.

Structural fragmentation affects the ability to *apprehend the other*. When the constitution of the other is compromised, not only is the perception of their value as a person impaired, but they are actually not even perceived as a whole person. This distortion of the constitution of otherness explains the paranoid intersubjective experiences of schizophrenics. In them, the other is an agent of a world of which the patient cannot partake and so cannot even understand. In this incomprehensible world, the other is twisted into a strange, alien and often hostile presence. They are sensed spectrally by the historical self of such patients, who are only able to refer to these experiences tangentially. However, this is simply because language lacks the words to communicate these alien experiences effectively. Yet even when these experiences are put into words, they cannot be shared. Indeed, schizophrenic patients may even make up words (neologisms) or use words idiosyncratically to indicate the isolation they feel from any primordial attunement with others and the world.

The zones of existence affected by structural fragmentation are resistant to the unification of the identities of the historical self. This means that only splinters of existence are lived, and it is the local manifestations of these splinters that constitute the specific clinical condition. For example, a shattering of the boundaries of the self-pole brings about what Schneider refers to as first-order symptoms, with experiences of thought insertion and withdrawal (Schneider 2007). In these, the historical self's sense of self-control (its agency), which depends directly on its integrity, is diminished.

This identity-level shattering deprives individual existence of the minimum level of confidence it needs to dwell in the world according to the social roles of its culture, translating them either into paranoid experiences or the disastrous execution of social identities, as seen in the case of mannerism (Binswanger 1957, case Jurg Zund; Binswanger 1992a). In mannerism, the patient acts awkwardly, perhaps being overly formal in their personal interactions, using formal titles when the occasion calls for informal treatment or acting informally when this is inappropriate. These behaviours, which appear contrived to the interlocutor, actually result from the inability of the patient's identity to adjust to the social protocol dictating the execution of these roles. Mannerism is ultimately rooted in an inability to base ipseity on the intersubjective co-constitution of the world: the schizophrenic's social originality does not come from an enrichment of their social identity with a personal touch, but from a blockage of this ipseic creativity. That is why it is so rare for schizophrenic patients to take on professional or parental identities. In general, the pathology prevents the historical self from incorporating itself into the regular precepts and habits of a social identity. This limits schizophrenic existence to a position prior to the world of collectivity (Kimura 2005). The historical self is then driven to seek intoxication to overcome this limitation, either by falsely elevating the horizontality of its experiences (drinking to feel like others, for example), or by dispelling the psychological pain of feeling like an alien in the world. Above all, this second element is crucial for an anthropological understanding of substance misuse in schizophrenics – and of the high rate of suicide in this population.

The manifestation of structural fragmentation in embodiment prevents the unification of its global meaning for existence in which the body is an instrument of signification (Zutt 1963c; Merleau-Ponty 1945; Fuchs 2005) and attunement with the world. Embodiment seems disjointed from the mind, setting up a pathological existential dualism, as if mental experience were disembodied (Stanghellini 2004). The fragmentation of embodiment is also manifested in the agitated and purposeless psychomotor movement of some schizophrenics and in their so-called somatoform delusions (McGilchrist and Cutting 1995). In some extreme cases, schizophrenic patients will walk for hours on end, covering long distances without seeming to know where they are going. When asked, they will usually respond evasively, making their behaviour appear to be devoid of any existential coherence. This lack of coherence is also visible in the bodily insensitivity of many of these patients to their environmental conditions. Often, even in very low temperatures, they will wear light clothing, or conversely they will dress up warm in high temperatures, as if their body were not attuned to the surrounding environment (Chong and Castle 2004). The sensation of pain may also be diminished in these patients (Stubbs et al. 2015). Substance misuse appears to be a way of sensitising their bodily experiences.

This shattering also influences the way temporal protention is lost in schizophrenia. Schizophrenic alteration can be seen in a stiffening of the organic joint that connects the three dimensions of temporality. Instead of living each present experience as a continuous flow into protention, there are sudden transitions, in which each temporal dimension seems disconnected from the others. A musical equivalent of this phenomenon would be a melodic line that is suddenly broken by a succession of dissonant chords which, taken together, do not form a musical composition. This disarticulation of temporality means experiences associated with the succession of time are always uncomfortable in schizophrenic existence. The schizophrenic person's basic experience is that anything that flows may lead to a total rupture of time, annulment and annihilation. In schizophrenia, the experience of void common to schizoid disorders – already terrifying in itself – is taken to its ultimate level. For example, a schizophrenic patient at my clinic begins to worry at 9 am about their routine consultation at 1 pm, although they will not be worried about any specific thing. Likewise, during the consultation they may begin to worry again when they realise that time is running out, even though they do not have a specific or pressing topic to deal with. This phenomenon makes sense if we see that every transition from one state to another is hampered by an articulatory difficulty, based on what Fuchs calls neophobia (Fuchs 2007b). Schizophrenic neophobia is not born from an effective psychological fear of the future (as occurs, for example, in the normal anxieties of life and especially in phobic anthropopathologies), but from the mere fact that temporal transitions exist. Every temporal transition is terrifying to the schizophrenic patient because it contains the threat of a complete fracture of time, as seen in catatonia. This is a very serious condition, which makes even the simplest of activities in schizophrenic existence very difficult. One of the central functions of substance misuse in schizophrenic existences is precisely to contrive some temporal articulation between the different dimensions of temporality (Mueser et al. 1995; Addington and Duchak 1997).

Fragmentation can dominate the temporality of existence with different levels of intensity, producing different clinical conditions. These range from a complete shattering of temporality – catatonic forms alienated from time – to situations in which temporality is held immobile in only a few areas – mild paranoid schizophrenia – to hebephrenic forms, in which temporality is inoperative, directionless, filled with correspondingly superficial and tormentingly puerile affections. In the (more serious) catatonic and hebephrenic forms, the structural fragmentation seems to definitively prevent any organisation of the temporality of existence, thereby preventing the development of a biography. In such cases, it is impossible to pick up any traces of the patients' professional identities or even their less intimate personal relationships. Temporality is so fractured that these patients' existences rest tenuously on old personal relationships (e.g. their parents), when they do not depend entirely on the pathological relationships of their own psychotic experiences. The historical self is diminished, debilitated, sometimes to the point of having to rely on changes in its state of consciousness to manage life. A typical example of this extreme case is the severe schizophrenic patient who spends most of their day in the bedroom smoking tobacco or cannabis.

The example below shows just how restricted temporality can be to a disconnected present in the case of catatonic schizophrenia. It also shows how this altered temporality affects other dimensions of existence. Dialogue with this severely laconic patient was possible only rarely; normally, there would not even be the kind of scant exchange reported below:

- Have you been coming to São Paulo often? [She comes once a week to have electroconvulsive therapy]
- I just came from the hospital, down the street, all the way here.
  …
- How are things in X [her town]?
- I just left this morning.
- Have you been going to your Y [family business]?
- No.
- Why not?
- Because I was here.

The temporality of the conversation is limited to the immediately preceding moment. My attempt to extend it – my questions about how often the patient visited the city or the family business, which implied repeated action over time – was not even understood and was answered with reference to the immediate temporality: "I just came from the hospital" or "because I was here". The question about the general context of the patient's life – How are things in your town? – was answered with reference to the immediate temporal dimension: "I just left this morning". Existence is narrowed to time intervals very close to the present, making any notion as broad as an opinion on the context of one's life meaningless.

4.1.2 Schizophrenic Intersubjective Fragmentation – Diffusion in Anonymity

One important element for understanding fragmentation in schizophrenia has to do with how the breakdown of structural unity affects intersubjectivity (Kimura 2000). With the fracture, the self-pole ceases to be whole, which leads to a concomitant change in the unity of the other-pole. This alteration is marked by a diffusion of the self-pole in the space of the other-pole, which is made anonymous (Sect. 2.3.3). Any change that prevents the self-pole from being constituted similarly prevents the other-pole from being a space of singularities. In interpersonal relationships, the historical self is manifested in an anonymous collective space in which the self-pole's capacity to participate is curtailed. One patient expresses this experience in the following terms: "I think some thoughts to myself, but it feels as if they're what everyone thinks … like everyone thinks the same thing about the world. I have to keep putting myself right about that". The diffusion of subjective experiences in anonymity reveals an other that is no longer able to constitute the historical self as the rightful owner and agent of its own experiences. The singular person is assimilated in a disturbed collectivisation that annuls singularity, as meticulously analysed by Binswanger in the classic case Jurg Zund (1957).

Paradoxically, this diffusion in plurality makes it impossible for any authentic collective intersubjective participation to take place. As the same patient puts it: "I thought I would not manage to take part in society because of the excess of meanings conveyed in people's speech. As if people were connected with each other, as if they could pick up on each other's thoughts without realising it". The domination of the self-pole by an anonymous otherness that can do anything and means everything quashes all existential dialectics and transforms existence into an outsider in a world in which it is dispersed.

4.1.3 Negative Schizophrenia as a Primary Pathological Form

From a semiological point of view, it is in the less serious negative conditions – in those where there are little delusional experiences – and the historical self remains relatively intact in its narrative capacity – that schizophrenic fracture appears in its original form. It is in this form of the syndrome that we see the deprivation of intersubjective sharing of the world which produces the loss of natural evidence, as in Blankenburg's classic case of Anna (Blankenburg 2012). In such cases, the patient often reports their experiences in terms of an inability to feel the world as real, to feel anything for others or even to feel anything at all. The situations in which there is a total breakdown of the existential structure, including the constitution of the self-pole, are rare and represented by catatonic-like psychoses. In them, as in the case presented above, the detachment of existence from the world makes it impossible for them even to communicate their existential condition.

4.1.4 The Existential Sense of Schizophrenic Delusion – A Secondary Structural Reaction

However, there is a pre-reflexive reaction on the part of existence to the fracture of primordial intersubjectivity, which functions as structural sealing. The phenomenological manifestation of this scarring is delusion. Delusion is an infra-biographical attempt by the structure of existence to offer a fixed point to which existence can cling to avoid total debacle (Cutting and Musalek 2016; Blankenburg 2012; Tamelini and Messas 2016). Therefore, in order to understand delusion, it is more important for the psychopathologist to observe the a priori world of the conditions of possibility than the experiential world as reported by patients. The themes of delusion are actually of secondary importance, psychopathologically speaking, since they are simply the superficial matter used to fill the cracks of the far deeper alterations (Blankenburg 2007a). They can vary without there being any change to the basic pathology. Therefore, the clinician's attention should not be focused primarily on the delusion per se, but on its meaning for the maintenance of existence.[3]

The words of a patient of mine with a rich array of self-descriptions who went through a short paranoid outbreak serve to demonstrate the importance of delusion for existence: "I completely lost touch with my family, I lost my profession", she reports (although actually she was actually going through a professional transition, which meant she temporarily lost her social role and related identity); "I had nothing left but the voice of Christ guiding my way. In fact, I succumbed a bit too much to His orders", she concludes, now on the other side of the psychotic outburst and able to re-examine it. The essence of what she experienced is typical of pre-reflexive in response to the imminent collapse of existence. The temporality of schizophrenia, I maintain, is shaped by a fragmentation of the structural co-constitution of existence and a correlated loss of protention. Nonetheless, it may be easier to discern from its reactive pre-reflexive sealing at a single point, usually taking a paranoid form.

Paranoid sealing has a reparative function. Experiences of persecution are only the tip of a whole iceberg of reconstruction in the face of existential devastation, which has to be traced back to the conditioning and a priori foundations of existence (Binswanger 1965). It is precisely because schizophrenic existence has such difficulty constituting its reality and its own self pre-reflexively (Fuchs 2020) that delusion becomes an ontological necessity. Another sentence from the same patient shows the ontological value of the delusional experience: "I need an anchor, I keep hopping around looking for some root to live". Her words clearly illuminate the foundations of schizophrenic vulnerability, namely, an inability to take root in the world of one's fellow men and thus to be temporalised (Levinas 2014). It is important to point out that these leaps over reality, as reported by the patient, in no way resemble the classic flight of ideas in mania (Binswanger 2000), which I will discuss below. What essentially distinguishes them is the fact that the manic person leaps over a reality within which they are imprisoned, while the schizophrenic leaps in hope of some genuine support on which to establish their authenticity.

Delusion thus functions like sealing in the structure of existence, which, in order to preserve its unity, halts the possibility of any movement or exchange. Delusion seals any leaks in the dam of existence. In the places that are sealed, there is no interchange or movement, but nor is there extinction. This pre-reflexive impermeability and immobility of delusion in the structure of existence is manifested as the irreducibility and dominance of delusional ideas in patients' daily lives. Delusional ideas do not change because their existential function is precisely not to change (Tatossian 2002; Tamelini and Messas 2016). Accordingly, substance misuse in schizophrenic patients should be perceived as an effort of the self-pole to maintain its paralysed and thus minimally integrated existence.

---

[3] This lack of focus on the themes of delusions is not generally shared by patients' relatives, which means that as far as the therapeutic relationship is concerned, the clinician must make suppressing the delusion their primary objective.

The same can be said of the feelings linked to delusional experiences. These tend to be monotonous and repetitive, although they can be intense, because of the dread of persecution. The feelings related to delusion do not derive from the intentionality of relations between the self-pole and the world, but from their impossibility. Therefore, delusional ideas often sound outlandish to the observer and do not prompt strong emotional responses. The delusional person inhabits their paralysed, repetitive world quite alone.

4.1.5   Existential Ambiguity in Schizophrenia – Deep Confrontation with the World

The life of the schizophrenic person is also permeated by some existential ambiguity. It could be argued that the disorder produced by the structural alteration brings about some existential advantage. Even in a textbook pathological condition, the complexity of human existence does not fail to reveal its contradictions. Pointing out something beneficial in the midst of the devastation wrought by schizophrenia should not be interpreted in any way as championing the disease as a manifestation of health. All I mean is that every human existence, in every situation, contains the kernel of great riches which, once identified and exploited, can enable the development of personal aspirations within community life. Thus, the need of the schizophrenic historical self to strive to grasp both rationally and profoundly a reality whose unity always escapes it empowers it to face up to the ultimate themes of humanity. This power of reason means its existence, even when it is sick, is guided by deep, stable, sincere values and principles unswayed by the frivolous seductions of the world. In a way, it could be said that for the schizophrenic person, truth is what matters above all else. The state of these existences takes on a constructive face in which their authenticity, their honesty and even their relational innocence become a boon for their credibility in the world of human relations.

The disorder forces them into close contact with the problems of the constitution of the world, attracting them to the most extreme themes of existence. Even their delusional experiences reveal the need to reflect on the fundamentals of reality. Schizophrenic delusions differ from other delusions in that they do not address the facts of the world, but the ways in which the world can become world for the historical self. These delusions, called epistemological delusions by Sass (2017), reveal how schizophrenic existence is completely permeated by enquiries into mystery and complexity. This pre-reflexive condition attracts schizophrenic existence towards the mysteries of the world, fostering a specific mode of substance abuse, which I will present below (see Sects. 4.1.8 and 7.2.4).

Likewise, the mysteries of the intersubjective constitution of the world do not escape the attention of the schizophrenic person's historical self, expressed in degrees of intellectual refinement that cause unending amazement and admiration. Let us look, for example, at the reflections of a patient about the connection between the appearance of her psychoses and her relationships with her sister: "if I had a substratum of relationship with her I would be able to control the psychoses that appear". With no specialised intellectual training, the patient manages, in one short sentence, to sum up the entire phenomenological understanding of the co-constitution of reality that I am developing in this work!

4.1.6 Anthropological Proportions in Schizophrenia

Structural pathologies such as schizophrenia are defined in terms of fracturing (or not) of the integrity and unity of the constitution of existence. Differently, anthropopathologies are shaped by the anthropological disproportions at play in a particular existential style. However, the two principles cannot be seen as mutually exclusive when it comes to comprehending structural pathologies psychopatho-logically. Structural pathologies can only be completely understood in the light of a dialectic that encompasses the whole of existence. To investigate schizophrenia from a psychopathological perspective requires understanding how the primordial fracture acts on the dialectic between the parts and the whole of existence. Any bid to understand schizophrenic psychosis psychopathologically therefore calls for the investigation of its meanings for an individual existence (Wyrsch 1949) and the values it actualises (Stanghellini and Ballerini 2007).

It is essential for the categories of anthropological proportions to be incorporated into the psychopathologist's investigative arsenal to grant them the capacity to record more subtle dimensions of the psychopathology of schizophrenia. From a dialectical-proportional perspective, schizophrenic experiences are not defined by the constitution (or not) of reality, but by the relative proportion, in each individual existence, of zones in which this constitution is incomplete and zones where it is intact. In this sense, proportional dialectical thinking introduces right into the heart of schizophrenia a dialectical relationship that enriches the psychopathological gaze and enables a better understanding of diverse clinical cases. For instance, it allows an understanding of the classical phenomenon of double-bookkeeping described by Bleuler, which is so characteristic of many schizophrenics. These patients will often present a primary delusion simultaneously with an unaltered world experience in several sectors and subjects unrelated to the delusional manifestation. This intrigu-ing phenomenon from the world of schizophrenia may be comprehended in rela-tively simple terms from the perspective of dialectical proportions, since there is a relationship of proportion between the experience of the delusion and the totality of the patient's existence, as we will examine now.

4.1.7 The Simultaneous Spatiality of Two Worlds: Double Bookkeeping

The classic phenomenon of double bookkeeping reveals how the structural frag-mentation of schizophrenia does not affect the whole of existential spatiality, deter-mining two coexisting worlds. I will use a clinical case to illustrate this condition. For the purposes of comprehension, I have chosen a case of chronic paranoid schizophrenia that is very typical pathologically speaking. The core of the patient's paranoia is a feeling of continuous, intense harassment from a supposed mafia organisation that wants to kill him and offer his body as a kind of sacrifice. As tends to happen in typical schizophrenic delusions, no clear reason is given for why this organisation chose him or what the offering would be for. The schizophrenic frac-ture is widespread, having damaged all his family and other interpersonal relation-ships, making it impossible for him to live in society. The patient mistrusts everyone and often sees signs of the organisation's activity against him on street signs. The theme has become consolidated and paralysed his life in a siege state. Simply put, the deep schizophrenic fracture is intense, overarching, but not absolute, and is experienced mainly in the intersubjective and visual perception dimension. To gain a dialectic-proportional comprehension of the effect the pathology has on the total-ity of his existence, it is important to recognise the conditions of possibility that are least affected by the schizophrenic fracture. In this case, the historical self is pre-served. It is precisely this self that manages to stand up against the harassment stem-ming from the intersubjective rupture of the structure. Therefore, this isolated, tormented self becomes the existential dimension upon which most demands are made to enable his biographical becoming to continue. From an anthropological point of view, the whole of his existence must therefore rely more heavily on the historical core of the self-pole.

This disproportionate elevation of a historical self partially removed from its intersubjective connection with reality makes the loneliness and discomfort it expe-riences all the more intense. The historical self feels even more isolated in its responsibility to give meaning to the world. There is, so to speak, a compensatory hypertrophy of the historical self. This hypertrophy of the isolated historical self is propitious for anthropological experiences of paranoia, expressing the discomfort experienced by a person who is isolated and does not feel safe in the world of his peers. There is nothing structurally pathological about it; it is no different from the way a foreigner, stranded in a hostile land with unfamiliar rules of behaviour, would have to protect themselves.

In this situation, there are two dimensions of spatiality at play: the structural pathological experience, which annuls temporality, calcifying it into ubiquitous, immutable persecution by anonymous agents, and anthropological disproportion, in which the historical self organises itself in a cohesive formation against a similarly cohesive anonymous world centred around a theme of anthropological value, which in this case is the theme of persecution. Persecution is at the same time an imposi-tion of the pathologically deformed structure and an irrefutably human theme. This existential condition cannot be credited exclusively to the structural pathology, although it is responsible for much of the phenomenal manifestation. The patient himself expresses this duality in an account he gives of an upsetting experience a few days earlier. Commenting on his experience of being treated disrespectfully in a bank after spending a long time in the queue, he exclaims: "Hey, what I'm telling you isn't because of my schizophrenia. It really happened". This shows how the experience of feeling belittled – which led to some altercation with the teller – came from a historical self very sensitive to aggression in human relationships; relationships that often place schizophrenic sufferers at a social disadvantage and result in their being treated with contempt.

However, on other similar occasions, this same patient has experienced purely delusional intersubjective discomfort, which stems from the overwhelmingly fractured spatiality of schizophrenia. At this point in treatment, the patient's powerful historical self is already able to help the psychopathologist discriminate between these two structurally different situations. And thus it shows how phenomenological investigations must be pursued on two planes when it comes to structural pathologies.

4.1.8 Dialectical Loosening and Decision-Making for Horizontality or Verticality

The fractured co-constitution of reality in schizophrenia leads to a loosening of the dialectical tensions typical of existence. This loosening, which is manifested in a loss of directionality of existence, can also be seen in the field of affectivity and psychological motivation. Since the world and otherness are not pre-reflexively constituted for existence in terms of relevance and differential values, the self-pole is faced with a bland, featureless world in which everything tends towards a similar degree of attractiveness. This flattening of the world makes it less interesting and produces the classic semiology of schizophrenic indifference and flat affect. This schizophrenic semiology indicates an impairment in the capacity of existence to organise itself in anthropological proportions. However, it says nothing about a person's value preferences. The historical self must continue to inhabit a world and make existential decisions in it, which inevitably involves choosing between seeking to induce relevance or surrendering, sometimes passively, to the convenience of alienation in its own pole. One of the most important decisions that the historical self must take is how to direct its life – in relation both to its psychotic experiences and to whatever healthy existential realms remain. Understanding the dimension of schizophrenic people's existential decisions is fundamental for understanding substance misuse as self-management.

It is important for the psychopathologist to identify whether the patient facing a dialectical loosening chooses to engage with the world or, succumbing to the tides of his/her pathology, moves further away from it. I call the first tendency horizontality and the second, verticality. These options do not necessarily alter the progression of the pathology, but they do modulate the way in which it is incorporated into their existence. It is up to the clinician to observe whether the patient, by moving too far away from the world (in a verticalisation of existence), loses even more of their ability to relate to their peers and tends towards a dangerous state of absolute isolation (Such is the case of schizophrenic patients who misuse cannabis). Although this misuse exacerbates the clinical condition of the schizophrenic person, it appears to the historical self as an anthropologically understandable means of succumbing to the condition in which it is immersed and from which it feels unprepared to leave. The misuse of cannabis in schizophrenic people has a recreational purpose (Mueser et al. 1995; Addington and Duchak 1997), as it does for anyone. However, the concept of recreation is far expanded here, because it goes beyond just a pleasant withdrawal from reality to the production of a high in an existence that is lost in the heights of solitude.

In these cases, the clinician should show the patient and/or their caregivers the risks inherent to verticalisation and the associated hermitic lifestyle. On the other hand, the risk associated with enforced horizontalisation should not be overlooked. Since the patient will already find it hard to participate in the rules of the shared world, this movement may exacerbate their psychological discomfort and increase the likelihood of paranoid experiences. In short, clinical decisions regarding schizophrenia should always be two-pronged: they should first be designed to reduce the extent of the primordial psychotic fracture as much as possible, but at the same time they should also aim to help the patient make decisions about how to behave in a world that will continue to be featureless or hostile.

4.1.9 Value Sense, Positional Sense and Structural Pathology – An Example of Clinical Decision-Making in Schizophrenia

The incorporation of schizophrenic fracture into the totality of existence respects the two fields of meaning that guide and organise existence hierarchically: value senses and positional senses. When it comes to positional senses – a person's typical anthropological proportions – schizophrenic experience should be seen in the way it mobilises the patient's anthropological proportions. Put simply, the psychopathologist will be interested in how the structural pathology is incorporated into the patient's personality. As for the value sense, it is important to examine what rational value the patient attaches to their schizophrenic experiences. This dual understanding is very important for comprehending the role of substance use in schizophrenia. To illustrate how complex this interaction can be, I shall present a clinical situation.

A 35-year-old patient who enjoys relative professional success comes for treatment because she feels she is losing control over her thoughts. Soon afterwards, her family contact me and confirm what the patient has said, adding that for some time now she has been acting strangely, especially with regard to social isolation. Despite this social isolation, her family say, she is doing fairly well professionally, but less well than previously. This worsening performance seems to have appeared in parallel to her increased isolation. They note some unusual behaviours, although these are not completely uncharacteristic of her personal style. Her personal relationships have always been a little distant, but not to the point of preventing her from getting married and having two children. She describes herself and is described by her family as emotionally distant and sometimes overly imaginative. After a few weeks of treatment and psychopathological investigation, I notice clearly the presence of active schizophrenic delusions, systematised into a network of meanings that could lead her to be a victim of a parallel reality. The patient recounts all her experiences with serenity and clarity, not noticing anything odd about them. She is only bothered when she loses her self-control when dealing with these attacks of parallel reality. The invasion of a parallel reality through telepathic actions is the point that most bothers her. She agrees with the interpretation that this loss of self-control is psychotic.

In her account, the patient states: "I want to maintain the autonomy of my acts". The meaning she gives the word is twofold. Firstly, in the sense of ontological autonomy, threatened by the recent schizophrenic psychosis, bringing a concomitant loss of self-control. This is the level of the structural constitution of reality. But she also complains that her mother does not give her personal autonomy, which she wants to preserve at all costs. Indeed, historically, she has had a difficult relationship with her mother, who used to disregard her privacy. She says that was why she always preferred to keep her distance from her family. At this anthropological level, autonomy has to do with the value given to an anthropological disproportion of a schizoid nature, which is the patient's primary way of existing. Thus, we have here a dialectic tension between the pathology (only when it comes to her loss of control) and the positional sense of the patient's schizoid existence, whose anthropological disproportion causes life to be experienced in terms of autonomy. It was because of this opposition that the patient sought me out for treatment.

However, the patient herself is able to establish a relationship between the pathology and her vocation to exist autonomously in disproportion. Her hypothesis is that her psychosis was triggered by her overdoing her (voluntary) withdrawal from her family in a bid for autonomy: "I have been out of the world for too many years. I think I went too far and then these telepathic things began". From the perspective of a rational value sense, the patient's quest for autonomy is also an orientation for her life. Sustained by a pre-reflexive anthropological disproportion, it is augmented by the rational value it is given, favouring a detachment of from the co-constituting intersubjectivity of reality.

In synthesis, this account shows how a case of schizophrenic psychosis can relate to a patient's personality and personal values, creating nuances in the meaning of the pathology and the function of its treatment in her life. The breadth and severity of the schizophrenic pathology does not bother the patient because in a way it is an extension of her peninsular style of intersubjectivity. This and the historical self's quest for autonomy are only bothered by the fracture in the intersubjectivity of reality insofar as it hampers the core of the historical self. Outside this centre, being away from the world seems perfectly coherent with who she is. Finally, autonomy as a rational value makes it easier to detach oneself from a world that is sinking into schizophrenic psychosis. The same logic of articulation between various dimensions is what guides the search for treatment. The clinician is only called on to help reinstate the autonomy sought by the vertical, isolated historical self. The experience of being harassed by a parallel reality that continually attacks it is not included in the request for clinical help, since it is unrelated to the value the historical self places on autonomy. The psychosis as a whole does not bother the patient, since it offers a makeshift form of anthropological autonomy.

Similarly, every clinical decision in schizophrenia involves the clinician recognising the meaning of the structural pathology to the patient's personality and, inevitably, the values that govern their life, including the value they place on the schizophrenic fracture.

4.2 Melancholia–Mania

Historically, the understanding of mania and melancholia has been guided by semiological psychopathology[4] towards difference in unity. They are understood to be semiologically opposed, but belonging to a coherent, independent nosological unit, namely bipolar affective disorder (BAD). This makes BAD a unique and fully fledged mental illness characterised by a bipolarity of mood experiences, which oscillate between pathological sadness and equally pathological euphoric or irritable elevation. The unity of the disorder stems from the fact that it affects mood and has its own evolutionary form, in pure cases. In mixed cases, the notion of unity is maintained since both states are understood to alternate so closely or, at times, mix their semiology to such an extent that the unity of bipolar disorder is easy to prove.

The phenomenological psychopathological understanding follows the same general lines, examining separately what, as a disorder, is part of a unity (Binswanger 1960; Sass and Pienkos 2013). However, the unity of the two pathological experiential polarities can also be understood in terms of the similarity of their structural foundation (Fernandez 2014; von Zerssen 1988). This is the basis for my approach in this section. In the following paragraphs, I will defend the position that both manic and melancholic experiences are secondary pre-reflexive organisations of the same primary fracture in the intersubjective constitution of the structure of existence, leading to an *existential retraction and a pathological elevation of engagement with the world*. This same interpretative principle guided the distinction

---

[4] In this section, I address melancholia strictly in the anthropological sense advocated above. Because, as mentioned earlier, a significant portion of the psychopathological literature does not pay attention to this essential difference between the two experiences, freely interchanging the categories of melancholia and depression (Sect. 3.9), the scientific papers I mention here are only those in which I identify a melancholic definition of depression, regardless of the term used by the author(s).

between negative (primary) schizophrenia and its paranoid form (secondary organisation). Before presenting the situation related to the primary fracture in the melancholia–mania polarity, I should make brief mention of the concepts. Unlike in schizophrenia, whose name already indicates the unity that exists in its different clinical presentations, experiences of mania and melancholia have never received a psychopathological name to unify them anthropologically. That is why I have given this section a double-barrelled term, melancholia–mania, to indicate the presence of unity in diversity. However, I will introduce them separately to facilitate the presentation of the secondary differences between them.

4.2.1 The Dense Retraction of Melancholia

Melancholia has been understood as depersonalisation (von Gebsattel 1966b), a collapse of temporality with consciousness being restricted to the past (Minkowski 1995), an invasion of the future in the past (Binswanger 1960), excessive embodiment of experience (Dörr-Zegers et al. 2017), embodiment of the mind (Stanghellini 2004; Fuchs 2005), excessive submission to social identity (Kraus 1996b), desynchronisation (i.e. an uncoupling in the temporal relation of organism and environment, or of individual and society) (Fuchs 2001), or a compromised existential feeling, the pre-reflexive layer of existence that underpins all emotional experiences (Ratcliffe 2015). Besides, melancholia (referred to as depression) also has a well-preserved self who watches over all the above-mentioned alterations (Tatossian 2002).

With so many phenomenological definitions, can we really define the core of melancholic experience? Unlike schizophrenia, melancholia has throughout the decades been refractory to a clear definition of its essence. Schizophrenia seems to lend itself more readily to a clear core consensual diagnosis by the corpus of psychopathologists. Nevertheless, I would argue that the differences in the understanding of melancholia expressed by the different authors reflect the structural characteristic of the disorder, which manifests syndromically in different ways depending on which conditions of existential possibility are more visible in each clinical case (Messas and Tamelini 2018). It is precisely this variety of clinical presentations that induces psychopathologists to give precedence to the observation of some of the manifestations (as presented below) to the detriment of others, causing some difficulty in reaching a single definition for structural, psychotic melancholia.

Psychotic melancholia bears some resemblance to the anthropopathological form on which it is based. Indeed, the characteristics of anthropopathological melancholia are responsible for the vulnerability of existence to an outbreak of structural melancholia. Classic authors such as Tellenbach and Kraus have demonstrated how melancholic psychosis arises from the inability of the melancholic personality type (typus melancholicus) to cope with new environmental demands due to its hypernomic identity and its conservative temporality (Tellenbach 1983; Kraus 1991a). Recent results have confirmed these intuitions (Mundt et al. 1997). There is therefore partial continuity between the two. What differentiates them is when the anthropological dialectics underlying melancholia are replaced by a rupture in the intersubjective constitution of reality. Every serious mental illness is essentially a loss of the dialectic tension of existence. When this structural fracture occurs, an analysis of anthropological proportions in motion is no longer possible, and must be replaced by a heuristic attitude based on the investigation of how structural change is distorting experience.

This alteration of existential totality also dictates that its constituent elements, the conditions of possibility, take on a particular existential position that differs from the one seen in schizophrenia. Now, the fracture determines a *structural retraction* in the whole field of existence. It is by observing the way this retraction dominates existence and relates to the co-constitutive distortion of reality that the main findings of psychotic melancholia can be understood.

To retract means to move backwards existentially in a way that encompasses all the conditions of possibility of existence. In psychotic melancholia, all existence is retracted and compressed, leading to a state of pathological densification. I call this phenomenon *dense retraction*. In order to show how it appears, I will compare it, whenever possible, with the anthropopathological categories of melancholia discussed above and will indicate the directions in which substance use serves the purpose of self-management in this situation.

(a) **Dense isolation of the historical self**

The hyperintegrity seen in the spatiality of melancholic disproportion is transformed by the pathological densification of the segment of existence associated with the primordial fracture. Broken off from the rest of existence, this segment experiences a total saturation in which temporality is impaired. This configuration corresponds to the experience of an isolated historical self that has broken away from the world and is paralysed within itself and completely absorbed by itself. What I mean by this is that the historical self is imprisoned by the presence of its own feelings, personal values and thoughts, and is incapable of moving away from itself and from its history to envisage a future to which it may head. The self-pole becomes completely immersed in its previous history, losing from sight the biography still to be pursued. This suffocating condemnation to live in the eternal plenitude of one's own presence is at the heart of this experience of the historical self as it looks on, disconsolate, at its disconnection from the world or from itself. This disconnection from the world then makes it impossible to experience any meaning that is not closely related to its own moral flaws and universal guilt.

The main consequence of this dense isolation of the historical self is the manifestation of one of the classic themes of delusional melancholia: guilt. Guilt derives from an excessive presence of the self-pole in the totality of existence. This overwhelming presence of the self-pole means it is implicated in all surrounding facts and therefore responsible for everything that occurs around it. In structural melancholia, the historical self is hyperresponsible (and hyperhistorical, too); a pathological condition that endorses the belief that it no longer shares responsibility for the world with others. In melancholic psychosis, the hyperresponsible historical self is paralleled in the increasing density of reality, which overloads all environmental events with meaning for which the historical self is responsible. Unlike schizophrenic paranoia, in which the historical self is experienced as a lack of cognisance of the world, in melancholic paranoia the historical self is overly cognisant of the world and thus overly responsible for it. Consequently, the historical self is also to blame for everything that takes place. That is why, in melancholic delusions, the patient will often feel blameworthy for some divine punishment that will decimate the employees of the hospital to which he is admitted. Or they may feel guilty for the economic ruin that will surely beset their entire family. Substance misuse serves as a foil for this endless torment.

(b) Devitalised embodiment

The historical self also remains whole in any pathological experience of psychotic retraction towards its own body; more specifically, towards a body that no longer participates in the world, as is the case in Cotard's syndrome. Here, the person feels as if their body was dead (or they may even feel dead). Death in this case means a disconnection of the self-pole from the existence of its own body. A rupture in intersubjective constitution imposes separation of the body from the subjective pole to which it once belonged. The body becomes an inert mass, devoid of the capacity to act as a centre of meaning and expression. Dörr calls this phenomenon crematisation (2017), inspired by the ancient Greek word, *khrema*, which indicates the flesh as matter, as opposed to *sarks*, the living mass present in the body of living beings. This divorcing of the self-pole from the world means embodiment ceases to be an organic instrument of the person to become an autonomous member of the world. The body's disobedience of its ego centre only goes to exacerbate the debilitated self-pole's experience of guilt, as is evident from the words of a patient suffering a serious and distressing bout of melancholia.

"I always say that tomorrow I will make it, but I can't [talking about having the energy to resume the manual activities she used to do] … I want to fight back but my body doesn't respond and then come the bad thoughts [of suicide]". It is the sense of powerlessness in the face of self-imposed duties that torments her and the only solutions that come to her are either guilt at not being able to perform them or exit by annihilation.

This disconnection of embodiment from its centre also makes the body a focus of risks, as if the historical self were inhabiting a large foreign body which it is unable to master, control or unify with its identity. The clearest manifestation of this is the paranoia of poisoning often seen in cases of melancholia. It is not so much the paranoia of someone who feels persecuted and suspects some hostile plot as a paranoia devoid of fear, agitation or a delusional system, which only goes to reflect how meagre an experience it is to possess a body that, isolated and embalmed, can only be a vehicle of contamination, degradation and death.

The structural retraction of existence is also manifested in the embodiment of the typical omega sign and precordial anguish of the melancholic patient. Both demonstrate a bodily expression of a restriction that runs counter to the natural expansion of life. In the clearest forms, this retraction appears as loss of biological cycles, as already mentioned.

(c) The total identity in melancholia

Melancholic densification can also be noted in the identity. The solitary hypernomy of identity which we saw on the anthropological level is transformed on the structural level into hyperidentity. Existence is trapped in the total presence of one of the social roles that compose it. Indeed, the whole historical self is transformed into this social role to the point that the person's singularity disappears and the "role-self" appears, which paradoxically feels completely responsible for everything around it precisely because it is no longer a historical self delimited by individual responsibilities and an agent of its own free will. The free historical self becomes the puppet of an identity outside itself, governed by social norms. The social role that invades the historical self is structurally disconnected from society, losing its vivacity and capacity to adjust according to social circumstances. This condition massacres existence because it prevents the social role from having a healthy relationship with social reality, from which it could be revitalised. Existence is invaded by a social role which is entrenched and incapable of any creativity. This existential condition appears in another important theme of melancholia, personal impoverishment. Impoverishment means failure in professional terms. Because the historical self is invaded by an unyielding social identity, the sick melancholic person always experiences themselves as professionally incompetent (although they may, of course, feel like an incompetent housewife, provided this is the main partial identity of their existence), and therefore at risk of professional ruin. They might be a family man who has ruined his children or a businessman whose dreams are shattered. The unity of a partial role identity is not lost, unlike what occurs in the fragmentary invasion of schizophrenia. In melancholia, the oppressive weight of society's values and rules on the historical self not only remains intact, but is exacerbated to the point of raising its commitment to the world intolerably high.

(d) Dominance of temporal retention

Structural retraction also affects temporality in melancholia, making its basic form of alteration a dominance of retention combined with a loss of protention. This loss of protention leads, above all, to a build-up of retention, since it is here that all biographical experiences are deposited, and is therefore the most likely to densify. As protention is virtual, it simply dissipates in the face of the structural retraction.

Typical experiences of temporal retraction involve pathologically digging up past facts and bringing them into present consciousness (Rovaletti 2014). In conjunction with the changes reported above, this dwelling on the past is propitious for feelings of guilt in relation to events that are long gone. Patients will often set about making amends for real guilt about things that have already been resolved (financial or ethical lapses) but which they find themselves obsessing over to their or their family's surprise; or else old issues that cannot be resolved, like painful recriminations over having missed a work meeting in their youth that would supposedly have changed their professional fate. Retention in structural retraction becomes independent from the present and inverts the natural temporal logic of existence. Instead of the present taking precedence and thereby regulating retention, a narrow retention takes over, invading and subjugating the present.

However, this dwelling on past events can also take on a jealous face. In this situation, the responsible historical self does not feel guilty, but is offended by a fact full of biographical significance. A clinical example would be the jealousy felt by a patient (in an acute melancholic phase) regarding a case of infidelity on his wife's part more than 20 years before the psychotic episode. In this particular case, the issue of infidelity had already been quite resolved by the couple. Indeed, both husband and wife (including the patient, after the psychotic state had passed) said that their life together was quite satisfactory, despite some everyday difficulties. However, during the psychotic episode, the patient feared his wife's former lover was stalking the couple and should therefore be hunted down. This experience actually led the patient to engage in dangerous acts to attack this past offender as if he were an imminent threat. After the period of melancholia passed, the jealousy also vanished into the dusts of time.

This time structure also provides conditions for patients to have experiences of ruin. The atrophy of protention and the dominance of retention means the future appears to the consciousness as an obscure and distorted field. This distortion stems from the fact that protention (marked by indetermination) is invaded by characteristics of retention (marked by saturation). "I already know where I can reach. Nothing else can happen", says a melancholic patient.

The future becomes a future preterite in which only two themes are possible: either regret at what has passed or recrimination over what should have been. All themes linked to "what will be" disappear. Therefore, this future, while it prevails, is like a painful repetition of a dense experience that cannot be dissipated in time. Deprived of protention, all that is left for existence is to do what has always been assigned to it. That is why the dread that psychotic melancholic persons feel at the certainty of being punished is sometimes ambiguous. After all, their lives are dominated by fear of some imminent punishment, which for them, in extreme cases, is both inevitable and fair.

(e) The unified other as creditor

The pathological condensation of the melancholic identity also restricts the potential identities of the other to a single role to which the melancholic person's condensed historical self experiences eternal debt. Generally, this unified and condensed otherness is transformed into a kind of merciless creditor just waiting to point out all their inadequacies. A cruel other who pre-reflexively denounces the patient as guilty and responsible for their or their family's ruin or even the ruination of all humanity (Minkowski 1995). A striking example of this transformed otherness was at play in our clinic during an interview with a 65-year-old patient overtaken by severe melancholia. I was the one conducting the interview, but the whole health care team of about 20 people were involved. The structural retraction meant the psychopathological dialogue was limited to the patient and myself, as if there was no-one else in the room. The patient's muted tone of voice made it hard for me hear her, even though I was sitting next to her. Yet at the end of this two-way interview merely watched on by the others, the patient, getting up to return to her room, addressed everyone and murmured, "I hope I have been useful to you". We were astonished as we realised that she had assigned us a single identity throughout – that of caregiver – which made us individually indistinguishable. We understood that the two-way dialogue between the patient and myself had actually been open to all, but we had all been condensed into a single figure that transcended our personal differences or roles within the institution. We were all her caregivers. And yet her attitude towards us was one of indebtedness, as if the interview was meant to serve us and not to relieve her pain. The structural unification of otherness affected equally the dense and indebted historical self and the supposed multiple selves of the therapists, placed in the role of creditors.

In the most serious cases, the other seems to disappear and the self-pole closes in around its pathological retraction. In these cases, the melancholic patient, detached from the world, listless and cognitively defenceless, stands before an inaccessible other, in relation to whom they can only express indifference. This condition is clear in some university clinics, where there is a high turnover of residents. In these advanced cases, the patients do not even seem to notice the change of personnel responsible for their treatment. Finally, the structural pathological retraction of melancholia can grow to such an extent that it annihilates the whole structure of existence, as seen in cases of catatonia. In a semiological evaluation, there may appear to be no difference between this and schizophrenic or somatic-caused catatonia, although they are born from different anthropological origins. Only by researching the clinical history can a differential diagnosis be made.

4.2.2 The Light Retraction of Mania

(a) The total-present of the manic person

I would like to use a contrasting strategy to defend my thesis of the pathological unity of melancholia–mania. I will therefore begin the presentation of manic pathology by examining the condition of possibility in which there is the greatest semiological difference between melancholia and mania: temporality. The semiologically oriented clinician will be quite aware that the temporal behaviours in mania are the opposite to those observed in melancholia. In mania, there is agitation, over-engagement with surroundings, high-speed decision making, lack of attention, haste, impatience, while in melancholia there is a generalised deceleration and tepid disinterest. In mania, there is euphoria and extroversion; in melancholia, sadness and introversion. When we examine them from a clinical point of view, mania and melancholia are so different from each other that it would seem impossible to put them under the same identity umbrella. In the following paragraphs, I will try to indicate, whenever possible, the points at which mania and melancholia can be compared, either by their differences or by their structural similarities.

I have defined the essence of melancholia–mania as *structural retraction* combined with pathological over-engagement with the world. I have shown how in melancholia, the structural fracture leads to a retraction of temporality centred on retention. I argue that the key characteristic of the dominance of retention is densification, because this is the dimension where there is the sedimentation of our biography, and so it is already denser by nature. In melancholia, temporality becomes denser because all personal history weighs on the self-pole. The opposite occurs in mania: while there is also a fracture in the intersubjective constitution of the world, resulting in pathological over-engagement with the world, this over-engagement with the world takes place in the present dimension. As the present, in mania, becomes a temporal dimension that is self-contained and fails to articulate either with the density of sedimentation of the biography or with a commitment to the future, all relative release from the present is marked by lightness. With the articulation between the three dimensions of time fractured, the manic present becomes prey to the attractions of the surrounding world, which take on a specific temporality which I call total present. The present is the dimension of temporality in which objects (including the psychological states of the historical self, such as feelings and ideas) appear in their maximum, actual and total presence. The manic historical self therefore interacts in a totally present world in which there are no mysteries, because all that is virtual is right there in front of them. As if they were in a great market full of new things for sale, the manic person skips around the various attractions of the world, leaping from one to the other without putting down roots anywhere, resulting in a sequence of isolated experiences which are not sedimented in the biography. The world becomes excessively attractive and bright to the historical self to the point of dissolving the hierarchies of importance in its appreciation of reality. Ordinarily, when we are having a professional conversation with someone, we focus our attention on that person's face and whatever they are saying. We relegate to the background any aspect of theirs that may attract our attention but is not pertinent to our immediate reason for interacting – maybe the quality of their attire – as it is irrelevant in the context. The ability to sideline value perceptions is given by the temporal structure. Say we are talking to someone in the hope of selling them a product in the future, then the consequences of our actions matter a lot, so we modulate our present because of its connection with that future. Similarly, we focus on what matters at that time, on our relationship with the person, because we have a habit of doing so, a habit that makes us have a good name to protect. With that, we anchor our present in biographical retention.

It is because we are able to pre-reflexively experience time as articulated and fluent that we have the power to put off making any comment, waiting for the right time to do so. A manic experience is not trammelled by this temporal hierarchy of reality, giving flow to all its perceptions in the total present. The total temporality of the present in mania means the enhanced engagement with the world reaches all manic existence at the same time. In our example, the face and speech of the interlocutor have the same present value as their suit or dress, so the manic historical self will be interested in all three at the same time and incapable of focusing its attention on the central purpose of the encounter. This is the root of all manic distractibility:

the destructuring of temporality resulting in a retraction of existence to a total present. The world of the manic person is only worth what is before their eyes: their historical links with the values retained in their biography and the future consequences of their conduct are impaired as they inhabit a present filled with an over-appreciated, attraction-filled world in which everything is endowed with the same value and in which they can only flit about, as in an amusement park. That is why manic conduct tends to be irresponsible or morally distorted in relation to the person's own previous patterns. This irresponsibility comes from their inability to perceive the results of their actions; the immorality comes from a temporary carelessness towards their own personal values, linked to their biography. The manic person's personal values do not disappear when they are caught up in the total present, but all those of greater abstract value that will take time to reach maturity, such as moral conduct, appreciation of the value of one's fellow man, appreciation for one's own property, for others, are superseded. Instead, experiences of immediate, concrete value take hold, such as someone's beauty (leading to inappropriate erotic conduct (usually read as hypersexualised)) or the attractiveness of some material good (leading to excessive purchases). Thus, manic existence is at the mercy of a sequence of jumps over reality, constituting a saltigrade present (Binswanger 2000; Moskalewicz and Schwartz 2020a) marked by flitting restlessness. The temporality of mania is one of dissipation, waste, purposeless abundance, where the density of biographical maturation is overtaken by overlapping, pathologically value-filled moments.

The disengagement with the density of retention in mania goes *pari passu* with an analogous disengagement with the characteristics of protention. I call this latter phenomenon protentive actualisation. The notion contained in this term is that protention is completely actualised, casting off its characteristic indetermination and becoming factual reality. For instance, the idea of being rich and powerful in the future is actualised to the total experience of being rich and powerful in the present. Protentive actualisation also results in a future that is total and bountiful. This future bounty can give the manic person great pleasure, because it lets them feel as if they were in a complete world. However, like a Midas who crystallises when they turn everything into gold, the manic person lives in poverty within the anti-historical abundance of temporality.

The manic total present is almost a phenomenological description of substance intoxication, as will be developed in Part III. Any modification of consciousness is ultimately the production of a self-sufficient present, surrendering to a world-turned-totality. Accordingly, any association of mania and substance misuse (Richardson 2013) is the highest of all comorbidities. The manic historical self seeks intoxication because of its synergistic effect in relation to the world it already inhabits, which, purveyor of such pleasurable experiences, it does not generally wish to leave.

(b) The mild restriction of manic spatiality – immediacy and horizontality

Similarly to what we have seen in terms of temporality, the restriction of spatiality experienced in mania makes the world immediate. The manic person experiences everything as possible, provided it is immediate. The manic person's spatiality, in apparent contradiction to a naive vision of reality, is quite restricted, although semiologically it may seem broadened because of the expansive manner in which they occupy space. The lightness with which the manic person experiences spatiality actually stems from the fact that to them, all objects appear simultaneously in their existential field. The whole world is at their disposal pre-reflexively. One-dimensional horizontality is the hegemonic dimension of meaning in manic spatiality.

This is why the manic person seems so at home in the world. However, what "the whole world" means to the manic person is paradoxically a tiny field of possibilities given in the present of their surrounding environment. Sometimes, it is just the world of the infirmary in which they are hospitalised. The ideas that inspire the manic historical self are therefore framed by an articulation between total present temporality and immediate horizontality. A clinical example could help clarify this statement. A patient who had recently entered a manic phase came directly from her home to the clinic, where she was seen. On the way, she stopped at a jewellery store and made a purchase of a value far beyond her means. When I asked her why she had made such an extravagant purchase, especially since she was not even a jewellery lover, she answered cheerfully that she had bought it because she had seen it in the shop window and thought it was beautiful. I want to point out here that the act of purchasing it did not represent for her a genuine personal idea, in the sense of a value-driven desire of the historical self which, in a moment of impulsiveness, she was unable to contain. Rather, it was a reaction to her immediate environment, a succumbing to a consequence-free present.

In the same way, the delusional manifestations of grandeur in mania do not express any sealing of the structure of existence in an attempt to gain a minimum of ontological security, as in schizophrenia. They are simply secondary expressions of a self-pole which experiences the whole world simultaneously as an open spectrum at its disposal. The spatial restriction of mania allows the historical self to feel like a God ruling over a reality that seems total to it and over which it believes it is free to act. It is no wonder, then, that manic grandiose delusions often relate to experiences of the divine.

(c) **Identity: the manic person's paradoxical isolation in the world**

As in melancholia, so in mania the historical self is isolated by a fracture in the intersubjective constitution of the world. As in melancholia, the manic historical self is pathologically drawn to participate in all the events of the world. However, differently from melancholia, this restriction of the self is characterised by lightness. To understand the psychopathological meaning of this lightness, I must briefly present the anthropological difference between lightness and density in a biography.

The process of biographical development is itself a process of existential densification made up of a sedimentation of experiences centred on a historical self. This sedimentation of the biography accommodates all personal experiences and decisions made along the timeline. For this reason, a pathology that densifies reality will lend the historical self an overly heightened sense of responsibility for the world. This densification compresses the historical self with regard to its decisions, mistakes and successes. With mania, the opposite occurs. In manic retraction, the pathological lightness also implies an excessive engagement of the self with the world, but with no corresponding increase in responsibility. The manic historical self experiences itself as the centre of the whole world, while also feeling that its engagement with the world has little or nothing to do with any personal responsibility. It is as if it had the world at its feet, which in turn produces manic inflation of the ego. This inflated ego is not, however, devoid of radical ambiguity. In it, the historical self paradoxically isolates itself in its horizontal amplitude, but at the same time mixes with the interpersonal world (Sass and Pienkos 2015). This isolation gives the sense of being master of the universe, superior to all fellow beings. The manic historical self does not identify with responsibility, only with power. However, at the same time it is oriented toward and attracted to the world, which is there to serve its every want. The fact that it acts irrespective of the needs of its fellow men and material objections, such as financial resources or moral obligations, has to do, paradoxically, with the fact that the interpersonal world is its own inspiration and source of power (Kraus 1998). As in Hegelian slave–lord dialectics, the lord can only lord over others because there are slaves who maintain him in this state. The lord exercises his power alone in a world of slaves whom he subjugates but also needs in order to remain in supreme isolation. The existential ambiguity of the manic person paradoxically isolates them in the world. While they are completely enraptured by that world, they are also unable to share it with others. Let us investigate this ambiguity from two angles. First, the experience of manic ego inflation.

The solitude of the manic person in the midst of his fellow men is at the root of two fundamental feelings of manic existence: euphoria and irritation. This euphoria reflects the anthropological state of an isolated historical self which is inflated, full of itself, with boundless power to influence the world and others. The corresponding irritation comes in response to the resistance the world puts up against manic euphoria. As manic isolation occurs within the world, it is natural for the manic historical self to encounter frequent obstacles to its actions. Unable to authentically tune in with their fellow men and feeling great and powerful, the manic person becomes irritated every time the world manifests itself as an objective reality independent of their will. In the light retraction of mania, the biographical historical self disengages from responsibility for any of its acts, while experiencing an augmented sense of power over the world. The psychotic form of the inflated and present-oriented self-pole is expressed in grandiose delusions, as mentioned above. These delusions indicate a loss of the co-constitution of reality; the content of the delusion, the thematic form it takes, is structurally grounded on a corresponding enlargement of this self-pole, which is secondary to the structural restriction per se. As suggested above, this light self-pole is disengaged from any continuity of its personal history – which is the opposite of melancholia. It is a self-pole whose delusional experience stems exactly from its lack of commitment to its history. It is a kind of absolute, bountiful self stuck in the midst of its fellow men with whom all dialogue is tiresome and conflictive. All those who have had the opportunity to treat manic patients will have experienced how abrasive relationships with them can be.

This, however, is only one of the forms isolated retraction takes in the manic world. Another is the paradoxical isolation in which the inflated self-pole is enthralled. In it, the absolute self is assimilated by the cultural community to which it belongs, taking on a false identity and totally absorbed in its actions by a partial identity role borrowed pre-reflexively from the community to which it belongs. This partial identity allows the isolated manic historical self (a) to retain its lightness, since a marginal identity is something like a carnival costume, indicating disengagement from the most deep-seated identity; (b) to acquire a minimally stable identity; and (c) to maintain some logical and psychological coherence in its manifestations.

In this variety, the historical self becomes assimilated by a partial identity, which takes command of its interpersonal relationships. It now inhabits the world as a partial totalised identity determined by the community's rules of conduct. The historical self becomes a puppet of an identity already constituted in society; in general, an identity that is already quite well consolidated, as I will exemplify below. An existential consequence of this condition is the complete imprisonment of existence by the community's values and modes of conduct. This is not a subjective experience of imprisonment, but a total subjugation of personal identity by one of its parts. Since this subjugation takes place in the absence of dialectic tension, the subjugated person's subjective experience is one of comfort and even plenitude. In subjugation, the historical self no longer resists its dissipation in a community identity; irritation with the world disappears and euphoria becomes the overriding qualitative state. In this state, substance use serves as a balm to accentuate the manic person's subjugation to the collective. An example serves to illustrate this phenomenon.

A religious patient aged around 50 was admitted to our clinic with intense euphoric mania. She was interviewed by the whole team, composed of about 20 people. The whole interview was overtaken by religious themes compatible with the patient's devout life. Animated, agitated and expansive, the patient would not sit still. She repeatedly got to her feet, and addressed all the interviewers individually, offering them redemption from the sins of the group and assurances of eternal life. Her manner was cheerful and ebullient, resonating affectively with the interviewers. She performed small ritual movements as she blessed each member of the group. At first glance, we might say that her egoistic expansiveness put her in the role of representative of the Divine on Earth, that her behaviour expressed the inflated isolation of the self-pole. However, as the interview progressed, we noticed that all her gestures, her general attitude, the intonation of her voice, the prosody of her religious discourse, the way she moved around the room – in short, all the manifestations of her existence – were carbon copies of the *modus operandi* of the ministers of her particular church. There was nothing in her behaviour to reveal the expansion of a singular, creative historical self; rather, what we observed was a miniscule self-pole absorbed in the sterile reproduction of a single social role without lending it any personal mark. The exuberance with which the manic experience took over her personal identity was expressed exclusively in the reproduction of a professional religious identity on which it placed great value. What appears to be an expansion of the self-pole is actually a reduction of experience to an identity form dictated by the collective.

(d) **The unfolding identity of otherness – the loss of the temporal hierarchy of partial identities**

The pathological totalisation of the present and horizontal immediacy in mania lead us to another of its structural characteristics, the unfolding of the identity of otherness. As temporality is out of joint, the present starts to reveal potentialities in reality and otherness which are not revealed under normal conditions of existence. Consequently, all things experienced as having value are appreciated at the same time; things from retention lose their historical density and things from protention are lent present value. Likewise, this world revealed in its entirety seems to be immediately available to the self-pole. As I have pointed out, distraction and inattention are typical phenomena in this state of affairs. Now, I shall discuss the intersubjective dimension of this phenomenon. In mania, there is a modification of the other as a personal identity, in the sense of an unfolding identity. For example, when we talk to someone hierarchically superior in our work environment, we address them from our social identity as a subordinate to their corresponding identity as a superior. In this setting, the work-related social identities take priority over our other partial identities. The other possibilities contained in our contact are momentarily sidelined until a social context appears in which they can be expressed. For example, when I get home and see my son, my identity as a father comes to the fore, overtaking my worker identity. The temporal–spatial constitution of reality imposes a hierarchy on the partial identities of existence. This pre-reflexive hierarchy allows one personal identity to be the protagonist at any given moment, giving way to another in a different moment and context. Temporality is what enables this succession of partial social identities in an existence, in attunement with the contexts in which they are authorised.

When the temporal constitution of reality is lost, this dialectic of multiple partial identities in each person is replaced by a manifestation and actualisation of all partial identities at the same time. The hierarchy of the partial identities is lost and the reciprocal relationship between each personal identity becomes adialectical, leading to inadequate behaviour. The ability of the various partial identities to organise themselves appropriately to the social setting depends on a continuous state of relational tension between them. It is this tension that allows the action of one social identity to limit the actions of the others (as in the example of a hierarchical conversation), resulting in the emersion of an appropriate identity for each context. When it comes to intersubjective relations, the existential retraction in time hampers this capacity to articulate a succession of identities according to the context and instead the whole diversity of identities contained in each person starts to become apparent. It is as if there was an overexposure of personal identities, putting all the partial identities of otherness within sight and reach. This pathology in the constitution of otherness is therefore quite different from the pathology observed in schizophrenia. In schizophrenia, there is a fracture in the very constitution of the other as a person; the patient relates to a personal spectrum, which often takes the form of a hallucination. In the case of mania, otherness as such is correctly constituted and so the manic historical self is able to perceive otherness correctly. Its problem lies in its inability to temporally organise the presences of otherness, which is necessary to perceive the particularities of the other hierarchically. With this loss of hierarchy, the manic person experiences a hyperperception of the other, while the schizophrenic perceives them only in fragments.

A classic manifestation of this situation is the inappropriate level of intimacy that a manic person, admitted to an infirmary, assumes with their interviewer. They may mock their psychopathologist or ask questions about their personal life, as if this was a friendship rather than a professional relationship, as if they were having some drinks in a bar rather than interacting in a clinical setting. This pathological intimacy may take the form of inappropriate sexual advances to the attending clinician. This invitation to multiply partial identities should not be understood as creativity. Creativity renews what is given within certain limits through relational enrichment or the observation of aspects of the relationship in an unusual way. Creativity extracts more than there is in a situation, it illuminates the alternatives from a particular perspective, it indicates ways out of a situation. In mania, although it can be playful and introduce unexpected content, provoking laughter, no renewal of the relationship is on the cards. There is no creativity in a giggle or a guffaw inside a psychiatric ward when a patient makes fun of how thin another resident attending the psychopathological interview is or when they ask the psychopathologist details of their sex life. In both situations, the humour does not bring forth anything capable of transforming or enriching the relationship. On the contrary, by invoking other partialities of the psychopathologist, the manic patient restricts the relational sphere precisely by proportionally reducing the scope for dialogue with the identity of the other they most need: that of the clinician. Mania does not create; it simultaneously actualises what is already created, saturating intersubjective reality. It suffocates more than it liberates, restricts more than it amplifies. The same could be said of the ipseic dimension of the existence who lives with mania. There is no creation of identity, no enlargement of their scope of action in society. On the contrary, the partialities of their identity capable of engaging with society narrow dramatically, limiting the person's existential options to the role of patient. Paradoxically, then, there is actually a kind of destructive creativity in maniac, where the excesses in capturing the other produce an impoverishment of personal and interpersonal potentialities. From what I have just pointed out, there is an obvious similarity between manic experience and intoxication, especially when alcohol-induced. From an intersubjective point of view, drunkenness induces temporary mania. This similarity is what makes substance misuse attractive to the manic person, as it amplifies their way of inhabiting the world.

However, it cannot be said that creativity is only restricted in mania. Indeed, the association between creativity and mania has been known for a long time (Kraus 2008). This creativity seems to be mediated by the same anthropological motives above, namely the ability to appreciate the present in all its immediate and simultaneous potentiality.

(e) **Embodiment: agitation and visuality**

In mania, embodiment is an expression of horizontal inhabitation of the world. The manic person's isolation in the world is what marks their motor expression, which is entirely directed towards objects of social value, people and situations in which human exchange is the central point. Likewise, the most immediate intersubjective dimension, visuality, is what determines the manic body's self-care procedures. It is not uncommon for manic patients to dress outlandishly or inappropriately for their social setting. A typical example of this is the excess of makeup manic patients will wear on the ward, as if they were preparing for some party they know will not take place.

4.2.3   Melancholia and Mania as a Structural Unit

As I have shown, mania and melancholia are dialectic moments of the same structural decomposition, marked by a rupture of the intersubjective co-constitution of the world and structural retraction. Both are manifested temporally by a destructuring of the capacity to arrange the dimensions of temporality in an articulated, flexible manner, resulting in each one being disfigured. In spatiality, both are manifested by narrowing. In intersubjectivity, they share an absence of relational creativity, characterised either by a paradoxical surfeit of personal identities (mania) or their scarcity (melancholia). And in identity, they are both marked by an abandonment of ipseity in favour of a saturated identity. It is this essential similarity that frequently causes manias to oscillate clinically with melancholia and vice versa. This clinical oscillation only indicates that different existential modes have been recruited for the secondary organisation of existence in the face of the same structural retraction of the pathology. The structural retraction can oscillate between being limited to the intolerable density of an existence infused, devastatingly, with the past and surrendering to the narrow lightness of a total present that is ultimately nothing more than a closure of existence itself.

In their surface manifestations, mania and melancholia therefore show an alternation between light plenitude (euphoria) and empty density (Cotard's syndrome, desrealisations and depersonalisations experiences), which reveals dialectically, at a deeper level, a restriction of the horizons of an existence that can no longer articulate itself in a world of equals based on the reciprocity of personal and community values. In fact, the lost melancholic–manic existence is crushed between two alternatives that are actually one. Euphoria is a plenitude that is, as it were, complete. Anguish is plenitude that is void. In both, the retraction means that the biography is unable to achieve renewal through the mediation of incompleteness and imperfection, necessary for existential renewals and rebirths. Crushed by absolute temporality and absolute spatiality, the apparent clinical differences between mania and melancholia are reduced to structural unity when examined from the perspective of their conditions of possibility. Similarly, substance misuse in melancholia–mania ultimately serves one purpose, which is to enable the isolated historical self some degree of management of its restricted world. In moments of melancholia, substance misuse serves to offset the harassment of historical reality; in moments of mania, its purpose is to elevate the barren land of bounty that is its imprisonment in a total world.

Finally, it is important to emphasise that both melancholia and mania can also coexist with or be followed by moments of depression, in the anthropological sense of the concept. The most typical case of this is a reactive depression after a manic phase. In such cases, existence suffers when it takes stock of the devastation it underwent during the pathological period, with its often ruinous results or with the long life span dissipated by the disease.

4.2.4   Clinical Decision-Making in Melancholia and Mania

As in all structural disorders, the clinician's first objective is to bring about complete remission of the disease. This puts the clinician primarily in the field of pharmacological decision-making, although environmental considerations may also come into play, such as suggesting the need for hospitalisation. Adventitiously, the clinician may make decisions designed to protect their patient from the risk to their own reputation or their life caused by some offensive behaviour. This primary clinical objective in mania and melancholia is marked by decisions related to the maintenance of life, making them inviolable in their essence.

It is when a patient leaves the active phase of the disease and returns to the normal path of development of the biography that the clinician is faced with more dilemmas and ambiguities. Now, the historical self has to deal with the remnants of the disease which, until this point, distorted its existence. It is at this point that the anthropological types related to melancholia and hyperthymia come into play.[5]

As above mentioned, the classical analysis by Tellenbach shows how specific personality vulnerabilities pave the way for structural melancholia (1983) and mania (1969). What these vulnerable personalities, respectively, called *typus melancholicus* (Tellenbach 1983) and *typus manicus* (von Zerssen 1996), have in common is their limited capacity to adapt in the face of stressors that require existential plasticity, that is, ipseity. These personalities are characterised by a marked influence of the anthropopathological characteristics of melancholia and hyperthymia. The limited ipseity of these vulnerable personality types means that in the face of stressors that challenge their personal identity, the wholeness of existence succumbs to structural pathology. The management of a restricted identity that is not able to transform creatively in the world, albeit highly functional and productive, is the main

---

[5] It is important to note that not all melancholic people have a melancholic typology (Kimura et al. 2000), just as not all manic people have a hyperthymic typology (von Zerssen et al. 1994). I examine here the conditions in which there is some continuity between melancholia and melancholic disproportion and between mania and hyperthymic disproportion.

challenge of existence in the moments after an acute phase of the pathology. Two conditions arise. In the first, the patient is able to return to their previous pattern of identity, meaning that they return to life exactly as it was before, managing to evade the need for some kind of renewal of their identity. In this alternative, the role of the clinician is restricted to managing the maintenance of stability by pharmacological means, above all.

However, the patient's preferred existential option of returning to their stable, solid identity is not always possible. Sometimes, the demands of life itself prevent an existential return to the status quo ante. The clinician's role in this situation is to rely heavily on the psychotherapeutic dimension of treatment. Above all, they must help the patient face the limitations and possibilities of their own anthropological disproportions. This inevitably includes profound reflection about their existential options and the viability of launching on the path of renewal of existence or closing off within the limitations imposed by their particular state or personality. In its deepest existential dimension, every psychotherapy of an existence vulnerable to mania or melancholia is a confrontation with the dialectic between pliability and rigor or between individual verticality and collective horizontality in the identity itself, which is put in terms of the dilemma of allowing oneself to be naturally caught up by the tendency to adhere to a particular social identity or to try something that runs counter to that natural tendency. In such a movement, the saturation of identity that is the natural vocation of manic and melancholic existence must be given up for something that gives a personal touch to life, but at the same time brings the risks of an existence defined by itself. For these existences, giving up this identity saturation, even if temporarily or in part, is fraught with difficulties. One example is a hyperthymic patient, who, after the manic phase, says she preferred the illness to sanity, because when she was in it she felt completely inside herself, while now she has to deal with the fact that she feels very inferior to others because she does not have any truly fulfilling professional activity. The manic phase had given her enormous vitality to take her identity role as a businesswoman to the extreme. This identity, successfully developed in the last 2 years, had never, she admitted, been for herself but for others to see her value. Her great existential dilemma in resuming the course of her life was to face the fact that she preferred to live in the total thrall of one social identity, but in order to maintain it she had to annul herself individually to the point of collapsing into a structural pathology. At the end of the day, resuming life means resuming the difficult and insoluble dialectics that interweave the history of human existence.

There is one last dialectical dilemma that lends mania a specific hue. This dilemma is of great value for the anthropological understanding of substance abuse. Although in anthropological terms, the manic state represents a restriction of existence, this restriction is inherently ambiguous, which in turn makes the historical self take an ambiguous stance towards its pathological state. The sense of subjective completeness that mania allows by presenting an unreal existence that is beyond the reach of the everyday grind remains attractive to the manic patient, even when they are not in a manic phase. Even when fully aware that the experiences during the pathological period were devastating for their life, the manic patient keeps harking back to the euphoria of each moment lived in the pathology, which has no equivalent in the range of feelings daily life can offer. In the same way, the intensity of manic pathology has no rival in the often repetitive reality of normal everyday life. The extreme horizontality of mania makes the world and others appear brighter, more vivid, imbued with maximum value. Meanwhile, daily life is by definition rooted in taking some distance, putting the world and others in perspective. The world is, I would argue, always about partial participation in things. Mania is a radical, total surrender that leaves marks on the memory of every person. The decision-making implied in this dialogue between nostalgia for the pathology and facing up to life as it presents itself is the equivalent to renouncing paradise. This leads us directly to the issue of substance misuse, to which I will now turn.

4.3 Temporality and Transition Between Anthropological Proportions – The Foundation for Understanding Substance Misuse–Specific Experiences

The set of pathological conditions presented above reveals existence's profound debt to temporality. Temporality, in its various dialectic compositions, is the bedrock on which biographical facts are based and therefore the fundamental condition of possibility for the development of the historical person. The dissolutive action of temporality determines a series of transitions between anthropological proportions throughout life. It is from the very vitality of existence that the constant need to reactualise the anthropological proportions of an individual existence springs. As existence, whether healthy or not, transforms and moves around in the world according to or even against its rational will, the same individual can, for example, present psychosis with schizophrenic characteristics at one moment and psychosis with melancholic characteristics at another. All it takes for the dissolving of temporality to take on the form of melancholia is for its primary effect to be the excessive cohesion of the self-pole and the social world. All it takes is the dissolving action of temporality to fragment the heart of the self-pole and distance it from attunement with the social world for it to be schizophrenic. The movements dictated by the rhythm of a personal history are organised by the continuous rearrangement of fundamental anthropological proportions and therefore subject existence to different existential formations. Like a cloud that is constantly changing shape as it moves, so existence is at the mercy of pre-reflexive proportional renewals of greater or lesser frequency, which make any psychopathological diagnosis non-exclusive and non-definitive. All transitions are thus possible, although they do depend on how long each pathological experience invades existence and how much harm it does. For example, the structural dimension of a schizophrenic experience is of a low dispersion capacity. In general, it irrevocably compromises the entire individual biographical; however, the anthropological stratum of a schizophrenic sufferer continues to move, which allows the emergence of other experiences, such as depression or phobia or other experiences typical of everyday life. Schizophrenia tends to be chronic and maintain zones of existential paralysis over time; however, the moving zones continue to take on new anthropological proportions, so it is never enough to simply say that a person is schizophrenic. Instead, the partial meaning taken on by the psychotic calcification at each existential moment should be investigated.

At the anthropological level, there is no definitive stiffening of the temporal conditions of possibility. The primary grounding of existence is preserved. Accordingly, disturbed experiences arise from a partial stiffening of the dialectical proportions of temporality, producing anthropological disproportion. It is the plasticity of these proportions that allows new temporal formulations to emerge, settle and disperse. It is this that guarantees the capacity for transition between the anthropological proportions on which healthy life depends. The capacity for transition between anthropological proportions is also what explains the succession of anthropopathological experiences over time (Messas 2014c). This is why, in a period of great professional uncertainty, an existence can, for example, manifest phobic anthropological disproportion and at a later biographical moment, when the same professional experience is already exhausted, express melancholic disproportion. Anthropological disproportions are existential styles that vary more or less according to the plasticity of becoming. The same existential content can be sustained by different anthropological disproportions according to their position in the course of time.

Transitions also occur from the anthropological to the structural level. For example, in a severely ill patient in our clinic, the symptomatology oscillated throughout their clinical evolution from an obsessive anthropopathology to a schizophrenic structural pathology without any significant variations in the manifest symptomatology. In this case, for some time during its evolution, certain obsessive thinking was experienced as alien to the self (ego-dystonic, in the language of descriptive psychopathology). In this period, the patient was clearly overtaken by an obsessive experience. However, they gradually started to question the source of this same thought and eventually began to wonder if it was not the voice of the devil whispering in their ear. This transition, occurring even between different existential levels, shows how pathologies are closer to each other than they may appear at first sight.

The longitudinal temporality of existence makes comprehending pathological experiences existentially a complex and ambiguous task. The existing dialectics between the transversal pathological form prevailing at a certain moment and the way it fits into the succession of sedimented experiences throughout life also influences the existential significance of psychopathological facts. Thus, a mature individual who has already experienced many frustrations in life will tend to assimilate a melancholic experience differently from a young, inexperienced individual, for whom this anthropological disproportion may have more serious effects. The capacity to identify a pathology, whether anthropological or structural, effectively depends greatly on gaining familiarity with the specific patient's experiences over time – something that can only be achieved after a long period of interaction. A pathological experience would only be discernible in absolute terms in a fictitious existence divorced from time, in which the pathologies could emerge in their absolute forms, uninfluenced by the specificities of each individual.

Finally, it is worth noting that the transition between experiences is also modulated by the rational freedom of the historical self. Even in its most distorted forms, existence is never subject to complete causal heteronomy, a situation in which the whole chain of causes unfolds irrespective of individual decisions. The freedom of the historical self, even if it is limited by the severity of a disorder, influences the way the dialectical movement between anthropological disproportions evolves. The historical self is capable of judging decisions that relate to the proportions that make up its own structure. Although this decision-making freedom is limited (it is not possible, for example, to freely decide to revoke a psychotic fracture), certain anthropological disproportions can be emphasised or reduced and so existence can be regulated up to a point. It is possible, for example, for mild anthropological disproportion to be circumvented by the strength of will of the historical self, which, reflecting on its own existence, marshals its powers to supplant the rigidity of its social identity and, in a bid for freedom, cast itself into professional renewal. The whole person, a mixture of inflexible foundations and a free and embodied spirit, also carves something out of the matter of which he or she is composed.

It is from this dual anthropological perspective – the continuous transformation and succession of anthropological proportions and the relative capacity of the historical self to manage this dialectical regimen – that we must understand the great theme of substance use, from which the problem of substance misuse stems. Substance misuse can only be understood if we understand substance use, since this is anchored in the decisions made by the historical self about its own existence. In this first anthropological dimension, the person's substance use is a free action ruled by free reason in a bid to achieve dialectic movement in the fundamental anthropological proportions of its existence. Every intoxication is, from an anthropological point of view, a modification of anthropological proportions and has some biographical purpose, serving a personal end. It modulates the transitions between the forms by which the world, the other and the historical self are manifested and relate to each other. It is from this point that I will proceed to examine the ambiguities and pathological experiences specific to the existential structures of substance misuse.

Part III
Psychopathology of Substance Misuse

Chapter 5
The Proportions of the Absolute – Introduction

In the third chapter of Genesis (3:1–7), the Judeo-Christian tradition puts newly created humanity, synthesised in the persons of Adam and Eve, to its first radical test by making it take a decision in the face of ambiguity. On one side of the conflict was access to wisdom about good and evil, the exclusive privilege of the Divine, curiosity about which was incited by the serpent. On the other was obedience to God, which would guarantee man eternal peace and communion (2:15). Adam and Eve's decision, surely misinformed by the serpent, cost humanity the perfect balance, immutable harmony and eternal perfection guaranteed by direct and unified presence with the Word. By putting itself on a par with the Divine, humanity breaks with Him, and from this fissure arises all its imperfection, incompleteness and finitude. The decision to know the oppositions of good and evil – of dialectics as a form of understanding reality – lies at the root of the Judeo-Christian interpretation of the destiny of humankind. Expelled from the Garden of Eden, humanity loses its capacity to integrate harmonically with the whole of the universe created by Him. And with this expulsion is born the hierarchy between man and woman, to the detriment of the latter (3:16), suffering through labour (3:18) and the finitude of life (3:19). Dialectics and Paradise are mutually excluded from each other and, by force of a decision taken by our primordial ancestors, we abandon our passive surrender to the absolute and find ourselves relegated to live in a complex world guided by dialectical principles in which the dynamics of proportions prevail. To know good and evil is to put them in proportion, to place them in perspective and, above all, to make decisions regarding these proportions.

In the earthly world, the absolute does not, however, cease to exist. Even outside the field of religion, the notion of totality remains as a reference for the dialectics of daily existence. Throughout this work, for example, I have referred to the whole of the existence or the whole of the personality. However, the imposition of temporality as a dissolutive force in the composition of existence means that existence can only be understood by understanding the parts that compose it and, simultaneously, the relations between the parts and the totality to which they belong. Since the expulsion from Paradise, comprehending humanity means understanding

G. Messas, *The Existential Structure of Substance Misuse*,
https://doi.org/10.1007/978-3-030-62724-9_5

proportions as opposed to the absolute. The changeable and progressive nature of the biography prevents the absolute from being a human criterion. Nevertheless, the field of possibilities of human existence is still inhabited by yearning for some absolute, some mythical time when man's conflicts with himself and with the world may be set aside in favour of an absolute which offers a perfect, bountiful, immutable world free of suffering, in which, a fortiori, no decision-making is needed. The search for this absolute, in its various forms, is what orients the use of psychoactive substances, anthropologically speaking. Through the action of certain psychoactive substances on its central nervous system, the human historical self manages, albeit only temporarily or at the cost of what we will see here, to dissolve the fractions that constitute it, to abandon the realm of proportionality and to inhabit an artificial paradise (Baudelaire 2007), in which the absolute reigns supreme and a primal re-union with the world seems possible. It is therefore in the dialectics between anthropological proportionality and experiential absolute that I will investigate the participation of substance misuse in the pathologies of existence.

Given the inescapable condition of existence as development in time, the yearnings for proportion and the absolute reveal an insoluble ambiguity. Whereas existential movement depends on a dialectic relationship of relative proportions of parts, the absolute only exists in immobility, in a definitive relationship, as a total unit in which movement and development play no part. Any nostalgia for some absolute Eden means seeking a solution that runs counter to the natural flow of temporality, wishing to change the very way temporality is articulated in the constitution of our lives. Yet the states in which the absolute absorbs all proportionality are rare, and are largely linked to patently pathological conditions. In the vast majority of situations, the regime of modifications of anthropological proportions inevitably involves conflict between a yearning for the absolute and the imperious presence of existence as a temporal proportion.

Therefore, every free and rational choice of a historical self to transform its state of consciousness must be understood, first and foremost, as a decision concerning temporality. What drives this decision is the search for new proportions of temporality, tempted by a yearning for an absolute, perfect, harmonious time devoid of dissolution and pain. However, as every anthropological dimension is constitutively interconnected with the others, each act of substance use envisages altering the anthropological proportions of all the conditions of possibility of the existential structure. For this reason, in this part, I will use the terms "consciousness modification" (or modified consciousness), "substance use" or "intoxication" to indicate any change in anthropological proportions achieved voluntarily – at least at the beginning of more serious clinical conditions – through the exogenous action of some psychoactive substance on the organism. As my aim is to define a general anthropological effect, this meaning ranges from the mild inebriation produced, for example, by a glass of beer to intoxication with psychomotor agitation induced, for example, by cocaine. Although these two experiences clearly alter the anthropological proportions of existence in different ways, they both fit into a more general framework of modification, which I will set forth below. Accordingly, the first object of analysis is to identify, in general terms, what consciousness modification means to an individual existence. Since there are great differences between people when it comes to how they are affected by a modification to their state of consciousness, I will deal with the general, average influences substances have on anthropological proportions. I should point out here that this part does not go into any detail on the different effects of psychoactive substances on consciousness. Rather, as I want to delve to a deeper and more fundamental level, my main aim is to examine the existential (mainly positional) senses of consciousness modification and substance misuse. Without disregarding the differences in the effects wrought by different substances, I will nonetheless concentrate on the description of the ones that are most prevalent internationally, at least in the West, and which therefore have a greater impact on public health, such as alcohol, cannabis, cocaine (and derivatives) and opiates (Degenhardt 2018). Whenever I want to indicate a specific effect of a substance, I will do so explicitly.

Aside from this introductory chapter, Part III consists of three chapters detailing different aspects of the psychopathology of substance misuse. Chapter 6 examines the general *anthropological functions of consciousness modifications*. The aim is to show the principles that make substance-induced modifications of the state of consciousness an everyday phenomenon, present for centuries in practically all cultures. In other words, I do not present substance use as being inherently problematic. In Chap. 7, I examine two perspectives together. First, I examine the *existential senses of the human situations in which substance use becomes problematic*, namely *existential vulnerabilities*. What I mean is that some existential situations (like adolescence and youth (Latimer and Zur 2010; Subramaniam and Volkow 2014) have a typical style of anthropological proportions that calls for a frequent modification of consciousness. This does not indicate a need that is inherently pathological; rather, it indicates, as we shall see, that the exogenous effects of substance use and different styles of anthropological proportion are intimately related, with the former serving the deep needs of the latter. This intimate relationship, like an inner dialogue, is why the exogenous modification of consciousness may become such an important existential alternative to some people that they make frequent recourse to it. Getting to know these persons' existential needs is the best way to assist them in clinical practice. In parallel to the presentation of these conditions of vulnerability, I will outline the existential characteristics of the *changes typically seen in substance misuse, addiction[1] and the psychoses secondary to substance use*. Addiction and secondary psychoses will be addressed as specific psychopathological entities. They are therefore typical anthropological disproportions in their own right, distinct from all the others analysed in this work, although in the name of textual fluidity, I sometimes include them in the broad category of substance misuse, as I do in the title of the book and in the title of this third part. (However, whenever I mention them, I will be referring to their specific sense.) It is my understanding that specific pathological

---

[1]Although nicotine addiction is a major public health issue, it is not covered in the psychopathological model I use here. The reason for this is that it produces little change in consciousness and so interferes very little in the dialectics of the conditions of possibility of existential development. It causes somatic damage, which falls outside the scope of this work.

states of substance misuse can only be understood in relation to vulnerabilities, since they are an evolution of them; that is, they are a typical style of anthropological disproportion that arises from other disproportions. As it is impossible to understand alterations induced by substance misuse without examining its profound interactions with all existence, Chap. 7 presents each of the conditions of possibility associated with substance misuse[2] individually. Since temporality is understood throughout this work as the primary condition of possibility of existence, the most obvious definition of addiction is to be found in temporality. Therefore, in the section that examines temporality, I have separated the psychopathology of addiction from the vulnerabilities and experiences associated with substance misuse. In the other sections, the distinction between substance misuse and addiction is not so clear, which is why no distinction is made between the two experiences. Nonetheless, wherever a clear differentiation is possible, this will be indicated.

It is important to highlight that the boundaries between the concepts presented in Chaps. 6 and 7 are not a given. In fact, my decision to divide the presentation in this way is guided exclusively by didactic considerations. At all times, the general anthropological sense of consciousness modification merges with its psychopathological expressions, often diluting the cause-effect relationships between substance and subjective states. Commonplace in people's lives, the act of modifying their state of consciousness and thus their anthropological proportions serves multiple functions, and the associated clinical alterations cannot be completely distinguished. However, the clinician must be aware that such differences do exist in clinical reality and should, whenever possible, aim to make a differential diagnosis of them. In Chap. 8, I outline some guiding principles for recovery based on the reflections in the previous two chapters. This chapter has only the function of indicating the rationale that should guide the treatment of substance misusers.

Although the operational diagnoses established by international organisations for substance use-related problems do not correspond exactly to the concepts developed here, since they follow different epistemological principles, they will not be disregarded. For the purposes of this book, the concept of substance misuse covers the phenomena listed in DSM-5 as substance-related disorders (APA 2013) and in ICD-11 as Disorders due to substance use or addictive behaviours (WHO 2019).

From a phenomenological perspective, substance misuse is understood as an attempt by the historical self to manage its conditions of possibility, yielding results that are harmful to its own positional or value senses.[3] In substance misuse, intoxication is the key element in this management of the dialectics of existence. When I refer to addiction, I mean the maintenance of existence in a single state of anthropological disproportion in which any dialectic movement is impeded or substantially

---

[2] The somatic changes wrought by substance use, such as increased risk of cardiovascular disease or cancer, fall outside the scope of this work. Although they are legitimate public health concerns, they are not within the narrow scope of psychopathological interests.

[3] As the constitution of existence is intersubjective, one of the consequences of substance misuse is harm to others, as seen in the association between binge drinking and driving under the influence, for example.

curtailed. In this case, intoxication no longer interacts with the themes of the dialectics of the existence. Similarly, the psychoses that are secondary to drug use are given special status, defined as altered experiences of reality in which intersubjective constitution remains intact.[4]

Any psychopathology of substance misuse must thus envisage an empirical understanding of the relationships between a state of anthropological proportions, the way the historical self reacts to them and uses them, and the evaluation made by the historical self about these dialogical relationships. It is at the indistinct point of convergence among these three core elements of the world that I will seek to introduce the phenomenological conception of substance misuse, with all its inevitable contradictions and ambiguities. This conception recognises how complex each act of exogenous consciousness modification is and how different levels of significance of reality are involved every time such an exogenous act takes place. Notwithstanding, the aim is to offer some conceptual instruments to enable greater understanding of this phenomenon.

---

[4] In a strictly phenomenological sense, as we will see throughout the text, the psychopathological alterations induced by substance misuse and said to be psychotic are not actually psychoses, because they are not based on any rupture in the intersubjective constitution of reality (Messas 2015–2016). However, I will use the term as it is already established in the psychopathological literature.

Chapter 6
General Anthropology of Consciousness Modification Through Substance Use – Instantaneity and Exogeneity in Self-Management

The use of substances to modify consciousness must be understood as a sub-set of the general theme of *self-management*, in which a person's positional and value senses are articulated. It is as an instrument of self-management, in which proportions and disproportions are paradoxically articulated, that substance use first appears in people's daily lives. In order to understand self-management by substance use, we must first be familiar with the existential instrumentality given by substance use.

Any modification of the state of consciousness is, first and foremost, an existential movement that starts out from a given state of anthropological proportions towards another (usually fleeting) state caused by the transitory action of a psychoactive drug (Messas 2014b). To understand this act of transformation, we must embark on a comparative investigation between the starting state of anthropological proportions and the transitory condition attained through substance use (Messas 2006) in order to observe the dialectic relationship established between them. This dialectic analysis is fundamental to make sense of the modification of consciousness, since only then can we understand any corresponding vulnerabilities to substance use. The dialectics of the use of substances shows that the central function of any consciousness modification is some form of "ecstasy". Taken in its strict etymological sense, this ex-tatic state reveals the potential for a human to leave itself, ek-stasis, to propel itself outward from a self that is continuous over time, even if this self retains time as a reference for the ecstatic condition itself. Momentary self-modification lies at the heart of substance use, whatever purpose it serves.

This escape from oneself by artificially manufacturing a new proportion is what permits us to identify the acute or synchronic meanings of substance use. *Meaning* should be understood here as the fundamental way in which the acute state of consciousness modification intervenes in the structured existential totality. It is this anthropological positional sense that the historical self seeks to manage by

© Springer Nature Switzerland AG 2021
G. Messas, *The Existential Structure of Substance Misuse*,
https://doi.org/10.1007/978-3-030-62724-9_6

modifying its state of consciousness. For example, the acute state of alcoholic intoxication at a work get-together may serve to reduce the relative value of professional social identities and place more emphasis on personal identities, facilitating people's interactions by diminishing the hierarchy of roles and the restrictions imposed by it. For an initial understanding of the meanings of substance use, a synchronic perspective is more important than a diachronic one. The acute meaning matters more than its chronic consequences, because these are no more than the gradual deformation of the acute meanings. The chronic results of continued substance use do not affect its synchronic definition, since they are nothing but new stable states of anthropological proportions – they constitute an anthropopathology in its own right – and thus no longer belong to the set of synchronic phenomena linked to the use. For example, although a state of alcohol withdrawal is evidently the result of the overlapping of countless experiences of intoxication, it is not a state of inebriation, anthropologically speaking. It lacks the essence of intoxication as I understand it here, which I shall present below.

The essence of consciousness modification as self-management consists of two simultaneous and associated elements: a *sudden shift* in anthropological proportions, which is brought about *independently* of the person's existential situation, their immediate context. It is an experience of the sudden displacement of anthropological proportions associated with the experience this brings about from outside of interpersonal relations and the surrounding world. By this, I mean that regardless of the psychological state, we are in or whoever we are with, if we drink an entire bottle of wine, for example, our anthropological proportions will change. I call this form of modification of anthropological proportions exogenous. I will now examine each essential component of consciousness modification separately.

The suddenness of the modification of the state of consciousness is what makes it so important in the historical self's management of its anthropological proportions. Of course, this suddenness should not be measured quantitatively in terms of seconds, minutes or hours. Rather, it should be understood as an existential movement that offers a maximum of response to the decisions of the historical self. Contradicting the conclusions that a moralistic conception may lead to, what generally prompts substance use is actually the speed with which it can render a change in anthropological proportions. In anthropological terms, substance use enables the historical self to see itself as a powerful self-manager, for with an act of free will (as long as it still is free), it can dictate its own fundamental proportions. The almost immediate relaxation provided by a benzodiazepine in the face of devastating news, for example, shows how much power is concentrated in the hands of the historical self to manage its own proportions with substances, reducing the retention linked to the bad news and proportionally increasing the hope contained in protention. The notion of sudden here must therefore be understood from its relationship with the state of anthropological proportions immediately prior to the act of consciousness modification – the point of reference from which the historical self wishes to diverge.

Consequently, two temporalities coexist for the substance user's historical self.[1] The historical self experiences the substance-induced modified state simultaneously with the characteristics of the prior temporality (which are maintained in retention except in very extreme cases of intoxication). Although the modified state may totally fill the experiential field at a given time, its position in the whole existence only acquires meaning in dialogue with the previous state, which still underlies it (e.g. someone who is drunk still knows what rules of conduct they are disrespecting). There is no modification of consciousness without a dialectic between a typical, relatively stable existential structure and an experience that modifies the previous proportions. The previous state of proportions modulates the way consciousness is modified. The most convincing evidence of this statement can be found in the well-known variability in the effects of drunkenness according to the individual's previous mental state (Ray et al. 2009; Franzen et al. 2018). The same intake that causes euphoria one day may only produce drowsiness on another.

This relationship between a state before and after substance use is the key to its self-management function, as the dividing line between healthy and problematic self-management (abuse and dependence) is intimately related to the dividing line between a significant relationship with a previous state and the loss of this relationship. Self-management by substance use is healthy only as long as it brings about a temporary modulation of anthropological proportions, affecting the person's habitual personality style. Inevitably, the personality style is what dictates the meanings of substance use in anthropologically normal situations. Once the effect has passed, the personality returns to its basic style of anthropological proportions. On the other hand, when the stimuli obtained from using a substance serve only to reduce the discomfort produced by its absence – classic abstinence syndrome, when a person drinks to avoid getting irritable because of a lack of alcohol – we can no longer say this is self-management in the sense I intend here.[2]

The notion of the exogenous origin of a psychic phenomenon has a long history in classical psychopathology (Bonhoeffer 1917), albeit being recognised more for the obscurity of its meanings than for the help it brought to the differentiation of psychopathological phenomena (Messas 2013). In synthesis, it indicates a mental pathology that does not originate from the internal logic of the mind itself and is therefore physiopathologically based on some somatic cause external to the mind and isolated from the body. In this sense, depression caused by hypothyroidism is seen as an exogenous disorder, whilst melancholia, whose somatic basis is unknown,

---

[1] The focus here is on consciousness modifications that have some meaning for the totality of existence, in its healthy or pathological state. As such, any pharmacological alteration whose physiological effect is so great that it incapacitates consciousness itself, reducing it, in its neurological sense, is of no interest here.

[2] It is true that in broad terms, this case could still be referred to as self-management, as the historical self becomes intoxicated voluntarily to reduce an unpleasant effect. However, in the stricter existential sense of a decision to regulate the anthropological proportions of existence, it does not seem to me to apply.

is endogenous. The notion of exogenous is usually defined by its opposition to endogenous rather than by some intrinsic characteristic. There is a clear dualistic simplification in the division of the origins of psychic phenomena between exogenous and endogenous. However, its distinction remains very important for comprehending the anthropological meaning of mental disorders phenomenologically, from melancholia (Tellenbach 1983) to substance-induced psychoses (Messas 2015–2016; Martinotti et al. 2015; Orsolini et al. 2019). Exogeneity defines a type of connection between psychic events which Jaspers called a causal relationship (Jaspers 1997). Causal relationships follow the logic of the natural sciences and allow the explanation of psychopathological phenomena. In the complex realm of psychopathological experiences, psychic events are explained either by causality or by motivation. In this second case, the relationships between phenomena are comprehended by the humanities, which investigate the internal, psychological meanings that exist between them. More often than not, the relationships between psychic events are guided by a mixture of relationships that are simultaneously causal-exogenous and comprehensible-endogenous.

It is essential to bear in mind the conception of this hybrid origin of psychological phenomena, whether pathological or not, in order to understand the meaning of modifications of consciousness. Given that every human experience is defined by a positional sense, an inescapable primal meaning, it is impossible for any consciousness modification not to have some overall meaning for all existence. However, the primal force from which this modification springs is exerted from outside the primordial attunement between the self-pole and the world-pole. The pressure exerted by the substance reaches the anthropological proportions of existence from its outer depth, transcendent to the intersubjectivity that constitutes reality. Therein lies the source of all its power: the self-management obtained by exogenous action provides each human existence a glimpse of semi-divinity, offering it a fleeting experience of supremacy over its own fate, inescapably bound to others, history and the society to which it belongs.

This primal exogenous force, however, within the limits in which there is consciousness, never reaches the structure of existence in a pure state, in the linear action of biological causality, untainted by the person's existential situation. All its consequences are modulated by the style of anthropological proportions of each individual existence, so the exogenous effect, in substance use, is generally limited to a tendency that is only moderately specific in terms of consciousness modification. The exogenous action of substances can only render a general tendency, which is complemented by the meaning the modification is given when it is assimilated by the totality of the existence. It is these exogenous tendencies that the historical self manages when it turns to substance use for the purposes of self-management.

In general, we might say, then, that alcohol tends to facilitate distension in interpersonal relationships (Sayette et al. 2012), cocaine tends to increase productivity in relation to the world (Frone 2008) and cannabis tends to decrease involvement with others and with the world (Janowsky et al. 1979; Wycoff et al. 2018). However, only by observing how they present to each person, with their unique types, can we ascertain whether this general trend is confirmed or not. Although one of the main purposes of employing the exogenous force of substances is to phenomenologically amplify the contact interface with the intersubjective world, enhancing personal relationships, for example, from an anthropological point of view, this force produces a movement of intersubjective enlargement that comes from outside the structure of existence. A movement whose origin means it is initially unreliant on any fundamental or profound synchronicity with otherness and the world. There is therefore an ambiguous and risky statement of individual independence in every act of intoxication. An independence which, whenever it affirms its unreliance on others for the full execution of life, denies itself vital contact with the lifeblood on which it intimately depends to exist in its own right. Self-management through exogenous alterations of anthropological proportions thus encapsulates several of the most dramatic ambiguities of human existence.

In the multiple formulations of the myth of Dionysus (Bacchus in Roman mythology), the god of wine and theatre, Greco-Roman mythology represents all the contradictions inherent to the power that intoxication (in this case, drunkenness) brings to the human being. The most paradoxical of the Greek gods deceitfully insinuates himself as a god in the midst of humans, embodying the opposites that appear in them and directly influencing their lives.[3] Dionysus is the god that leads to the expansion of human horizons but also their destruction. He is a god (and therefore immortal) who rarely appears together with other gods and only tolerates the company of mortal mythological figures, half human, half animal (like satyrs and sileni), or wild and irrational ones, like nymphs and maenad, but always human. He is the simultaneous vehicle of human ascension to the dimension of the divine, to enthusiasm (literally, "possessing the god within oneself", "carried by a divine fury"), and his fall into the deformity of the pure beast. The Dionysian myth visually expresses, in the full sight of humans, the wealth of complexities they must orchestrate in themselves, the riches and flaws inherent to the *conditio humana*. Indeed, Dionysius is the Greek god who is most visual in his manifestations, a *deus praesentissimus*. The self-management that substance-induced consciousness modification enables is thus Dionysian in its nature, inasmuch as it makes explicit, as the Christian myth already foretold, the radical nature of human life, divided between irreconcilable extremes, between its participation in the divine, capable of fully managing itself, and its reduction to the animal, under the sway of natural instincts, blind to reason.

The Dionysian dimension of existence is therefore the one that encapsulates the dialectics of all the possibilities of managing anthropological proportions we have seen up to now and which underpin the possibility of any existence. That is why a psychopathology of substance misuse only makes any sense if we know the conditions of possibility of all pathologies, anthropological and structural: it is inherently a modification of anthropological proportions, sometimes self-imposed, sometimes

---

[3] This brief interpretation of the Dionysian myth is based on Carpenter & Faraone (Carpenter and Faraone 1993) *Masks of Dionysius*. Cornell University Press, 1993, especially the chapter "He has a God in Him: human and divine in the modern perception of Dionysus". Heinrichs A, pp13–43.

automated by the needs of the pathologies themselves and only acquires deep meaning when the disproportions that feed the pathologies and with which they relate are known. A psychopathology of substance misuse that is limited to the description of the associated behaviours – quantitative (quantity of substances used), qualitative (narrowed repertoire), pragmatic (relational or social losses due to substance use) or somatic (tolerance and withdrawal) – will only touch on the complexity of the anthropological phenomenon that is substance use and misuse.

Chapter 7
Specific Anthropology of Vulnerabilities, Substance Misuse, Addiction and Secondary Psychoses

7.1 Temporality

Temporality is fundamental for understanding all experiences related to substance use, and, *a fortiori*, misuse (Messas et al. 2019b). From a temporal perspective, the main purpose of a voluntary act of substance use is to remove oneself from the habitual conditions of biographical temporality. Consciousness modification therefore reflects a search for new proportions of anthropological proportions, a new expression of existence (Messas 2014b) in which the dialectics between present, retention and protention might be modified by the historical self. For example, say somebody has a few drinks with friends after a demanding day's work. Their purpose in doing this is to temporarily release themselves from the worries of their job. By engaging in an experience that is intense and isolated in the present, they temporarily cut off any connection with the recent past, which, from an existential perspective, may be salutary. However, if retention is reduced to such an extent that all sense of social protocol is lost (e.g. a person who drives under the influence and thereby breaks the law and puts third parties at risk), this self-management can be defined as harmful.

The possibility of instantly managing the dimensions of temporality interacts ambiguously with existence itself, sometimes enabling its expansion, sometimes its deconstruction. The capacity to move one's own temporal foundation grants the historical self unusual Dionysian powers over the plasticity of temporality – the ways the dimensions of retention, present and protention are articulated. And, as we will see below, this power extends through temporality to affect the other conditions of possibility of existence. It is the existential meaning of this self-mastery of the proportions of temporality that makes it harmful, productive or ambiguous.

© Springer Nature Switzerland AG 2021
G. Messas, *The Existential Structure of Substance Misuse*,
https://doi.org/10.1007/978-3-030-62724-9_7

7.1.1   The Management of Existential Imbalance – Longitudinal Temporality in Youth as an Example of Deconstructive Creativity

It is well known that youth is one of the stages of life that is most vulnerable to risky and harmful substance use. Most substance use disorders begin between adolescence and early adulthood (Poudel and Gautam 2017), although their consequences may extend throughout life. While there are some clear existential differences between a 12-year-old boy and a 25-year-old adult in terms of their ability to decipher the world, I will examine them together because, in terms of the style of anthropological proportions that bring existential significance to their modification of consciousness, they are each at one end of a spectrum. The adolescent can be understood as the entry point to this spectrum and the young adult as the exit point. They are, respectively, the least and most mature representations of a style of anthropological disproportion that I will call *temporal imbalance*. Temporal imbalance is best understood from the longitudinal perspective of temporality, as it is a mode by which existence experiences the style of longitudinal proportions I call dawning (part I). (It also overlaps with flourishing, but, as it is mitigated at this stage, here, I focus solely on dawning.) It is in this existential sense that I want to explore it here, above all to indicate that one of the main existential vulnerabilities concerning substance use is inherent in the natural process of biographical development, and in this sense is part and parcel of the risks of being. Let us see its characteristics.

Temporal imbalance occurs during the triumphal but unstable stage of entry to a new cycle of potentialities and multiple forms of life. Essentially, the imbalance of youth is the abandonment of childhood anthropological proportions for a new temporal proportion. In the anthropological state of imbalance, existence weakens or abandons the centre that has been its anchor until then and seeks to extend the possibility of existing to the utmost. This movement of excessive protentive plasticity leads to a weakening of the rooting of existence in the present. Existential protention and creativity – everything that is to come – become more valuable than anything there is in the present moment, leading to increased instability and the oscillation of existence. And so we have adolescence as irreverent, unstable, passionate, deceitful, surprising, flippant, cruel and romantic.

This weakening or abandonment of habitual anthropological proportions opens the door to a wide gamut of possibilities of existing. For the young person, protention is a wide, almost unlimited territory, so vast that it does not seem to connect with the present. This vastness allows them to imagine themselves doing any job or living anywhere in the world. The fundamental disproportion of temporal imbalance is hyperprotention. Hyperprotention means excessive openness to new existential possibilities in conjunction with excessive plasticity and openness to new anthropological formations. When this imbalance is at play, the forms of existence become volatile, which can be expressed by extreme inventiveness and the capacity to renew life projects, leading to the successive abandonment of incorporated identities and relationships in the name of new relationships and identities with limited involvement in the personal history. For example, a young person may quickly change their life plans, giving up some acquired skill or turning their back on a network of social relations, all for the sake of a new dream. They may flow seamlessly into devotion to new, previously unfamiliar activities and identities. They are swept along by the seduction of the new, turning their back on their historical roots.

However, this loss of historical roots leads to greater existential vulnerability, since existence itself is no longer guided by any existential thread (a role usually played by the family or parents in childhood or adolescence). The loss of the external element as a guide for behaviour differentiates the anthropology of imbalance from the anthropology of borderline disproportions (Sect. 3.1). Individuals with this latter disproportion will always be guided by an all-powerful other, while, in the temporal imbalance, there are several alternatives for conducting life, ranging from group membership – typical of youth – to no guidance at all, passing through great passions of an amorous, political or other nature which illuminate the biographies of young people. The imbalanced existence may not allow either the values of the historical self or the action of an important other to serve as a guide for their biographical development and may thereby face enormous existential risk, including the risk of substance misuse. Indeed, there are strong indications in the literature that the absence of parental influences or membership of a cohesive group increases the chance of substance misuse (Baker 2005; Dingle et al. 2015). However, it is important to point out that a state of imbalance that needs a powerful other around which to orient itself is anthropologically reminiscent of borderline disproportion. It is no coincidence, then, that many borderline behaviours are passed off as childish.

The great instability of the relations between what one is rooted in, where one intends to go and what must be done in the present moment makes the exogenous modification of the state of consciousness extremely important existentially. As the existential state is extremely pliable, the power of exogenous action to engender existential alterations through intoxication is very great. In other words, what a young person in a state of temporal imbalance is capable of experiencing when intoxicated – elated about their future, or appreciative of their peers at a party – differs from what an adult person is capable of in the same situations. I do not mean that an adult does not experience euphoria when they are intoxicated with friends; I merely mean that because the young person does not yet have sedimented layers of experiences that will give density to their biography, the alterations they can achieve from intoxication affect their existence far more radically than they do in adulthood. There is an unparalleled overtone of potency in the young man who gets drunk to approach women, for example. There is something attractive in testing oneself in this radical experimentation with a life that is still more about learning than refining, with its tenuous levels of commitment, that the adult cannot match. The imbalanced person's capacity to invent their own identity makes the exogenous modification of consciousness a real, effective attraction for a life in which everything is possibility, experimentation, plasticity and innovation. The existential function of substances in the temporal imbalance of youth is therefore ambiguous. This ambiguous influence of substances on youth is what also makes them risky.

(a) **Synergy and Antagonism of Self-Management in the Instability of Existence**

There are two basic ways in which self-management by substance use can affect the instability of existence: either in synergy with the basic anthropological proportions or against them. I will give an example of each case.

The first example demonstrates how great an effect substances can have on the anthropological proportions of a young person through synergic action. Paul, 19 years of age, had problems with substance abuse in early adolescence, but in the last 2 years he has recovered completely and is able to reflect on the existential function of its use: "I really liked drugs because they cleared my mind of worries. They gave me more space to find out things, new ideas, new interests. Drugs drove me to be better" because they "helped me to focus on my interest; I didn't think about life, I thought about the moment".

From the perspective of the value senses of the historical self, the patient felt that the balance of substance use in his life was positive for some time, despite the associated problems. Between losing control of himself from time to time and being able to handle his own sense of the world as he wished, the patient did not hesitate to value the second option, since it provided him with an anthropological disproportion that foregrounded the novelties of the world. This possibility of producing novelty is a fundamental aspect of the self-management of states of imbalance[1] and one of the main reasons why exogenous modification is so attractive to people who live under this temporal influence. By modifying their anthropological proportions, they can be better than before, as the whole range of experiences available to them is enriched. There is a synergy between the interests and values of the historical self and the exogenous effects caused by the substance. And not only does the substance enable novelties to emerge, but it also shines a spotlight on this novelty in consciousness, allowing life to centre around these new objects, as the patient puts it. The power of renewal of the historical self and the force granted to it by a simple exogenous act are so strong that, despite the potentially hazardous consequences of excessive use, living Dionysically continues to be this young man's option of choice. Between the creative force which these experiences spawned and their deconstructive power, this young man understandably opted for the former.

The second example allows us to identify a typical situation of self-management in borderline people, where antagonism is sought in order to alleviate the sufferings inherent to this form of disproportion. Lucas, 28, was recognised as borderline when he was 16 years old. At the time of the interview he was hospitalised, having attempted suicide after a break-up. He had repeatedly slashed his wrists when he had gone through strife in his relationships. He explained that by cutting himself he could replace the diffuse psychological pain with the focused pain of self-inflicted physical injury. His sentimental life had always been turbulent even though he had good social relationships, was intelligent, and had a close group of friends. He

---

[1] We will see later how the opposite occurs in other temporal forms, such as exhaustion, when the essential function of exogenous modification is to maintain existence or to produce some value for the exhaustion wrought by the repetition of similar experiences.

usually lived well and enjoyed life, but then he would suddenly be taken over by the pains of life and get carried away in emotional outbursts. He stressed that it was the suddenness of his pain that made it unbearable. He was open about his liking for cannabis, saying it relaxed him like nothing else could. Accordingly, he used it frequently and was unable to report any social loss resulting from it; indeed, he claimed that it made his world more stable and enjoyable, regulating the excessive oscillations of his disproportion. For Lucas, the effect of cannabis was stabilising in the face of the excessive temporal malleability of his conditions of possibility. The exogenous effect of cannabis served to counterbalance the intense value with which Lucas pre-reflexively experienced the intersubjective world. By reducing the value of otherness, intoxication paradoxically enabled Lucas to live in this world with a degree of ontological security to develop as an autonomous person. The antagonism of anthropological proportions is a self-management mechanism widely used by borderline people, and is consistent with the epidemiological findings which frequently associate borderline personality disorders with substance misuse (Lane et al. 2016; Trull et al. 2018).

(b) **Risks of Consciousness Modification in Temporal Imbalance – Biographical Indifferentiation and Psychosis**

The transformative action of substances on anthropological proportions joins forces with hyperprotention in states of temporal imbalance, exacerbating existential instability. Here, self-management takes on its most Dionysian face, permitting the historical self to modify temporal proportions in such a way that there may not be enough structural stability for the experiences to be sedimented in the biography. Paradoxically, too much experimentation with oneself turns existence into an endless testing ground where no conditions for personal historical cohesion arise. Seen from this perspective, engaging in chronic intoxication means shutting oneself off from vital temporalisation and becoming prey to an existential instability which, from a certain point on, is warped into the annulment of genuine temporality. The deconstructive nature of acts of consciousness modification will, over time, prevent the sedimentation that is needed for historicisation. This sedimentation is fundamental for preserving the dynamics of the dialectical regime of anthropological proportions and ultimately enabling the maturation of the individual's personality traits. Thus, paradoxically, the various welcome attempts to temporally readjust the imbalance are, as it were, washed away every time they occur, culminating in an inability to retain even the healthy innovation embedded in the disequilibrium itself, as if all existence was stuck in de-historicised disequilibrium. The abuse of Dionysian power turns against the historical self, stripping it of the capacity for biographical maturation.

The result of this refusal to engage in the personal history is *biographical indifferentiation*, which manifests in the difficulty many substance misusers have in maturing, seen in their inability to maintain stable professional or love relationships (Frone 2004, 2008; Wilson et al. 2019), to adhere to treatment (Sansone and Sansone 2008; Brorson et al. 2013) or to take on many responsibilities in life. Maturation is a typical form of expansion, marked by the continuous, gradual transformation of the human's basic configurations of temporality, spatiality and intersubjectivity (Messas 2010b). From the perspective of temporality alone, for this to happen, certain elements of retention must be abandoned so that new experiences can be admitted and so that the proportions of temporal dimensions can be rebalanced. For example, the dimension of protention is more powerful in adolescence than in old age, when the dimension of retention is more pronounced. It is this capacity for rebalancing that allows human beings to go through each phase of their life effectively. Substance misuse can prevent this structural remodelling of existence, hampering entry into different phases of life and resulting in an existence that falls short of its potential, becoming lost in inauthenticity. An immature person is like someone who did not get the right costume to be invited to a party. They are sure something good will happen at the party, they appreciate it, they would like to be part of it, but they remain on the outside, dejected and hoping that one day they can join in.[2]

In their relations with longitudinal temporality – an inevitable source of differentiation, which requires irreversible decision-making, the abandonment of certain potentialities of life so that it can be set in a particular biographical direction – the substance misuser chooses not to decide, to refuse temporality, to approach existence as if it were a suspended state of complete surrender to indefinite potentialities (Zutt 1963a). This state in which there are more potentialities than realisations, more alternatives than decisions, marks the dilemmas of the youthful existence where self-management is warped into eternal ambiguity. In this paradoxical option for non-decision-making, substance use is of enormous value. It is an effective instrument for giving material form to this holding back of the biography by transforming it into a succession of unconnected moments. The excessive malleability that consciousness modification gives the historical self in a state of imbalance contains within itself the kernel of annulment of all longitudinal temporality because, while each act of intoxication creates a new world, it prevents this new world from being incorporated into the real world, for which existing inevitably means making oneself in history.

Likewise, this pre-reflexive incapacity for historicisation is the key to understanding the elevated risk of suicidal ideation and suicidal acts in early cannabis (Clarke et al. 2014; Carvalho et al. 2019) and alcohol users (Bagge and Sher 2008; Wang and Yen 2017). The alternative of suicide stems from an overly unstable temporality, where protention is not maintained strongly enough for the historical self to continue on its path. In moments of existential difficulty, the historical self anchors onto the possibility of glimpsing a future – the prerequisite for the human capacity to experience hope. Continued temporal imbalance resulting in dehistoricising timelessness reduces the capacity to experience hope. It is very important to point out that this phenomenon is not the result of a depressive state. In this, the meaning of existence is lost (see Sect. 3.8). In a temporal imbalance involving protentive instability, what is lost is protention but without any corresponding loss of

---

[2] Indifferentiation by immaturity is therefore different from the fossilisation of existence, which we will see below (7.1.3). In this case, there is no such experience of a valuable world in relation in which the historical self is insignificant.

meaning for existence. In this curious psychopathological formation, the historical self does not see any perspective that justifies living on, even though it knows what senses move life. In clinical practice for adolescents and young adults, it is not unusual for suicide attempts to occur in the absence of a depressive background mood (Simon et al. 2001). When interviewing the patient, the psychopathologist is told that the idea was transitory, opaque even to them, sometimes motivated by some break-up but sometimes with no clear reason. This mysterious type of suicidal ideation can be understood by the volatility with which protention disappears in existences that, due to early onset of substance use, present problems in their historicisation processes.

This imbalance, lacking even a minimum of support for the maintenance of a stable state, is also a potential precursor for the psychoses that arise in states of temporal imbalance. For example, it is in this existential period that the two major structural pathologies, schizophrenia and bipolar affective disorder, tend to be manifest. Since temporal imbalance of itself destabilises the temporal articulations of existence, substance use does not necessarily have to be chronic to generate psychosis, although more often than not it is associated with a continuous state of use (Marconi et al. 2016). For substance use to harm the structure of existence, it is enough for the broken forms of hyperprotention it stimulates to collide with a weakness in the intersubjective constitution of reality. This weakness, whose causes and reasons have not been established by science, makes the integrity of existential temporality particularly weakened in its capacity to accommodate the sedimentation of experiences in personal history. Substance use in this existential period, especially cannabis (Radhakrishnan et al. 2014; Thorpe et al. 2020), has the same kind of effect as this structural weakness, potentiating the effects of the atemporalising pharmacological action. Taken to the extreme, this synergy damages the integrity of the experience of reality, which is manifested in (often irreversible) psychosis (Kawohl and Rüssler 2008; Mustonen et al. 2018). It cannot be said that schizophrenic psychoses that appear during times of temporal imbalance are caused by cannabis use (when it exists); however, the frequent association between these two elements suggests that cannabis has the anthropological function in this pathology of propitiating dehistoricisation precisely at a time when it should not be stimulated.

(c) **Temporal Balance and Substance Misuse**

Although in this section I have emphasised how temporal imbalance influences self-management via substance use, there are existential conditions which, even if there is a proportional balance between the dimensions of temporality, may nonetheless culminate in potentially serious substance misuse. These conditions are observed primarily in social groups for whom substance use is common practice. In this case, the positional sense that inspires the historical self to repeatedly use substances is quite simply (and appropriately) the acceptance of and participation in the values of a group. Peer pressure is a factor often associated with substance-induced self-management (Bot et al. 2005; Chan et al. 2017). The continued effect of intoxication, fruit of this sociocultural practice, can lead to changes in anthropological proportions that gradually take on a dimension which is incompatible with the biographical development according to the person's own value senses of the person themselves.

7.1.2 Longitudinal Temporality in Existential Exhaustion – Management of Isolation in the Present

From a longitudinal point of view, a second existential state which substance use is often associated with is exhaustion (Sect. 2.1.2). As I mentioned earlier, longitudinal exhaustion is typical of the most serious pathologies, such as schizophrenia – in which there is a complete exhaustion of existence – or critical existential conditions – where an entire partial identity ceases to offer any meaning to existence – which are identified semiologically with anthropopathological depression. Although structurally speaking there is a clear difference between schizophrenic exhaustion and exhaustion associated with serious depression or existential crisis, for the purposes of the discussion in this section, they can be examined together. The reason for this is that they are both comparable in terms of how the dimensions of temporality are articulated with each other. Therefore, the focus herein will be on examining how the historical self handles substance use when faced with a typical temporal configuration of exhaustion. Exhaustion presents a circular relationship with substance misuse. While it is a longitudinal state that results from severe mental disorders and for that reason requires consciousness modification as self-management, it can also arise as a sequela of substance misuse. We have already seen how substance misuse can modify the capacity of existence to direct the development of its own biography. One of the ways in which substance misuse in imbalance evolves to an annulment of biographical temporalisation is precisely by the exhaustion of existence. Thus, in serious cases of addiction (see below), it is not unusual to observe clinical conditions typical of exhaustion, such as indifference to life or inability to structure a life project. In such cases, substance use starts to function circularly as an element in the management of harm caused by substance use itself. To understand cases like this better and to understand the significance of substance use in these existences, it is necessary to know the temporal articulation of exhaustion.

As already defined above, exhaustion is characterised by the isolation of the present in relation to retention and protention. With this dismantling of the form of temporality, there is a loss of the capacity to find any meaning by which to exist and, consequently, a living historical basis to which to belong. This limitation of existence to the present time means self-management is restricted to the operationalisation of phenomena belonging to the present. Therefore, in order to understand the meanings of consciousness modification in exhaustion, it is first necessary to understand the temporal characteristics of an existence limited to the present, since this is what has to be managed.

An exhausted existence has lost its capacity to project itself into the future. It can no longer experience anything beyond the circle of things already experienced, which lends all experiences a sense of suffocating and vicious reproduction, in which the freshness of novelty inherent to each experience, even recurring ones, is not felt. To be exhausted means to no longer experience the world as a field of possibilities, since the present, cut off from its protentive and retentive projections, loses the capacity to renew itself through the influxes of the future and to lean on the reliability of the past. To be exhausted also means having nowhere to escape to in memory and tradition. Frequently, severe substance abusers manifest the feeling of not belonging to anything else: to their family, their society, their historical era (Flores 2011; Dingle 2018). They spend their lives in their rooms, devoting themselves to minor activities that they feel are unproductive or irrelevant not only to themselves but also to others. Or they imagine other worlds, generally happier and fairer ones but do not engage in their construction. Although they want to break with reality, they remain impassive and alien to it. They move away from the world, only to recreate it in their imagination. An example of the latter can be seen in the story of a patient in our clinic, a serious cannabis abuser. Although he has abstained from the drug and wants never to use it again and to change his life completely, all he does is pass his time in his bedroom and take part in activities at the clinic. During treatment, he prepared a complex plan for a fairer world. In it, money would no longer be needed because people would be able to get around by taking free rides. Although this elaboration did not present any psychotic traits, it did not lead to anything during treatment, either. He talked a lot about his plan, presented it in its every detail but never lifted a finger to execute it.

This phenomenon of radical narrowing of the range of available experiences correlates with the *tedium vitae* of these patients. Imprisoned in the present, in a way neither guilt nor nostalgia can they experience. Their exhausted existence can only be maintained by the repeated production of the same, identical experiences, images and ideas, without these connecting with the other temporal strata of life, neither taking inspiration from the reserves of retention nor functioning as impetus for protention.

Since existence is anchored too strongly in the present, the main force capable of keeping it unified – or artificially maintaining it with a modicum of unity – is exogenous stimulation. In this case, the exaltation of the present is sought out not as a force to galvanise existential possibilities (imbalance) but in the absence of alternatives. The exalted present of exhausted people is neither euphoric nor relaxed nor happy. It simply is. The intention of an exhausted existence does not extend beyond achieving a modicum of life, for which intoxication is particularly effective. It is for its function in the maintenance of the structural unity of existence *tout court* that we understand the apparently contradictory – but very frequent – use of cannabis (Green et al. 2005; Hunt et al. 2018) or alcohol abuse (Subramaniam et al. 2017; Hunt et al. 2018) in schizophrenics, for example. For these people, as existence flails in the quicksands of exhaustion, intoxication remains the last route to some vital stimulus, even though it may worsen the pathological condition (increasing experiences of delusion, for example). Staying alive as an existential unit is, after all, more important than staying healthy.

In the existential conditions of exhaustion, the historical self fights a difficult battle with itself. Self-management is faced with the extreme situation of having exogenous modification at its disposal as an ultimate tool to maintain some unity of meaning for existence. The decision-making that the historical self has to face is thus radical: either filling existence by artificial means or resigning itself to annul-ment in a voided present. Usually, this radical alternative leaves the patient with little choice but to opt for the artificial exaltation of the present. However, in several situations, continued substance use compromises the decision-making capacity because the exogenous exaltation of the present is accompanied by (sometimes sig-nificant) clinical deterioration. The decisions are then restricted to choosing the lesser of the evils. Now, it is up to the clinician, together with his/her patient, to find a way to choose some alternative from the available options, either undesirable or inviable. This clinical assistance for patients in exhausted situations is perhaps the most difficult activity any mental health clinician has to undertake, since it is no longer based on technical knowledge, but on sharing with their patient the extremes of existence, limit situations, as so well examined by Jaspers (1960).

7.1.3   The Present Continuous of Addiction (and Its Distortions)

The anthropological disproportion that I examine now, along with its typical distor-tions, is the pure psychopathological form that derives from the continuous modifi-cation of consciousness through substance use. The result of continuous substance misuse is substance addiction, whose temporal essence I present below. In addic-tion, there is an anthropological disproportion characterised by a densification of the present, so that the present continuously prevails over the other dimensions (Kemp 2018). I will call this condition *present continuous*. In this state, the present dominates temporality, modifying the participation of retention and protention in each moment of experience.[3] Existence is fixed in this prominence of the present

---

[3] This continued prevalence of the present clearly differentiates addiction from the disproportion of imbalance. In this latter case, the present may prevail at a certain time, say, when a group of friends get together at a party, where they use substances such as alcohol or cannabis. Let us imagine that at that moment, each consciousness completely surrenders to the collective celebration of the pres-ent moment. Everyone involved in the celebration forgets the complexities of life and fraternises in a gesture of unification with a present that may seem eternal. This is in fact an expression of a hyperpresent. However, in imbalance, this is only one of the ways of managing temporality. The same young man (or any other person whose temporality is particularly malleable) who manages temporality in this way may use a substance the next day to forget the present and, in a state of relaxation, experience hope for the future, transporting himself imaginatively to a time of achieve-ments yet to come. This contains a postponement of the fruition of the present in favour of a condi-tion that does not yet exist, but which is envisaged. The self-management of imbalance is about

experience, which absorbs the two other temporal dimensions. Although the retentive and protentive dimensions of existence remain dialectically connected to the present (we are not talking about exhaustion in which the present cuts itself off), they are subordinated to its essential characteristics.

The aspects of distance and virtuality particular to retention and protention are replaced by actualisation, the essence of the present. In its original sense, present means that which is before us ("*prae est*" in Latin). This means that the present offers a stream of actuality, a direct, immediate, unbroken relationship between the self-pole and the world-pole. This form of relationship does not exist in the mediated virtuality inherent to retention (what once was no longer is but still influences what is) and to protention (what is not yet but which attracts the intentionality of what is). In addiction, everything that exists for the subjectivity converges to manifest itself spatially before the "eyes of consciousness" of the historical self.[4] There are no gaps in the experience; it is always about filling and presence. In the same way, as will be seen below, this presentification of the virtualities of temporality impacts not only the spatiality of Dionysian experiences, but also their materiality, since everything that is present and visual is also sensorial and perceptual, to the detriment of the intuitive and imaginative.

As this seamless immediacy characteristic of the present extends to the other dimensions of temporality, it affects their characteristics, making them more likely to appear actual (making them active). If the past normally supports us from afar like a solid, silent buffer that is continuous in its operative virtuality, and if the future normally acts as an active virtual magnet that moves us forward, dissipating somewhat the solidity of the present, now the two dimensions tend towards the centre and by so doing tend to be dilated according to the dictates of the present. A protention that is dragged into the present becomes a hindrance to an experience that wishes to be total, complete, seamless, which wants to do without any independent, creative and, above all, virtual future. This is how we can understand the actualisations of life plans seen in so many patients who abuse substances, particularly stimulants or alcohol. The patients project themes and situations for their future but behave as if this future was already a reality. During hospitalisation, for example, they may talk through with the clinician everything they will do so they can get money to live. As soon as they leave the clinic, they immediately behave as if they had already earned that money, spending more than they can afford and

---

managing a wealth of alternatives. In addiction, it is about the management of restriction, the absence of alternatives and continuously leading life in this temporal style.

[4] Here, it is worth noting that Dionysius is also regarded as the Greco-Roman god of epiphany, that is whose manifestation is marked by visuality (insight). This makes him the least abstract of the gods of this pantheon, the one that depends most on his materiality to be approached by humanity. This is an aspect of the myth that cannot be overlooked when we consider the phenomenon of hyperpresentification in addiction, which focuses all manifestations of the temporal complexity of reality on its present visuality, where all multiplicity is revealed in one fell swoop, literally before the eyes of the one who experiences it. Similarly, it is impossible not to associate this *deus praesentissimus* with the characteristics of the total temporality of mania, whose manifestations closely resemble those of ecstatic intoxication.

disregarding everything they had organised during hospitalisation. The future imagined as something still to be done is warped into something that has already been done, as a continuity of the present, enabling only a relationship of immediate, sensory, physical, material enjoyment and pleasure. It is this assimilation of the virtuality of protention by the actuality of the present continuous that also explains the Dionysian hedonism typical of substance abusers. A life that is only present is a life to which nothing is owed and for which nothing needs to be constructed. Nothing needs to be prepared or awaited, renounced or postponed. Since everything is present, everything is already ready and all that remains existentially is to enjoy the moment.

This *carpe diem* approach is existential decision-making based on a temporality in which the continuous present is indivisible and thus, adialectical, a present that is, in short, paradisiacal. The dialectic that leads existential decisions from the composition of parts is warped in the absence of choice because the absolute whole is always accessible. It is therefore partially misleading to understand addiction in terms of a problem in the free decisions of an individual based on their personal values. Although personal values, spiritual freedom and personality are naturally always in play when we think about an existence, it is important for the psychopathologist to keep in mind that there may be only limited alternatives pre-reflexively available to their patients. The notion of self-management, so helpful for understanding how important intoxication is in substance misuse, loses its *raison d'être* here, since the historical self is now managed by a temporality crushed in the present. A person whose temporality pre-reflexively offers their historical self a continuous present is presented with the possibility of returning to a lost paradise preceding the moment when the human beings, in their curiosity and disobedience, had to start making their own decisions about their life. The option to return to the lost paradise is so clear to the historical self that it is not manifested as a paradox, as doubt or as decision-making tension. The person simply lets themselves be absorbed by the absence of any need to take decisions, which they obtain in the artificial paradise of substances. This comfortable endowment helps us to understand the habitual lies of substance abusers, as well as the guilt-free way they behave when they ignore what they just agreed with their relatives or their clinician, the indifference with which they justify certain acts of violence against people close to them or strangers, the coldness with which they put others at risk when they drink and drive over and over again. The long list of irresponsible behaviours by addicted persons has its anthropological roots in the ease with which they can renounce the dialectics of anthropological proportions for the sake of the present continuous of a paradise rediscovered. For these existences, the future as a field of consequences for behaviour is an undesirable, scary intruder, but one that can be banished with a minimum of effort.

This almost adialectic immersion of the historical self in the present is not, however, without its internal contradictions. Almost always, the historical self is quite aware of the social meanings of what it does. More often than not (as is also the case in the actualisation of retention), it may even be quite immersed in the temporality of the society in which it lives. Thus, it experiences very clearly which social and historical values it must obey. That is why patients who are severe substance abusers or addicts repeatedly justify their irresponsible acts before their family and clinician, often (even sincerely) ask for forgiveness for what they have done and readily submit to the punishments dictated by the society they damage. More than anyone else, they know they have made mistakes and they know what is at stake for those who make mistakes. Nonetheless, the power to dissolve the rules of the dialectical game of life is too close at hand for them to resist indulging in this almost divine capacity. The seductions of the absolute tend to make the decision to choose paradise almost a categorical imperative of renunciation to earthly, partial and ambiguous life. The presentification of retention is also shown in the inflexibility with which addicted existence is linked to its most traditional personal relations, especially the family. When retention becomes solidified in this way, the overall capacity for transformation, for a person to move forward in their biography, is diminished. For example, for us to leave an abusive relationship, not only must the memories of the period be forgotten as much as possible, but also all the influence of this period on our present life (retention, in its broad sense). We have to lose something in order to reconstruct the biography. The retention-turned-actuality in the present continuous is because retention is always being actualised and is overly inflexible, as if existence was stuck in that same past from which it cannot rid itself. In this sense, one could also say that in addiction, retention is stuck in the present. For good or for ill, there is a sclerosis of the dialectic capacity of temporality, which results in the shackling of existence to proximate retention. The main clinical manifestation of this sclerosis is the way addicted patients often remain deeply dependent on their original family, especially their parents or siblings, even in advanced adulthood. It would be mistaken to attribute this behavioural dependence to the idea that only the family will still tolerate the patient after a long trajectory of substance abuse. Although there is some truth in this, it cannot explain the dimension of the issue. Often, the traditional family bonds actually remain too active in the patient's life. For example, the mother's feeling of guilt at what has happened to her child appears extremely vividly in her consciousness. Likewise, the son's feeling of duty towards his parents or his family, even in old age, remains too active, as if the relational style between them had not changed at all over the years. This is not about immaturity, a refusal to enter time, as we saw above in anthropological imbalance; these are patients who do not display juvenile or immature behaviour. Rather, it is about a rigidity in the forms of interpersonal dialectics, which is the only way to explain the extremely conservative dynamic, allowing very little creativity for the parties involved in the relationship. Indeed, it is important to note the strongly conservative aspect of vulnerability in the present continuous. This conservatism runs counter to the hedonistic indifference with which the historical self indulges in the densified present of their addiction, indicating that there are dialectical ambiguities in human existence even in conditions in which the historical self feels empowered to suppress them. This ambiguity stems from the fact that the continuity of the eternal time of paradise encapsulates both indifference in relation to the future (because it does not exist) and slavery in relation to the past (because it does not dissipate). It is because of this indissoluble ambiguity that the same type of person who surrenders themselves Dionysiacally to earthly pleasures without apparent guilt is also one in which suicide rates are high (Yuodelis-Flores and Ries 2015; SAMHSA 2017).

(a) **Present Continuous and Cognitive Losses – Evolution Towards Exhaustion**

In extreme cases, the restriction of existence to the present continuous drifts into exhaustion, or isolation of the present. This state also explains how often cognitive alterations are related to addiction (Domínguez-Salas et al. 2016; Ramey and Regier 2018; Verdejo-Garcia et al. 2019) in its more advanced stages. The capacity of cognition to decipher the meanings in which it is immersed is what enables the historical self to direct itself towards a future in which it is actualised as a person, with all their ambitions, values and strategies. The reduction of protention to the actuality of the present makes the cognitive apparatus superfluous, if not outright undesirable. "What do I need the complexity of the executive functions for if I can remain in a continuous state of pleasure by using cannabis?" these persons seem to think (Crean et al. 2011; Schoeler and Bhattacharyya 2013). What is the point of episodic memory if, by maintaining a drunken state, I can banish from my mind's eye everything that upsets me and only see I want to? (Gunn et al. 2018).

(b) **Distortions of the Present Continuous – Fossilisation of Existence and Psychosis by Condensation**

The existential logic of a life lived in a continuous present is that it rules out the chance of any absence; it is a total time from which the dialectic modifications produced by the flow of time (dissolutive temporality) in the proportions of present, retention and protention are abolished. This is the paradise lost that this existential form envisages. This excessive stability of the temporal structure of existence saps its capacity to transform itself temporally. The blocked mobility of the anthropological proportions produces an existential stiffening in which life is only worth whatever is before the eyes of the historical self or the identity it has always been marked by. The maintenance of this lack of movement over time has psychopathological consequences.

These consequences, often seen in addicted persons, include the maintenance of the same forms of family relationship, the same preferences, the same ways of dressing over the years, even the same forms of behaviour, which may have been edgy decades before but now seem outdated and pointless. At times, they keep telling the same old jokes. This is all indicative of a kind of fossilisation of existence in a certain period of life, which reveals, in a static mode, a particular form of life that was once dynamic and vibrant. This *fossilisation of existence* appears in varying degrees of severity.[5] In its mildest form, it can be seen in chronic substance abusers who do not even cogitate a life project. They are hyperstable. They usually attend alcohol and drug clinics, even after long periods of abstinence. There, they demonstrate a certain abulic indifference to what is going on around them, participate in

---

[5] In a quest to depict a similar experience, Di Petta describes the world of the addict as a frozen world (Di Petta 2019).

the discussion groups, occasionally voice some personal opinion but do not seem engaged with their life or that of their peers. Their temporal dimensions remain locked in the same relative proportion. Their discussions about their future are always the same, their world views do not change, they always react to certain situations the same way, always use the same range of topics and choice of words. The teams of carers may change, the residents responsible for their case may change, but they continue to have the same life projects with no actual starting date. With some metaphorical force, it could be said that the contact with such patients suggests that they just "are"; they are the same, through and through, as if there was no flow to enable some differentiation in their lives. Their identity, such as it is, is similarly immutable over time. It is not that these people are immature, which would mean they would be unable to penetrate a world they feel to be too valuable, beyond their reach. Rather, the hyperstable person inhabits a world in which both they and those with whom they engage do not seem worth changing.

However, in more severe cases, this same phenomenon of fossilisation can have the same disruptive power that a schizophrenic psychosis has over the dynamics of existence. What distinguishes fossilisation from schizophrenic psychosis is that the latter acts secondarily as an anchorage for an existential structure that has fragmented, while fossilisation is the result of the *overstability of segments of existence*, which become calcified simply because they stop moving. The root of schizophrenic psychosis is a rupture of the co-constitution of reality; the root of fossilisation is *excessive condensation*. The psychotic clinical conditions stemming from the fossilisation of existence are therefore different from those of schizophrenics. They are psychoses with a less elaborate content because they are not new significations of reality, admitted with the function of giving it some unity of meaning; they are more hallucinatory and less delusional, precisely because they derive from a densification of reality and so tend to manifest materially, not imaginally. We can therefore refer to them as *psychosis by condensation*.

Psychosis by condensation is mainly hallucinatory, for the following anthropological reasons. A hallucination is a form of perception and is therefore based on present reality, while a delusion is a non-shared form of apprehending the meaning of reality (or lack thereof). It is from an intersubjective perspective that pathological experiences of condensation can be most clearly distinguished from schizophrenia. Typical cases of psychosis by condensation (at least in its milder forms) are those patients who report strange experiences which they credit to their substance use. A patient at the clinic asks me directly whether the images of a saint he has seen during the night in his bedroom are real or are caused by the alcoholism for which he was admitted. Another patient with severe cocaine addiction tells me he was hospitalised because he had started hearing night-time conversations in his kitchen between people he knew were not there. As he knew that every time he took too much cocaine these voices would come back, he realised it was time to go to hospital again and get treated. Patient and psychopathologist share the same world, constitute reality together and are able to discuss on these common bases what happens in the patient's field of perception. In milder cases of *psychosis by condensation*, patient and clinician discuss an event almost in the third person, neutrally, both being similarly qualified to express an opinion on it. In the words of a patient who was trying to explain his evidently altered experience to the clinical team, "it's just like magic, a mix of hallucination and reality".

In more serious cases, the change of perception is associated with a lowering of consciousness, making it appear as if the shared aspect of the world described above is lost, and giving it a delusional-hallucinatory appearance (Di Petta 2014). The most dramatic case of this situation is *delirium tremens*, in which illusions with animals (snakes, spiders) can be accompanied by an atmosphere of persecutory dread which may on the surface resemble delusional schizophrenic persecution. However, even under these conditions, it cannot be said that the ability to grasp the primordial sense of the world has been lost (Binder 1979). Rather, what occurs is that the consciousness of the person suffering from delusional hallucinations is flooded with biological forms, a distortion caused by the overpresence of the usual senses of the world. What explains these experiences is the extreme stimulation of the materiality of the world, not its reduction, as seen in schizophrenic fractures. The psychopathological phenomenon of illusion is based on a modified perception of the world. For example, in the alcohol-induced illusion of the alcohol-dependant person, the intravenous cannula may turn into a serpent. This perception is consistent with the perception of its sinuous cylindrical shape, which is transposed into a sinuous, cylindrical animal. This involves the vivification of a perceptual experience whose foundation is the mutation of inert matter into living matter. It is from the extreme intensification of perception itself that this warped perception is born. (Likewise, it is from the hyperpresentification of existence that perception gains such relevance in consciousness.) The psychopathological kinship of these radical conditions is with epileptic psychosis, not schizophrenia.[6]

Similarly, although they are not linked to perceptions, the hallucinations provoked by LSD or MDMA, for example, have the same pattern of mutating the material density of the world with experiences populated by visuality (colours, tones) or volatility of reality (moving closer and further away) (Di Petta 2016; Orsolini et al. 2019). In these hallucinatory experiences, the historical self is not alone in the world, disconnected from its peers; rather, it has the experience of inhabiting a world that is so material, so full of intense sensations and objects, that the relative value of otherness diminishes. Someone who sees the colour of a lake they are in front of turn violet and an alligator flying out of it towards them cannot devote much attention to the friend who is at their side at that moment.

(c) **Exit from the Present Continuous – Intense Contrast-Induced Reaction**

Although the lost paradise may often seem to be recovered with each act of intoxication that induces a present continuous, this is not a state that can last indefinitely. The action of intoxication is limited, from the perspective of its physiological dynamics. Consciousness modification depends strictly on the causal potential of

---

[6]This work does not intend to go into the extent of the psychopathological kinship between epilepsy, alcoholism and psychosis by condensation. However, there is a wealth of phenomenological literature on this matter: Tellenbach (1970), Dörr (1995) and Minkowska (2007).

the pharmacological act on brain physiology. Exogenous consciousness modification is, from a natural point of view, an acute physical-somatic state that induces temporal alterations. Given that repeated, intense physiological action is needed for it to be maintained, the acute densification of the present does not last for long, dissipating quickly and having to be restored artificially so that the present continuous can continue to be experienced. This biological temporal limitation of exogenous action has consequences that directly interest us here.

Even if the acute pharmacological action is repeated very frequently and intensely, as is seen in addiction, at some point it ends. When this happens, the present continuous is inevitably left and the historical self must submit to the dialectics of temporality that govern human life.[7] Structurally, giving up exogenous action implies giving up a tendency to immortalise oneself in the present continuous and returning to the habitual temporality of the everyday biography, albeit disturbed by a densification of the present. These two temporal forms are diverse. Exiting pharmacological action is therefore a state of *contrast* in the temporal dimensions of the existence, a path back from quasi-atemporality to temporality.

No matter how long the historical self may have been marooned in the annulment of self-management, as long as there is life, sooner or later it must face and deal with the uncertainties of the future. However, while held in thrall by the present continuous, the historical self will have grown accustomed to going to any lengths to obstruct protention and prioritise a paradisiacal stability rooted in a total present. The historical self loses its capacity to manage its biography in the face of the turbulences coming from protention. It is precisely because it has immersed itself in an artificial continuous present, fixing existence in a single temporal form, that the hyperpresent historical self unlearns how to manage the complexities of temporality. Its existence ends up being divided between a present continuous and its total negative, a world of absolute instability that is far too complex to be managed. Renewed contact with this temporalised world is therefore experienced as terrifying contact with chaos, prompting extreme reactions marked by agitation, irritability or even aggression and paranoid experiences. It is worth mentioning that these reactions appear in people apparently qualified to deal with even more complex and difficult situations. Usually, catastrophic reactions are seen in patients with dementia who are unable to understand the world because of their cognitive impairment and so become agitated and aggressive, as if conjuring up the dread of a stranger they often know they were once able to overcome. But the cases I want to point out here are different and less dramatic than these more advanced cases of dementia because they occur in patients with no substantial cognitive impairment. In these cases, the catastrophic reactions originate in existential temporal restrictions (although typical catastrophic reactions, with cognitive deficits, also occur in addiction).

---

[7] It is important to note that this return to the dialectics of temporality takes place in an existence densified into a present continuous. Thus, when a patient exits an acute state, they will enter an existence that is stiffened, not fully temporalised. Nonetheless, there is still some return to a reality rooted in the dimensions of time.

These are, for example, situations in which patients without any apparent phobic disproportion in their personality react with dread at the slightest stimulus. For example, a 50-year-old patient who was successful in his professional area but had a history of severe alcoholism decided to admit himself to hospital. The attending physician accompanied him to the clinic, prepared his hospitalisation, and observed that his mental state on admission was perfect, with no lowering of consciousness nor any acute sign of his problem with alcohol. When everything was prepared, the physician was made to leave the clinic. The patient then suddenly became agitated, shouting that he felt threatened, that she had left him in a dump and that if she did not get him out of there he would kill her. The physician went back in to the clinic and as soon as she encountered the patient, he immediately calmed down and apologised for what he had done minutes earlier. He said that he did not know why it had happened, but that it had occurred all of a sudden (and was inconsistent with a panic attack). The moment of exiting the present continuous is extremely dangerous, for it brings forth the *contrast* between a temporality that is densified in the present and the three-pronged temporality that remain in the existence of addicted persons. I believe that contrast is the central experience that explains such excessive behaviour. It can therefore be seen as an *intense contrast-induced reaction.*

To better understand this experience, it is important to establish how it differs from fear, for which it may be mistaken. As we have seen in phobic disproportions (Sect. 3.2), fear springs from the excessive amplitude of the world and from otherness, leaving the self-pole feeling too weak to deal with the challenges of daily life. For there to be fear, there must be considerable pre-reflexive spatiality in a field of experience; the world must be felt as something too big to be inhabited safely. That is not the case here. An intense contrast-induced reaction is not triggered by the vastness of experience or even the experience of a powerful otherness (in the example given, the patient bullied and threatened the doctor, not without an air of superiority); it is based merely on the fact that time is now rolling into the future again and the historical self has to deal with this new element, time, which terrifies it because it no longer knows how to live in a zone of indetermination, where things are ambiguous, probabilistic and cannot be captured in a single sensory moment, as occurs in the present continuous. The experience an addicted person has when they exit the acute state of intoxication is like the experience of a person stranded compassless in a totally foreign land, although in their case rather than facing an unknown space and its terrors, what they have to face is time and its unpredictability. But the intense contrast-induced reaction does not have to be exemplified using such a dramatic case. Another classic case of this anthropopathological state typical of addiction is that of the patient who, faced with a new endeavour in life that is important for their recovery, has a major relapse and returns to point zero of treatment. The new endeavour, usually discussed with the clinician, team and family, is often coherent with the patient's life plans and often nurtured for a long time. It is simply the fact that it is new, based on the virtuality of an as yet non-existent future, that produces such great existential instability.[8] Launched directly into contact with a temporality

---

[8] In this sense, this imbalance is similar to hyperprotention, examined above.

that is no longer only present, the historical self feels an overwhelming need to return to the continuous, dense, all-encompassing present it is used to. This it achieves by *relapsing* into substance use. The ease with which addicted people relapse into substance abuse in the face of any difficulty in life is thus explained by two fundamental, intermingling anthropological conditions acting in synergy. I have just presented the first of them, the contrast-induced reaction. We will see the second below.

(d) **Ambiguities of the Present Continuous – Dialectics of Unstable Stability in Addicted Persons**

The extended permanence of temporal stability in the present continuous sought in a Dionysian existence has the paradoxical effect of leading to *existential instability*. This instability originates in the distortion of the temporal vocation of existence. With the excessive stimulation of an extended present and the assimilation of protention to the characteristics of the present, existence loses its power to launch itself into the future and gradually becomes unstable, in much the same way that a plane stalls if it loses its propulsion or a cyclist wobbles and falls if they do not keep moving forward. There is no middle way for human existence: advance or sink. Instability and reduction of the capacity of temporalisation are therefore two sides of the same coin and are the common general aspect of the chronic states of substance use. This fragility is manifested in many individual forms, but wherever its appearance is verifiable, we can say that what we are dealing with is addiction. An addicted person is an individual who, after a lengthy period of abusively amplifying the relative importance of their present, inevitably moves into the realm of existential instability. Living in a world where everything is present, the addicted person ends up condemned to live in a futureless world where their ideas and projects never transition from virtuality to reality. Every genuine actualisation of a personal dream in a biography depends entirely on opening up possibilities, where we gradually sow and cultivate the ideas little by little to harvest them later. The absorption of temporality into the present in an addicted existence means these dreams remain dreams and nothing more, precisely because they are experienced intensely as if they were real. Disconnected from authentic protention, the existence of the addicted person flows into an unstable situation in which the alternatives are a total present or nothing.

This existential instability is manifested as impulsiveness, a key factor in the relapses of substance misusers. Relapses often operate by enabling a return to an existential safety zone, the state of present continuous. A relapse is directly related to impulsiveness, itself a very specific mode of existential decision-making born from the addicted historical self's lack of practice in examining the alternatives posed for its existence. Any return to temporality in its trinary form forces the historical self to reflect on the dilemmas reality imposes upon it. It is obliged to face the set of imperatives of its construction as a biographical person, with its renunciations, its personal choices laden with personal responsibilities, its routines and its plans, which inevitably run into difficulties.

Faced with a world that appears unstable, impulsivity is a way of resetting the stability of a historical self used to the absolute temporality of substance use, for which its cognitive apparatus is not necessary. Existence in a Dionysian regime does not require reflection, since exogenous pleasure enables a state of stability without the need for any cognitive effort. So, for the addicted person, existential reflection is synonymous for existential instability and therefore often rejected. This banishing of reflection means impulsiveness often becomes the overriding feature of the substance misuser's modus operandi. Any rational appreciation of impulsiveness tends to hamper progress, since it adds a component of voluntary rejection of the principle of biographical historicisation.

(e) **Value and Positional Senses in the Present Continuous – the Limits of Free Will**

The way an addicted person values their own surrender to substance use is what determines the dual relationship with the mode of valuing the capacity of biographical development. Two extreme conditions may occur within a spectrum. Either, the historical self may adopt the present continuous as a lifestyle, as a value sense by which to govern itself and its relationships with its surroundings. Avoiding the dilemmas of the temporal dialectics of life, the oscillations between freedom and determination, tradition and innovation, between the doubts and certainties of existence, may be a rational option for a historical self that submits to its Dionysian face and surrenders to artificial paradises. This surrender is in a way facilitated for those historical selves whose vulnerability to substance use or whose continued excessive substance use determines a positional sense in which the present continuous predominates. For these people, the original dilemma they face is to choose between their natural inclination, given in the Dionysian positional sense, and the value sense they observe as important to their fellow men, such as the construction of life as self-differentiation, as personal work of affirmation and individualisation. For them, this personal and ethical differentiation is not a value in itself. Therefore, some decide on the path of artificial paradise, indifferentiation and renunciation of the complexities of dialectics. These people do not exactly face an ethical dilemma in their substance use, since in a way they act according to some implicit notion of internal nature. The historical self decides to throw itself into whatever its temporal and spatial foundations indicate. With this, they affirm their agreement with this mode of conduct. It is ultimately a theme of human freedom that, only in its most extreme cases, can be understood as straying into the field of psychopathology. However, society tends to reject those who opt for a Dionysian suppression of dialectic reality. In his Nichomachean Ethics, Aristotle calls this genre the ethical vice akolasia (intemperance), which literally means the impossibility of a person to be corrected by punishment. The akolastikós does not believe that their behaviour should be transformed. In psychopathology, such a mode of existence is catalogued as a personality disorder, especially in its antisocial form, for which society's opinion regarding the effects of its behaviour matters little.

At the opposite extreme, value sense and positional sense come into conflict in the individual consciousness. The historical self understands the historicity of human life as a destiny that should be taken on and is dissatisfied with the positional sense in which it lives. This historical self is upset when it is carried away against the flow of biographical differentiation. In this condition, the historical self perpetually faces the dilemma of having to face a temporal form for which it is not prepared and which often causes it intense discomfort. These are the people who inhabit our substance misuse clinics. They are the ones who ask us for help every day to remain, albeit painfully, within the limits of existence as a proportional dialectic among the anthropological conditions of possibility. Aristotelian ethics indicated that these people's ethical vice lies in a-krasia, in the difficulty of governing themselves. For them, there is no correspondence between what free reason leads them to and what the foundations of existence call for. These people experience what is arguably the most distressing of all human difficulties: the dialectics between the historical self and its own conditions of possibility, between rational values and pre-reflexive choices. Ultimately, in each clinical case involving substance use, this central dilemma indicative of the limit of human power over oneself is re-actualised. Only in this second condition is it fair to say that addiction is weakness of will (Radoilska 2013; Schlimme 2010) because only here is there in fact any conflict of forces between a person's positional sense and his or her value sense.

7.1.4 The Dionysian Temporal Circle and Its Associations with Psychopathological Experiences – Synergy and Antagonism

From the perspective of temporality, the psychopathological states related to substance use are part of a circle called the *Dionysian temporal circle*. This circle of experiences related to substance use comprises the three forms of temporality associated with substance misuse we have seen so far. From the excessive instability of anthropological proportions to its excessive stability, passing through a fossilised form of stability, substance use exerts a dialectic relationship with the structured totality of existence. The exogenous effect of consciousness modification therefore affects human existence in all its temporal possibilities, determining distinct, successive and even contradictory existential meanings according to the main sense it is given. Self-management through substance use can serve different functions in each of these temporal possibilities. Sometimes it helps in the passage from one temporality to another, sometimes it accentuates the disproportion characteristic of a particular temporal style, sometimes it reduces it. In other words, self-management by intoxication cannot be said to have just one existential function; rather, it is an ambiguous agent that sometimes enables a transition from one formation to another, sometimes maintains a particular formation, sometimes engenders it. Substance use can therefore begin with the healthy purpose of enhancing existential malleability, only to gradually collapse into the complete exhaustion of existence. A typical case of this condition is heavy cannabis use at a young age, which can degenerate from the fun, innocent testing of one's own potentialities into an irreversible structural pathology such as schizophrenia. Substance use can also start with the aim of stabilising temporality only to end, after a long period of abuse, by destabilising it. To exemplify this condition, let us cast our minds back to borderline personalities, with their typically restless and unstable personalities, who use the stimulating effect of substances to achieve greater stabilisation for their relationships and thereby improve their permanence in the world. As their use progresses, the stability rendered by the present continuous gradually deteriorates into instability, making their lives even more unstable, with sudden mood swings and even suicide attempts. Thirdly, substance use may initially serve to heighten the colours and flavours of the world for exhausted existences (schizophrenia or enduring melancholia, for example), functioning as a mechanism of self-medication (Potvin et al. 2003; Bolton et al. 2009), but may gradually lead to transformations typically rendered by instability of embodiment, such as alcoholic withdrawal syndrome. section Finally, self-management by intoxication may initially be associated with a style of temporal proportion typical of an anthropopathology or a structural pathology, potentiating their experiences. One example would be the use of euphoriants, especially alcohol, in association with manic phases. Both produce an analogous temporality constituted by a totalised time. Here, Dionysian self-management serves to increase the disproportion of this total time at the service of the historical self (which enjoys this state of plenitude – I will return to this in Sect. 7.2), to the point of making life in society unfeasible.

It could therefore be said that self-management by intoxication is associated in multiple ways with anthropopathologies and that only in individual clinical cases can we identify the exact original meaning and the personal progressions that made such a person become prey to substance misuse. The two extreme situations that imply problematic substance use are usually excessive instability or excessive stability. In them, the development of the biography is hindered either by an inability to cope with the dilemmas of life or by an incapacity to leave a hyperstable addicted state and resume interaction with the world-pole. At either point, the circle closes and the psychopathological modes of presentation linked to self-management by intoxication begin to resemble each other in anthropological terms. What the unfavourable outcomes of substance misuse have in common is the impossibility of all personal potentialities being fulfilled in the development of the biography. The fundamental anthropological disproportion of substance misuse is a disorder of time restriction, spatial limitation and constrained personal autonomy.

But this is the most extreme outcome of the Dionysian circle. Fortunately, there are several situations that can be exploited to avert it. As a rule of thumb, the best approach for the psychopathologist in cases of substance misuse is to attempt to identify how their patient's substance use fits into this Dionysian circle in order to better understand it and prevent the most extreme outcomes. There are two basic functions the historical self may seek from self-management by intoxication. As we have already seen (Sect. 7.1.1), the exogenous modification of consciousness can act in *synergy* with the basic proportions of existence, enhancing their characteristics, or in *antagonism* towards them, mitigating the unwanted effects of these proportions. Between these two possibilities, several other intermediate actions are possible. In other words, the synergy-antagonism duality should be seen more as a general principle that actually encompasses an infinity of intermediate forms.

7.2 Spatiality (Plenitude, Self-Management and Addiction)

7.2.1 The Spatiality of Anthropological Plenitude – Compression and Exclusivity

It is in the association of temporality with spatiality that the historical self rekindles the biblical hope of humanity to once again experience paradise. The Dionysian handling of spatiality allows the historical self to nostalgically build a world that came before all dialectical divisions and decision-making complexities – to regain a paradise lost, as expressed poetically in the poem by John Milton (Paradise Lost 1976). Existentially, substance misuse consists of replacing the typical anthropological dialectics of proportions with complete surrender to the absolute, fusion with the whole (Kimura 2005; Messas 2015). In this world, the spatial dialectics of compression–relaxing, individuality–collectivity and horizontality–verticality particularly come into play for the construction and management of a world that would offer *anthropological plenitude* (Messas et al. 2019b). Plenitude is summed up by a polysubstance abuser in the following words: "it's a feeling of perfection that lasts 15 seconds". (S. 36 years old).

The aim of all experiences of intoxication is ultimately to manufacture a total experience, a homogeneous subjective state from which all heterogeneity is expelled (Messas 2014b). In a way, the intoxication-seeker wants to suppress the natural complexities of human experiences for the sake of simplicity and security of a full experience (which makes them the opposite of the obsessive person's yearning for perfection). In general, this experience is one of joy, well-being or relaxation. Below, I will examine which modifications of spatiality are indispensable for this paradisiacal plenitude to be achieved. Some of these conditions were examined in the first part of this work (see Sect. 2.2) and will be taken up here only as required for the clarification of the idea. Similarly, some reflections on the anthropological characteristics of spatial plenitude remain incomplete until they are complemented by reflections on intersubjectivity and identity, which I will do shortly after the examination of spatiality.

For a state of plenitude to be reached and maintained, some form of spatiality is needed that allows only the state of plenitude to be experienced and nothing more. There must be as little interference as possible in the Dionysian experience for it to fulfil its task of retreating from time and encountering eternal paradise. I would argue that the spatial preconditions for the experience of plenitude are *compression* and *exclusivity*.

What I mean by this is that the experiences which emerge in states of plenitude should have a maximum of homogeneity, so that ideally there is only a single experience, nothing of what contrasts or distinguishes it from others. Emptiness is something that self-management by substance use seeks to banish by every means possible, since it constitutes an invitation to the emergence of dialectics and things that are new – mortal enemies of the desired paradisiacal state. When someone tries to numb life through substance use, all they want to experience is numbness, whether through relaxation or through rapture. They do not want to increase the complexity of the world, but to reduce it in all its ambiguities, inconsistencies and uncertainties. In a formal definition, it could be said that the spatial plenitude of intoxication is a state in which experiences are homogeneous, intense, cohesive and compact in relation to each other, leaving no scope for anything unexpected to emerge that may be incompatible with the mood achieved.

This is why, for example, if we are celebrating something with some friends and we get drunk, we want to be overtaken entirely and exclusively by the emotions that are consistent with the occasion, usually the pleasant ones, like euphoria, conviviality and an appreciation of the qualities of our peers. However, dialectically, the compression and exclusiveness of the experiences may also cause unpleasant feelings like anger to take over. This also applies to experiences rendered by substances that lead to subjective distension[9] or self-absorption, like cannabis. These subjective experiences are both states in which an attempt is made to banish all tense, negative or in any way heterogeneous feelings and ideas from the state of plenitude rendered by the action of cannabis. This is how the aspect of exclusivity of the spatiality of plenitude should be understood: not as an impediment of any experiences whatsoever, but only of those that do not chime with the experiences sought by the act of modifying consciousness. This characteristic of Dionysian spatiality is summed up by one substance misuser thus: "The drugs fill my void, they make me interested in life".

Acute and chronic substance-related behaviours and disorders such as binge drinking and cannabis dependence, respectively, demonstrate clearly this one-sided dominance of a single aspect of psychological experience. Binge drinking is one of the principal causes of alcohol-related morbidity and mortality (Plunk et al. 2014; Schoenborn et al. 2014). Its main experiential characteristic is the rapid onset of a state of plenitude which is rid of all ambiguities. In this state, the historical self will experience *only* the agreeable aspects of others and none of their flaws, or vice versa. This latter case may lead to interpersonal violence, such as is seen between rival football supporters (Boles and Miotto 2003; Ayres and Treadwell 2011). The historical self sees the other only as an opponent, not as a whole individual person with both good and bad traits. Another consequence of binge drinking is high-risk sexual behaviour, in this case because the person's experience of the other is limited to their sexual desirability, and fails to take account of any of the potentially harmful consequences.

The second example is of cannabis misuse and schizotypal personality disorder (Davis et al. 2013). For some people, cannabis can induce a state of satiated plenitude that is free of conflicts and also of personal desires and anxieties. When this use turns into chronic abuse, these people's entire existence may start to be identified

---

[9] Psychological distension, experienced as affective relaxation, should not be mistaken for the (pre-reflexive) spatiality of relaxation. In this, the complexity of experiences, sentimental or ideational, is enhanced for a period of time. In the relaxation of psychological distension, what is pursued is a homogeneous emotional and ideational state filled only with good contents.

with a feeling of sated indifference, which blocks out any urge to face the challenges of life or pursue a personal project (Kemp 2018). In the words of one patient, "when I use cannabis, that's all I want to feel, nothing else". This pattern of misuse may equally be understood as well as a loss of retention, in which not only does memory lose its strength as an instrument (Auer et al. 2016), but a whole segment of personal habits and values is abandoned.

7.2.2 Experiences of Enhanced Materiality: Elevation of Raw Sensoriality, Sensorialisation of Feelings and Sensory Precipitation

One of the manifestations of spatial plenitude most closely linked to the psychopathology of substance misuse is *enhanced materiality* (Barthélémy 2013). What this name is designed to designate is an experience of compression and exclusivity which is so great that it leads to an altered sensory perception of reality with no corresponding alteration of the intersubjective constitution of reality. I mentioned this phenomenon earlier when discussing hallucination as a pathology of condensation. At this point, I just want to complement the point by indicating three modes in which this excessive materialisation of reality is manifested: elevation of raw sensoriality, *sensorialisation of feelings* and *sensory precipitation*.

I will give some clinical examples including the first-hand accounts of severe crack cocaine addicts to help explain these pathological experiences, which are very frequent in abusers of stimulants, especially cocaine and crack cocaine. The increased materiality may lead to:

(a) **Elevation of raw sensoriality**

A 35-year-old patient says "My hearing gets a lot more active ... my nerves get agitated. And you get really spaced out. You don't have any idea about anything. I would see stuff."

Reality as a whole is picked up more acutely, manifesting itself as a full, total present whose excessive sensory perception means the historical self loses its self-control and its command of the facts.

(b) **Sensorialisation of feelings**

This is how a 37-year-old patient expresses herself:

"At first, it was euphoric... Over time, that changed... From euphoria, it went to... it was sort of, kind of unexplainable, I dunno... How can I put it? I'm trying to find the right word for it... It was like you felt the compulsion... *tactile*! [emphasis added] You know, like you get the compulsion and you can't let it go." The patient's difficulty in expressing her experience in words is indicative of the originality of this kind of experience in which something that the historical self formerly experienced as a feeling became a hybrid mosaic of sensation and feeling, an embodied feeling that takes on the materiality and objectivity of tact.

(c) **Sensory precipitation**

Two self-reports describe the sensory precipitation of substance misusers:

"Dude, I've even seen a bug. I've even seen animals, I've seen monsters, I've seen guys kill me... But that never happened, right? But I've seen every kind of thing you can imagine, I've seen it, bro. Then I dream, I sleep, I have these weird dreams, right..." (B., 19 years old).

"I hear voices, I look sideways and it's like there's someone watching over me, a spirit, a woman in white clothes. Sometimes there are these *exu*[10] around me, I see them all around me. But it's like I see them, it's hallucination from the drug. If there's someone talking to you, you immediately think they want a fight, they want to fight you. But all that anger's from the drug." (D., 22 years old).

In chemistry, precipitation is the formation of a solid from a chemical reaction. It is in an analogous way that precipitation is used in meteorology to indicate that the gas (water vapour) has turned into a liquid (rain) or a solid (snow), which reaches the ground and affects human life directly. In precipitation, the solidity of a direct perceptual, sensory, tactile manifestation is associated with a volatile form prior to the appearance of the precipitate. This change in the state of the matter, from a less dense to a denser state, is used here metaphorically to indicate these hallucinatory images associated with the misuse of stimulants. The perception of reality is densi-fied and is physically imposed on the historical self, inducing the appearance of objects which it knows do not actually exist in their own right. Both of the above accounts show very clearly the experience of composite perceptual distortion on the basis of spatial compression. The pre-reflexive addition of materiality to visual space causes living figures (monsters, animals) to appear out of nowhere, without the historical self losing the awareness that they are not shared by those who listen to the account.

7.2.3   The Dionysian Spatial Circle of Addiction – Plenitude, Kenophobia, Repersonalisation and Reinstatement

Dionysian spatial plenitude is by definition a transitory state. It is therefore crucially important for the psychopathologist to identify everyday situations where existence must abandon this state of fullness and re-enter the dialectics of anthropological proportions. Absolute and proportion – anthropological plenitude and anthropologi-cal proportion – are irreconcilable, mutually exclusive opposites which nonetheless undergo a dialectic regime of alternations and suppressions, which explains a great many of the disorders directly linked to substance misuse. The continued mainte-nance of plenitude may lead to irresponsible behaviour, mood swings, depression, suicidal ideation, cognitive losses, hallucinations and acts of violence. All these behaviours and experiences are rooted in the spatial suppression of the complexities

---

[10] Exu is a spirit that is believed to be incorporated in followers of the Candomblé religion.

of each experience. This annulment leads to a spatial stiffening of existence, which in turn, dialectically, leads to a weakening of the existential structure which is analogous to the instability I identified when analysing temporality. This fragility derives from the difficulty an existence has in knowing how to deal with complexity once it is accustomed to plenitude. I call the central phenomenon that defines this difficulty *kenophobia* (*horror vacui* in Latin). This term comes from combining the noun "kenós", which means "empty" in ancient Greek, with fear, "phobos".

Kenophobia is an existential movement of resistance against the return of the historical self to a complex, uncertain world. Its hallmark is the invasion of consciousness by emptiness. The addicted historical self, surrounded by the plenitude of frequent intoxication, puts up great resistance to the fulfilment of its human destiny, inevitably insufficient, incomplete and empty. One patient with a psychotic presentation due to cannabis use put it in these terms: "I thought that it [cannabis use] would fill the void, but the void just comes back again. Crap. That's when the anxiety sets in". The euphoria of plenitude is replaced by the dysphoria (anxiety) of finding her personal history at exactly the point where she left it.[11] Therefore, the dysphoria that follows acute substance use in addiction must be understood as a contrast between the plenitude of euphoria and the partiality of dialectics, composed of voids and incompleteness. The feelings of anxiety, restlessness, irritation, impatience and depression that define dysphoria are not so much psychological states caused directly by the biological effect of any substance as the anthropological position of re-encountering the voids of existence, against which the historical self is placed, sometimes against its own value senses. Kenophobia imposes itself on the Dionysian existence because wherever there is void, there is also ambiguity; wherever there is ambiguity, certainty is no longer possible and the historical self must again take personal responsibility for decision-making. By taking on this responsibility, the historical self is implicated with each utterance, each manifestation, each act and each renunciation of an act. Re-encountering the void that exists in each experience means facing the uncertainty that lurks within them and the consequences that stem from them. The historical self is faced with itself every time it gives up the plenitude of intoxication and reencounters itself as a person. From this reencounter comes *repersonalisation*[12]: the person as a unit of experiences, values and decisions is born ontologically with the expulsion from Paradise. Repersonalisation literally functions like expulsion from Paradise, both in the

---

[11] It does not seem accidental that in ancient Greek the word "euphoria" is composed of the prefix "eu" – well, easy, comfortable – and the verb "phoreo". "Phoreo" indicates both state of mind and the act of carrying, bearing something. The ancient Greek culture already saw the state of mind as a mode of bearing the world. Euphoria, then, is bearing the world comfortably, while dysphoria is difficulty in bearing the world. More than an individual psychological state, the Greek language envisaged with this contrast an existential position that I identify here as the exit from a fulfilled world and entry into a world that is burdensome because of the difficulties and ambiguities of its dialectics.

[12] I use here the broad notion of person, as indicated in Sect. 2.3.

renunciation of a perennial state immune to pain and in the inevitable perspective of taking responsibility.

That is why experiences of repersonalisation contain the most dramatic ideas of guilt, remorse and shame (Sawer et al. 2020), sometimes in conjunction with intense depression and suicidal ideation. The contrast between plenitude and dialectics only accentuates the intensity of individual responsibility not only for decisions taken during the period of intoxication but also for life as a whole. The most characteristic phenomenon of the pains of repersonalisation is the moral hangover, in which the historical self stands before the court of itself, evaluating and judging its option for plenitude, often very harshly, as we shall see from the statements of this patient, hospitalised for crack cocaine abuse: "For me to be here it's also because I'm no angel. That's the real truth. But I sincerely regret a lot of things I've done, especially getting involved with drugs and not listening to my parents." (C. 29 years old).

Kenophobia and the difficulties inherent to repersonalisation make the phenomenon of *reinstatement* a seductive existential alternative. Reinstatement is a radical experience, which consists of a rapid return to plenitude. It is not, therefore, an unlimited concession to the use of some substance, from which some transitory pleasurable effect is sought, but total surrender to the original state of paradisiacal plenitude. To understand this, it is necessary to keep in mind the force of attraction that a consolidated habit has in the configuration of the structure of existence. I support my argument on the persuasive power of a classic work of medical philosophy, The Problems (Aristotle, 1957), which I will use again later in this work. The inherent ambiguity of deciding between remaining in a harmful state to which one is accustomed (here, plenitude) or abandoning it in the name of something better, but new, should not be underestimated. In book XXVIII of the aforementioned work, which deals with self-control, continence and incontinence, Aristotle states that "those who alter their mode of life suffer from the change, and their only safety lies in returning to their usual life, like a return to nature" (Problems 949a 30–32, trans. Hett). Thus, reinstatement cannot be understood as the fruit of a rational decision (or absence thereof) by the historical self that is free and outside of its own history, which can make a balanced choice between good and evil. This excerpt shows how the very decision taken by the historical self depends on a pre-reflexive ambivalence of a different order, which sets in opposition not right and wrong, but something as strong as a habit transformed into second nature and health, which is somewhat artificial insofar as it runs counter to that nature. The complexity of reinstatement as an existential alternative for substance misusers does not absolve them from all the responsibilities arising from relapses and their consequences. Nevertheless, it allows the clinician to judge more humanely the excruciating tension the addicted person experiences in the face of the pressure to relapse into substance use.

With reinstatement, the spatial circle around which the existences vulnerable to substance misuse or addiction gravitate completes a loop. From a psychopathological point of view, these existences can be understood from their involvement in some point of the Dionysian spatial circle. Sometimes, we find them in the disorders of plenitude, sometimes we find them in the management of kenophobia and repersonalisation (asking for help to quit a substance or to tolerate day-after guilt), sometimes struggling with the reinstatement brought about by genuine, pre-reflexive, unequivocally human nostalgia for Eden.

7.2.4 Substance Misuse and Excesses in Self-Management: Horizontality and Verticality as Primordial and General Anthropological Directions

Anthropological plenitude is an existential state guaranteed by the compression and exclusivity of experiences in consciousness, allied to an exaltation of the importance of the present. This plenitude, however, does not occur in one fell swoop, out of the blue, as if some divine power displaced human dialectics and enthroned in its place a fully fledged state of absolute present. To reach this transitional state, an existential movement is necessary on the part of the historical self, which voluntarily alters its anthropological proportions through two main directions: horizontality and verticality. The dialectical progression between the proportions of horizontality and verticality is the biographical path that may finally lead to the hyperpresent plenitude which characterises the most advanced cases of altered experiences. There are, however, several conditions resulting from excesses of self-management by substance use which, if identified in time, prevent life from descending into the Dionysian circle.

The horizontal direction uses the exogenous effects of substances to enable more engagement with the world, both material and intersubjective; it is a decision for increased socialisation and increased engagement with the world of existence (Binswager 1992a; Chamond 2005). On the other hand, the Dionysian option for verticality invests in the disproportionate valuation of the self-pole in relation to the world, guided by the values of individuality, autonomy and independence; it is a decision in favour of the idiosyncrasy of the individual in relation to the social. The notions of horizontality and verticality have already been addressed elsewhere in this book, both as fundamental axes of the dialectics of spatialisation in general (Sect. 2.2.6) and as typical spatial modes of certain anthropopathologies (schizoid disproportion in Sect. 3.7). I will not repeat the definitions of the concepts here. The function of this section and the next is to identify how the use (horizontal or vertical) of the exogenous effects of substances can distort existence, leading to a state of substance misuse. It is always useful to remember that over time the relationships between these spatial options and disorders enter into circularity, to the point that, at a given moment in the life of a substance misuser, it is no longer known whether substance use caused the alteration of spatiality or altered spatiality determined the modes of substance use.

As both notions describe a spatial movement that always relates the self-pole with the other-pole and the world-pole, its application simultaneously relates to spatiality and to intersubjectivity and identity, since the latter two are fundamentally relational conditions of possibility. Thus, the presentation of the role of the two fundamental directions of existence in substance misuse will begin in this section in terms of their spatial implications, and will be detailed in the next in terms of inter-subjectivity and identity. I will begin by investigating a specific form of obtaining anthropological plenitude in relation to the world that is characteristic of a culture in which productivity is a fundamental value, then I shall turn to the more complex question of intersubjectivity itself.

7.2.5   Horizontality as the Preferred Anthropological Direction – Plenitude as a Form of Efficiency

Plenitude can be achieved through the extreme expansion of the world as a field of efficiencies. The main pharmacological tools to enable this form of self-management are stimulants, from the licit ones, such as methylphenidate or lisdexamfetamine, to the illicit cocaine and crack cocaine. These substances, whose use is growing world-wide (Sweeney et al. 2013; Piper et al. 2018), differ from others in that the target of their horizontal stimulus is the *world of labour*.

The realm of work is marked by a repudiation of waste. However, the notion of waste here takes on a rather broad conception, covering the inherent waste of medi-tative reflection, devoid of immediate purpose, and the mere experience of pleasure for pleasure's sake. At its heart, this repudiation of waste is based on an elevation of horizontal directionality. With this, worldly objects become more interesting. With a stimulant, the historical self takes away the emphasis on subjective states geared towards itself and resolutely turns towards the world-pole. The virtual bonds that tie the self-pole to the world are pulled in, reducing the range and flexibility of the spatiality of existence. From the perspective of the global state of consciousness, there is an increased level of vigilance. When consciousness is highly activated and clear, the world becomes more interesting and engaging with it becomes the main purpose of life. Consciousness becomes, so to speak, pure vision directed towards objects. The historical self seeks out this state of consciousness voluntarily for its ability to raise productivity. With it, the historical self predisposes itself to the manipulations of the world required by work. For maximum efficiency, the histori-cal self must experience the world of work as the most interesting mode of dwelling in the world.

Nevertheless, when the self-pole is brought too closely into contact with the objects of the world and consequently experiences heightened interest in them, the basic figure-ground form of perception is distorted (Zutt 1963b). The first conse-quence of this is a loss of relevance of objects: as everything is interesting to the historical self, there are no objects of lesser value that are unworthy of attention. All objects from the world tend to attract the same level of interest, leading, paradoxi-cally, to a *de-differentiation of value* wrought by the excessive value placed on everything.

The historical self is overwhelmed in this de-differentiated world where all hierarchies of value are lost because it is forced to concern itself with whatever appears in its field of consciousness. This leads to a flattening of the values of objects, rendering of equal value to those things which ordinarily would appear to be of different value. When it comes to moods, overinterest in a world made equal flows into *dysphoria* (Zutt 1963d). The plenitude that the stimulating substance produces cannot, given the spatial conditions mentioned above, translate into a form of pleasure because genuine pleasure depends on some flexibility of the self-pole in relation to the world, lending experiences their particular authenticity. All genuine pleasure lies in a harmonious proportion between the self-pole and the world-pole. Similarly, every pleasurable activity also presupposes a differentiation of the world, a gap in the self-pole that it seeks to fill by interacting with the objects of the world.

The plenitude of a self-pole that is entirely geared towards a world de-differentiated by excessive value prevents it from enjoying habitual experiences of everyday sociability, such as a party, a rest, a catch-up with friends, a concert. The impossibility of enjoying this packed world distorts the mood baseline into dysphoria. Marked by instability and irritability, dysphoria is evidence of how a loss of differentiation in the world makes it appear barren, devoid of anything of genuine value. A world where everything is equally valid inevitably leads to demotivation and repetition; in short, tiredness.

Trapped in the full and evident space of a world where everything is of interest – from the perspective of productivity – the historical self loses its capacity to experience the genuine novelty and freshness of life. The horizontal effect of stimulants exhorts the historical self to repeat what it already knows, to perfect something that is already automated (Zutt 1963d). The authentic possibility of renewal is replaced by the automatic repetition of what is known; the experience of creation gives way to the technical management of the world. This is how stimulants like smart drugs are able to enhance memory and increase the number of hours effectively focusing on a work activity, while reducing the need to change the focus of attention to other subjects and objects or even the need to eat or sleep. The option for total efficiency replaces the vertical depths of existence with the explicit horizontality of the world, bringing with it the threat of the transformation of the human into an automaton, an administrator of objects. Rather than engendering renewal, excessive interest in the objects of the world mutates into a conservative barrier, denying space to what is existentially new and needs patience and contemplation to germinate. However, for the very same reason, plenitude enables the historical self to achieve maximum potency, at least for a while, in something that is more consolidated in itself. Plenitude in the space of work raises the labour identity to maximum participation in the whole of existence, bringing the totality of the person closer to the partial nature of a single role. In the medium term, this submission of the whole identity to a single role brings the risk of producing melancholic or hyperthymic disproportion (Sects. 3.3 and 3.4).

Likewise, the self-pole's overproximity to the space of labour may, when taken to the extreme, lead to hallucinatory psychoses associated with condensation, as shown above. As a rule, these are accompanied by behavioural modifications which tend to involve over-adherence to the world of interest, such as psychomotor restlessness, distractibility, irritability, excessive concern with reality. This last experience is described by a patient who was a homeless polysubstance user: "I have a mania for picking up [objects from the ground], thinking that I dropped a piece".

7.3   Intersubjectivity and Identity – The Masks of Dionysus

Dionysus, the god of wine and drunkenness, is also the patron of the theatre. It could not be otherwise, given the flexibility of his apparitions and the multiplicity of forms in which he reveals himself to worshipers. Dionysus manages his identities by means of the different masks he wears, and so he controls the forms his interpersonal relationships take. The multiplicity of his masks corresponds to the variety of ways in which he relates to humans. Dionysian versatility affects identity and intersubjectivity at one and the same time. Dionysian masks are the theatrical representation of human power over the free management of one's own identity, the identities of those with whom one relates, and the mode in which these identities are articulated dynamically among themselves. Master of disguise and invention, the *deus praesentissimus* instils in humanity divine nostalgia for the creation of ourselves and the way we relate to others. It is an ambiguous form of creation, for while it reveals the truth that is hidden in relationships, by the same token it distorts it. It is again from this Greco-Roman god of ambiguity that I take inspiration to analyse self-management through the use of psychoactive substances and their associated risks. To understand intersubjectivity, I will use the same two anthropological directions I have just employed, horizontality and verticality. To understand the dialectics of identity, I will base myself on the above reflections about the modes of *intersubjectivity* (see Sect. 2.3.3). The separation of the analysis of intersubjectivity from the analysis of identity is mainly didactic, since in reality, as the reader will see, there are many overlaps between the two. It is impossible to separate them clearly without losing sight of the complexity of the object. However, I will try to separate them whenever this makes the arguments clearer and more distinct. Ideally, the two should be interpreted as parts of a whole. I will start with intersubjectivity, introducing, whenever necessary, considerations about identity.

7.3.1   Self-Management of Intersubjective Horizontality

The great and oldest instrument of Dionysian horizontality, at least in Western societies, is alcohol. Astonishingly, contemporary intuitions about its function in the management of human relations already appear in Greek philosophical literature, especially in Hippocrates (Messas and Andrade 2018) and Aristotle. It is Aristotle's school that is credited with the most elaborate reflections on the effects of alcohol on human identity, in the Problems. The most famous of them is Problem XXX, which is so up-to-date and insightful that I will use it to begin this section on the management of horizontality. This problem first examines of all the polarities between singularity and plurality, from the effects of wine:

"For wine in large quantities seems to produce [...] a *variety of qualities,* making men ill-tempered, merciful or reckless" (emphasis added) (953a 33–36, trans. Hett).

In other words, drunkenness has a definite role in humans; it transforms their nature, producing ek-stasis, an exit of the individual from the habitual state of their identity, introducing the multiplicity of natures contained latently within them. Above all, wine is a revealer of qualities, or a de-differentiator of the qualities consolidated in sober life. It is impossible at this point not to associate the anthropological conditions of wine-induced drunkenness with the temporality of mania, where all the partial identities contained in a person are similarly revealed at once through the loss of the relative hierarchy between them. It would therefore be no exaggeration to state that when it reaches a certain level of intensity, the Dionysian act of drunkenness has the same anthropological meaning as a manic phase. The difference between the two resides in the direct causal link between the subjective state and the pharmacodynamics of alcohol, which does not exist in mania. It is no coincidence, then, that manic conditions are often associated with the abuse of alcohol and other substances (Richardson 2013). In most cases, intoxication acts in synergy with the patient's anthropological disproportions, reinforcing the tendency of the manic person to develop all their partial identities in the present. Mania and alcohol therefore have great existential affinity, since they bring plenitude to the horizontal dimension of existence.

The multiplicity of qualities in the terrain of identity does not, however, explain the whole phenomenon triggered by drunkenness. The most important has to do with the dialectics between individual and otherness in its horizontality. The pre-reflexive articulations that bind the individual to him/herself and to others are not endowed definitively to the human being and can be modified by the historical self via the use of alcohol. Alcohol acts on one characteristic of human nature: the indeterminate nature of identity, bringing about two main movements: a movement towards otherness (potentially leading to its loss), which has to do with disproportions of horizontality; and an overvaluation of the self-pole, which has to do with disproportions of verticality, and will therefore be examined in the next section (Sect. 7.3.2). I will now attempt to point out the harmful consequences of these movements to existence.

(a) Harmful Consequences of Excessive Horizontality – Proximity and Horizontal Dysmetry

Substance use accentuates horizontality, bringing the self-pole closer to the other-pole and the world-pole. One example of this is the experience of heightened sexual desire during substance use: the other – actually, one desirable aspect of the other – becomes more relevant than it would have been without intoxication. Another example is the feeling of belonging to a group of friends after a few drinks at a bar, which is accompanied by an elated feeling of camaraderie. The distances and differences between the members of the group seem to disappear and are replaced by a fraternal closeness, as if the relationships were old and already consolidated. For example, all the intoxicated people become admirers of a particular football team and begin to coalesce around the partial identity of the football fan, whose relative value is temporarily raised. If before the drink there were two employees from the same office who did not feel very comfortable with each other, after a few drinks something mysterious happens. The mystery consists of the development of the employee's identity into the identity of a fan. Now, because of the similarity with the analogous identity produced in the partner, the two can already feel like brothers. This fellowship originates primarily in the capacity of alcohol to dissolve consolidated identities, quickly offer a new partial identity, and facilitate proximity between the two, leap-frogging company protocol and the time needed to build an intimate relationship. However, the extreme power of alcohol to mould identity has its risks. Dialectically, horizontal proximity to the other can lead to interpersonal violence, since the undesirable aspects of the other are also perceived more markedly than they would be in a state of sobriety. The subjective states typically produced in this proximity associated with alcohol use are joy, carelessness, eloquence, disrespect, irreverence, irritability, aggressiveness, mockery, etc. although they can also be obtained by other substances. This set of subjective states results from what I call *horizontal dysmetry*. Horizontal dysmetry is defined by the loss of the ability to measure appropriately the proportions between closeness and distance which are typical of a society, a group of people or a person. Horizontal dysmetry is often seen in compulsive anthropopathology, in which there is a structural tendency to become too close to others and reality (see Sect. 3.5). This is why dysmetry appears either as exaggerated curiosity about others, a desire for intimacy that was not authorised by the other, or as inattention to the other, since attention quickly flits elsewhere. Horizontal dysmetry also explains the difficulty certain people have in separating or even partially distancing themselves from the group to which they belong. More clearly, dysmetry is a common phenomenon in hyperthymic disproportion and especially in manic structural pathology (see Sects. 3.4 and 4.2). The dysmetric world is inhabited by an excess of human presence, which substance use only goes to increase, but in the absence of a strong enough basis of retention for the dysmetric alterations to lead to a deepening of intersubjective relations. Dionysian dysmetry is false in its origin because it is an existential movement based on exogenous pharmacological effects. Usually, the dysmetry person's self-management by substance use is designed to find synergy between the effect of the substance and their own anthropological proportions. The exogenous effect fits the person's typical style of being, accentuating the disproportions that they already have. For example, people who are addicted to alcohol will find any excuse to incorporate a daily happy hour into their life, where they exercise their dysmetry exacerbated by drunkenness together with friends who share the same experience. The eloquence and euphoria of these events sustain the state of plenitude by bringing closer together identities that have become fictitiously equal. However, whenever there is a condition of dysmetry, the intimacy and values of the other are put at jeopardy because they may not be given due attention by the historical self. The dysmetric self-pole's movement towards the other is based on value criteria determined by their lack of perspective. So it is, for example, that a drunken man at a party will try to approach a girl, even if she is not interested in him. Horizontal dysmetry is at the source of many of the behaviours of human disrespect, personal devaluation and interpersonal violence, especially marital violence against women (Fals-Stewart et al. 2003) seen in our culture. The state of dysmetry arises from the ease with which the partial identities of the historical self are dissolved by alcohol or other substances, leading it to live in an ambiguous state from which it cannot escape. On the one hand, it takes pleasure from the fact that it possesses so many partial identities; this makes it feel enriched, strong, interesting, funny, liked and powerful, something that in its habitual daily life it cannot feel. However, precisely because it can produce so many identities so easily, it weakens as a historical self because it becomes a stage on which diverse superficial identities are played out. There is a paradoxical and gradual emptying out of the historical self behind the ease with which it is able to don and doff its own identities (which makes it somewhat similar to the borderline case).

In horizontal dysmetry, however, the self-pole and other-pole's proximity may, at least at first, accentuate the value of the self-pole. We saw examples of this egoic dysmetry when we examined hyperthymia and, more specifically, endoxia. It is very important to point out that this enhancement of the self-pole's value comes about through the dialectics of horizontality, namely, an overvaluation of the self-pole *in relation to the other-pole*. The historical self inevitably feels more important or valuable *within* an interpersonal relationship. This leads to arrogance, impatience at the other or mockery of some weakness of theirs. A polyuser of stimulant substances notices the alteration he experiences in these terms: "a sensation of supremacy... of looking down at everyone from on high". The self-pole affirms itself in strict contrast with the direct, immediate and continuous presence of the other. The self-pole is worth more because the other-pole is worth less. It is a zero-sum game, which is what distinguishes this appreciation of the value of the self-pole, for example, from what we will see later, which arises from the management of verticality (Sect. 7.3.2).

a1) *Forms of Dysmetry by Proximity: Intersubjective Extrusion and Emptying in Intersubjectivity*

When there is increased horizontal proximity, the existential movement triggered by the action of substances on anthropological proportions has the effect of moving the self-pole too close to the other-pole. This closeness has ambiguous consequences. On the one hand, there is a contempt for social protocol, which is born from the presumption of intimacy that horizontal dysmetry produces. This presumption causes the other to be targeted beyond the identity roles that regulate interpersonal relationships. On the other hand, this contempt leaves the self-pole overexposed to otherness, making it transparent. This transparency is because the private sphere of the historical self is spread across the public space of the collectivity. I call this phenomenon *intersubjective extrusion*. With this term, I want to indicate that the substance misuser's psychological contents undergo pre-reflexive pressure to be exposed in the space of intersubjectivity. The unity of the historical self is not jeopardised by intersubjective extrusion. Indeed, the maintenance of unity is what differentiates intersubjective extrusion from schizophrenic experiences, where feelings are also exposed in intersubjectivity. In schizophrenia, this happens because the self-pole and the other-pole are not mutually constituted, which is not the case in extrusion due to substance misuse. In schizophrenia, the identity of the other is twisted into the impersonality of a mysterious stalker, but in the experience of extrusion it remains intact. Private matters enter the public domain, sometimes mimicking certain hysterical behaviours, as was noted in Bilz's (1956) classic work on the psychopathology of alcohol. This exteriorisation of first-person subjectivity to collective spaces is manifested, for example, in untimely and inappropriate accounts of personal facts, the embarrassing revelation of private secrets, or an incapacity or disinterest in preserving from public scrutiny unseemly facets of one's own conduct. Conversely, it also manifests in a sometimes promiscuous and inappropriate interest in the privacy of others or in attention to personal facts that are not necessary for the good development of relationships. Intersubjective extrusion is summed up anthropologically in the Latin sentence "in vino veritas" and its Greek equivalent "oinos kai aletheia" (wine and truth). Both show how intoxication is paradoxically committed to the presentation of truth, but of a truth that is often socially inappropriate and contrary to the interests of those whose truth it is. Complaining about the poor opinion her family had of her, a patient who was a severe abuser of alcohol put into words this involuntarily excessive expression of truth, which seems so transparent as to be false: "I'm totally transparent and nobody believes in me".

The self-pole's transparency makes it self-evident to the other-pole. One example of this is the pronounced predictability of addicted patients' behaviour. A relative, a peer, a person they know or their clinician is often able to predict a relapse in their substance use long before it happens. The substance misuser begins to behave in a familiar way, making it easy for those who are close to them to identify their intention to relapse precisely in the extent to which they attempt to hide it. What is popularly termed manipulation by substance misusers is actually the opposite of this: it is the establishment of a chain of conduct prior to a relapse which normally does not pull the wool over the eyes of anyone who knows them well. Their intimate space dissolves in intersubjectivity, as it were, to such an extent that they become transparent to others. When the person is particularly socially vulnerable, this becomes even clearer, as a homeless chronic substance abuser explains "sleeping on the street is appearing in society". In this case, the social transparency is complete because the effect of extreme social exposure (being homeless) is compounded by the extrusion caused by substance misuse.

In its most harmful forms, the intersubjective extrusion generated by the act of intoxication takes the form of complete weakness of the self-pole in relation to the desires of the other-pole, constituting a relationship of social and interpersonal vulnerability that is at the root, for example, of the association between substance use and gender violence (Boles and Miotto 2003; Choo et al. 2014). In the words of one patient, it is clear how vulnerable her intoxication made her to the marital violence of which she was a victim: [referring to the husband who assaults her] "when I drank, he'd beat me black and blue. When I didn't, it wouldn't happen".

However, the most dramatic form of intersubjective extrusion can be observed in the delusions of jealousy associated with addiction, especially alcohol (Soyka 2006). This received considerable attention in classical psychopathology in the work of Lagache (1997). The typical intersubjective situation in which this pathological experience emerges is that of the humiliated historical self (usually male), already weakened by years of alcoholism and biographically dependent on the spouse (usually female). The humiliation is often compounded by low sexual satisfaction (Shrestha et al. 1985). When in a state of drunkenness, this historical self has the experience that the spouse betrays him sexually, with many people, near and far. The phenomenological understanding of the delusion of alcoholic jealousy suggests that there is an exteriorisation and spatialisation of the internal conflict in which the person lives. This conflict arises from the original experience that, being devalued as a person because of the addiction and as a sexual partner because of the impotence, the historical self fears its spouse will have a sexual life with someone else with the existential means and potency to satisfy such an arrangement. This subjective fear, experienced as a personal feeling under the intense influence of alcohol, dissolves in the collective space, invading intersubjective reality and gaining colours of reality. It is a kind of prolapse of private life into the collective space. The individual's emotional conflict takes on a three-dimensional, cinematographic aspect, fruit of the extreme exposure of the historical self to the intersubjective world. This dissolution of intimacy in the intersubjective space is rooted, as in other pathologies stemming from substance misuse, in the material condensation of experience. When condensed, experiences are precipitated, transforming a psychological dynamic into a sensorial reality.

In intersubjective extrusion, there is ultimately an *emptying of the historical self into intersubjectivity*. Its autonomy is gradually replaced by a heteronomy in which it becomes very difficult for the historical self to define itself biographically in its own terms. An existence extruded in intersubjectivity has great trouble directing its biography autonomously. Often, the best way to help a person in this state is to help them constitute an asymmetric intersubjectivity in terms of power, in which the other-pole takes control. From this position of power, the other is able to guide and help them to find the best possible autonomy. It is mistaken to think that people with such difficult and distorted life stories can overcome the emptiness in which they live only by an act of free and rational will or that they have the strength or interest to do so. In fact, the overexposure of the self-pole to the other-pole makes having a relevant other take over the management of the life of those who have lost themselves in this form of dysmetry an important therapeutic strategy. That is why mutual help groups are fundamental in the recovery of substance misusers, yielding the best therapeutic results (Chappel and DuPont 1999; Lo Coco et al. 2019). Through this associative form, the emptied person is able to find someone who, having experienced the same emptiness, is able to take the place of a strong person to lead their life (see Sect. 3.5.6). The emptied and transparent historical self, excessively exposed to the intersubjective world, needs a strong other in order to maintain minimally harmonious and sustainable intersubjective relationships.

a2) Forms of Dysmetry by Proximity: Submission to Collectivity and Identity Dysnomy

Another form of anthropological disproportion by proximity is the compression of the self-pole into the other-pole and world-pole, resulting in existential submission to the collectivity. This imbalance is manifested most in the most serious clinical cases of substance misuse, particularly cocaine and crack cocaine. Too close to the world-pole, the historical self is imprisoned in the elevated (negative) value perception the collectivity has of it. In this dysmetry, the self-pole is too sensitive to how it is perceived by the collectivity, a condition that leaves existence two alternatives: adhere to collective values unconditionally or remain in debt to its prescriptions. There is thus a direct link between the frequent experiences of guilt of misusers and their submission to the social, even in those who do not feel depressed and even take pleasure from the experience of marginality (Messas et al. 2016). Submitted existences are pre-reflexively conditioned by set social duties whose values they cannot relativise. They are too exposed to what is prescribed to them and unable to find enough distance to reflect on this condition.

This form of submission to the collective makes it possible to understand, now from the perspective of intersubjectivity, the association between suicidal thoughts and acts and the abuse of stimulants (Roy 2009). The experience of depression arises from the excessive incorporation by the historical self of the depreciative evaluation that misusers are normally given in society, constituting self-stigma (Matthews et al. 2017; Crapanzano et al. 2019). As the historical self can no longer move away from the world to reflect on this condition, its extreme proximity leaves it no choice but to take action against the environment, which is witnessed in hyperactive motor behaviours, impulsiveness, aggression and violence. This historical self is determined by a heteronomous way of existing, dictated by a duty to the collective which it is generally unable to fulfil. The more it tries to do so, the more submissive it becomes to the collectivity and the more it exposes its weakness. In anthropological terms, it could be said that this submission to collectivity is an intersubjective form typical of situations of substance misuse, in which an extremely weakened self-pole finds existential balance through an attempt to assimilate the habits, practices and values of the collectivity to which it belongs. In this submission to the collectivity, not only is the historical self transparent in its exposure to otherness, but it is also worn down by basing its own emotional experiences and values excessively on the collective. A clear manifestation of this condition is the "ready speech" (Adorno et al. 2013) often sensed in substance misusers. These are individuals who seem to say exactly what they think their interlocutor wants to hear, regardless of their own personal opinion, making them seem false. For individuals with this existential form, it is as if obeying was more important than being.

In order to understand how a historical self can weaken to the point of submitting to the collectivity, emptying itself out into otherness and extruding itself into intersubjectivity, an incursion into the theme of Dionysian identity is necessary. Although the substance misuser is submissive to the collectivity, they are not melancholic; although they are exposed to the other, they are not borderline or phobic; although they need a strong other, they are not compulsive. The anthropological disproportion that marks the debilitated historical self of substance misusers is *identity dysnomy*. Identity dysnomy is a specific form of disproportion in the articulation of the historical self with its partial identities, which results in its weakening. It is easier to describe by making a brief comparison. The melancholic person submits to egoic assimilation by the social identities with which he/she unites: their historical self takes on the identity provided by the social role as its total identity, a phenomenon known as hypernomy. Its suffering comes from its inability to operate this identity which it takes on in its entirety. Meanwhile, the borderline self departs from the identities prescribed by society, acting in too singular a way. This is hyponomy, whose suffering lies in a lack of attention of the other. Different again is dysnomy, which means a difficulty in incorporating the norms (nomos) to which one is exposed and which are held up as appropriate. The dysnomic person experiences intensely the modes in which they must act, but their partial identities are incapable of executing this task. The excerpt below, taken from the testimony of a homeless substance misuse patient, is eloquent in communicating this experience:

> I love my son very much. I feel really useless, really down as a man when I think I can't be with my son. It makes me feel ashamed. I die of shame, I die of fear, ... I'm not afraid of the police, I'm not afraid of anything. It kills me to think of some relative of mine coming through this door and seeing me here like this. It would be absolutely mortifying. It'd be so embarrassing that I think I'd walk out of here and stop in the middle of the street, you know? (...) I think I ruined my son's life because I'm not around and I can't guide him. (B., 30 years old)

In dysnomy, there is a proximity between the self-pole and the collectivity that cannot be completed. The historical self feels bound by values it cannot take on as its own, although it thinks they are the right ones and should be its own. The more it experiences these values, the less it can live up to them. The dysnomic historical self thus remains aloof from the partial identities it wishes to actualise, unlike the melancholic historical self, which is capable of being assimilated by partial identities. The testimony cited above gives us the chance to make an imaginary differential evaluation of the two disproportions. If the substance misuser were melancholic, they would tend to experience their failure as a father, stressing their failure to perform that role. They would feel that even when they made their utmost effort, they were incapable of fulfilling the duty allotted to them by social prescriptions. The experience of the dysnomic person is different. The self-reproach comes from the fact that they did not perform the identity role they should have. In the first case, failure stems from incompetence; in the second, from neglect.

Identity dysnomy is a source of shame and humiliation on the part of substance misusers, as it reveals that the identities by which their mode of existence is actualised are not consistent with the values they themselves hold dear. An insoluble impasse paralyses their dysnomic existence because, while they do not try to comply with behavioural norms, they still hope the results of their life will be coherent with the normative system. This contrast with the norms coupled with the recognition of their value and compounded by the need to act according to these rules makes dysnomic people cause considerable disturbance in their surroundings.

7.3.2 Harmful Consequences of the Management of Verticality – Indifference and Isolation

Substance use may lead in the opposite direction to the one we examined above. Instead of prioritising engagement with the world and others, self-management by substance use may envisage independence for the self-pole from the world-pole through verticalisation. In normal situations, this independence may lead to an enhanced capacity to grasp otherness while not losing direct contact with it or the world. Verticalisation raises the position of the self-pole in relation to the world-pole, which enables greater perspective, just as someone on a mountain peak is able to appreciate more expansively the valley that unfolds before their eyes. Otherness remains valid as such, although it gains new dimensions. The everyday, non-pathological phenomenon most related to this form of self-management is caricature. In caricature, the artist deliberately deforms the features of their subject, with the paradoxical result that they are perceived by observers for whatever it is that most marks them. The emphasis the caricaturist puts on this feature does not stem from a cold distancing from the subject, but quite the opposite. The laughter that a good caricature causes is a sincere response to the unexpected revelation of multiplicity – a multiplicity that the hurly-burly of everyday life prevents us from seeing. The laughter provoked by caricature is indicative of an enrichment of social life through the mediation of a new perspective introduced by the caricaturist. I understand the laughter prompted by cannabis use as having a similar cause. The association between cannabis and laughter has to do with the way it changes the habitual mode by which the self-pole interacts with otherness. The hilarity of cannabis indicates that we are all more than just the social identities of our historical person. We are also too tall, too fat, too shy or too bald. This merriness of cannabis-induced laughter lies in an exogenous enrichment of the complexity of the world and its people. Up to this point, this revelation of multiplicity does not lead to scorn, but merely an exaltation of others' characteristics from a new vision of the whole. It is precisely because the self-pole and world-pole are articulated in new ways that the historical self is no longer so involved in the intersubjective relationship and is able to enter the general mood of contemplation that gives rise to episodes of cannabis laughter. This verticality is the anthropological direction traditionally associated with this substance use. Indeed, everyday language picks up the importance of this anthropological direction by associating the effect of the altered state of consciousness with a high.

Nevertheless, ongoing excessive substance use can lead to an anthropological disproportion that is detrimental to biographical development. In its quest for verticality, the intoxicated historical self becomes wrapped up in itself and neglects other components of the world, weakening its pre-reflexive bonds with intersubjective reality. The primordial attunement between the self-pole and the world-pole is impaired, the psychopathological consequence of which is an emptying out of existence, as is seen in the schizotypal transformation of personality. Here, existence becomes outlandish and incomprehensible to the eyes of the world, as if it had plunged into a solitary, isolated universe.

This phenomenon has much in common with the emptying out seen in schizophrenia, although in theory Dionysian verticalisation does not shatter the structural unity of the world, only distorting it by reducing the relative value of the world and the other and thus isolating the self-pole. It is definitely a schizoid anthropological disproportion (see Sect. 3.7). Consequently, in this form of pathological verticalisation, the world and otherness both lose value simultaneously. The isolation of the self-pole does not correspond to an elevation of its value; on the contrary, it leads to an emphasis on personal ideas and projects that are not necessarily shareable with (or feasible in) the world and therefore remain unrealised, in a larval state, drifting over the world. Substance use is fundamental in the production and maintenance of existence in this state of ethereal elevation, as it enables a state of satisfaction that is refractory to the demands of the world. The emotional states that characterise this verticalisation are tinged with indifference. The self-pole and other-pole are mutually irreconcilable, unable to communicate effectively because of the limited verbal expression, the eccentricities of the person's behaviour, or simply a general emptying of intersubjectivity (Binswanger 1992a). A person who loses themselves in verticality often ends up being termed a "weirdo" for their difficulty in experiencing the shared values of the world and their idiosyncratic behaviour. This closure of the self-pole in on itself also results in disrespectful behaviour towards others and the collectivity, with antisocial attitudes such as damaging family assets, abandoning parental functions or even callous violence.

The reduced power of intersubjectivity combined with vertical isolation can also manifest itself in affective instability. This occurs because the intersubjective support that each feeling normally has is reduced. The harmony with which we experience a feeling is what assures its stability. Say you are going through a difficult moment in your life and often feel sad, downcast or even hopeless. One way you may try to pick up your mood might be through an interpersonal encounter. If you go to a psychotherapy session or even meet up with a close group of friends, you will gradually be able to recoup your typical personal style of feelings. It is thanks to the other (in the case of psychotherapy) or the others (in the case of the group) and their support and attempts to buoy us up that we are able to recover. This is because our affects are in tune with the affects of others and so can be brought into harmony with them. In isolated Dionysian verticality, this possibility is impaired or even lost. The historical self is left at the mercy of itself and its oscillations, not to mention the instabilities that the intoxicated condition itself can promote. The emotional lability seen in addicted persons is indicative of a historical self incapable of engaging intersubjectively in a way that would help it produce an alternative mental state to the one imposed upon it from within. In more advanced situations, the vertical isolation of existence may lead it to inhabit a floating world (Di Petta 2019), in which not even the value senses of the historical self seem to be under its domain. In this floating world, existence loses even its general direction and its capacity to organise in any anthropological direction, which means interest in the world becomes intermittent. The floating world is an extreme condition of verticality in substance misuse, whose temporal result is biographical indifferentiation.

The vertical direction can also be explored at its lower end, as an existential fall (Binswanger 1992b). The fall of existence is manifested in the loss of the perspective and independence provided by spiritual height and a corresponding restriction of existence to its impulsive and instinctual components. This form of earthly materialisation accentuates the more animal and primitive facets of man to the detriment of the spiritual values of compassion and comprehension. The material fall of existence is manifested in the baseness of certain aggressive and spiteful behaviours which accompany substance use.

7.3.3   The Historical Self and Its Engagement with the World – Alternatives to Personal Freedom

The plenitude of intoxication is brought about by an experience of exclusion that involves supplanting the dialectics of the world by yielding to totalisation in the absolute. This state inevitably forces the historical self to face the very plenitude it has built or within which it has become imprisoned. Decisions regarding the maintenance of plenitude – the voluntary act of intoxication – always include a moment of decision-making when reason deliberates on its foundations. Even fuzzied by dependence and the craving caused by substance use, the rational aspect of the historical self continues to be decisive, even if only to plan the acquisition of more substances. The ways in which the historical self behaves in relation to plenitude therefore matter beyond psychopathology. It is at the crossroads between the rational component of the historical self and plenitude that individual responsibility lies. Except in the most severe and advanced cases of dementia linked to substance use or in serious psychotic alterations, the historical self continues to be responsible for the world it inhabits and for its conduct therein. This means that there is an implicit or explicit value sense underlying everything it does or fails to do. In this value sense that governs decisions, there always remains a concept of the world in which individual freedom, the free spirit, acts. To understand substance misuse as a problem of individual freedom, it is necessary to understand what positional alternatives are within the reach of a given historical person in the world, as it is these that are impacted by the power of plasticity of the value sense. It is about this world that the rational aspect of the historical self is or is not free to act, is able or unable to enforce its will.

There are two possible alternatives in this field: increased or decreased engagement with the world. Plenitude with *high engagement with the world* corresponds partially to the disproportions of horizontality. By opting for this, the historical self is stating that its conduct will be guided by others, by the objects and the attractions of the world, mainly in their material and sensory facets, as well as the values of society and what it produces. The free decision that must be made in this situation is whether to remain in this extreme immersion in the world or to seek a balance which can only be reached by giving up some of the intensity of the world. This form of decision about plenitude is existentially similar to the disproportions of melancholia, hyperthymia, compulsiveness and mania. On the other hand, the historical self may opt for *low engagement with the world*. This form of self-management corresponds mainly to the disproportions of verticality. Here, the historical self merely flies over a world in which the alliances that are the hallmark of human engagement no longer make sense. The alternatives that present themselves to this historical self are either to surrender to this derailed bliss or to take individual responsibility for oneself, others and society. The choice is between investing in a world that can or should be worth more or being taken in by the idea that the world – and ultimately, people themselves – are irrelevant. This is an option for nihilism, as we can see from the words of one patient who was seriously ill due to polysubstance use:

> You want to know why I got like this? I don't even know. I think it happened by accident. I'm not sure. It's just a phase I'm going through. I don't know if some kind of test, maybe, only God knows, I don't. It's by accident what's happening to me. I'm not that bright. He's the only one who knows anything. He knows what pieces are placed on each... life is a chessboard. He knows which piece to put where. He'll move the pieces. (N. 34 years old)

7.4 Embodiment

In embodiment, the specific modifications produced in anthropological proportions by substance abuse are focused on the experience of *craving*. In this experience, typical of states of addiction, existence is visibly subjugated to the need for the substance. Craving indicates that embodiment has become a significant material support and instrument for relating to the world in a mode of existence swallowed up by detemporalisation and plenitude. In order to understand the distorted nature of this phenomenon, we must first briefly examine the polarity of *necessity–saciety*, which becomes distorted in craving.

This relationship is marked by the appearance of a specific need, which is to be met by a particular object, which in turn leads to satiety. For example, the experience of hunger makes consciousness uneasy and impels embodiment, through a specific sensation, towards a corresponding action in the realm of food, namely, the act of eating. Once the need encounters its object of desire, this pressure is undone. The bodily sensation disappears and the specific transitory link between the self-pole and the world-pole is unmade. The historical self is satisfied, freed to continue in its endeavours. The state of satiety therefore leads the increased corporeality – hunger – back to its baseline style, even if temporarily, until a new need is established. Over time, it is common for the relationship between need and satiety to undergo a qualitative alteration, leading to enhanced taste. It is natural that as the years go by, we are capable of refining the hunger–satiety relationship, transforming it into a sophisticated act of appreciation of flavours, combinations and textures.

Temporality allows this development to occur. Indeed, it is strictly down to this evolutionary temporal chain in which hunger remains hunger and satiety remains satiety that the articulation between the two can be refined. In short, a temporally enhanced relationship between need and satiety offers the conditions for continuous learning in its fruition.

However, this relationship can be disrupted. When a substance is craved, it is because the relationship has ceased to respect the dictates of time. In fact, it acts in the opposite direction from time. By detaching itself from the temporalisation which sustains it and gives it balance, craving for a substance indicates the loss of the capacity to maintain a need–satiety type of relationship. The addicted person's need cannot be compared to hunger or even to other experiences of need, such as sexual need. The force with which craving affects them bodily is demonstrative of its existential role, which is to bring about a paralysis of temporality by coagulating the self-pole and the drug-object. This coagulating force prevents the relationship between user and substance to deepen or be enhanced. In addiction, there is no progression of a relationship between historical self and substance over time; on the contrary, there is a *de-differentiation* of this relationship, most tellingly described in the following terms by patients: "I don't know why I use anymore. It doesn't give me any pleasure any more, but I need to use". It is precisely this inability to establish a progressive, differentiated relationship with the use of a substance that sets it apart from healthy substance use. In healthy use, the relationship is refined over time with the inclusion of new experiences from the intoxicated state of consciousness in biographical development. Therefore, in theory, every substance can be used without it being detrimental.

When temporality is disrupted, the distance between the self-pole and the drug-object is also disrupted, leaving no chance for a fertile relationship between the totality of existence and intoxication. Successive experiences of proximity and distance are needed in every fertile relationship so that it can be enhanced, as described above. Craving forces the self-pole into adhesive contact with the portion of the world of which it is deprived, resuming the movement towards plenitude. In its most extreme form, craving calls for embodiment to commit to an existence stripped of temporality and spatiality, dense and immobile. In addiction, there is not so much desire as a deformation of desire, which is fossilised in the distorted form of overwhelming embodiment. Nor is the essential memory of pleasure maintained, for this depends on some perspective between the poles being reinstated, where pleasure is the point of contact through which the self-pole can celebrate life. The addicted person continually abuses a substance because they are no longer able to even recognise its otherness. They become one with it, in a mortal embrace which takes them bodily back to the almost mineral form of relationship with the world I referred to above.

Chapter 8
Resumption of a Personal Biography: The Dialectics of Recovery

I've got nothing to lose. I've got nothing. I've got no dignity, no family, get it? It's just me for myself. Just me for myself. Just me with my problems, get it? From here I could get worse, it's easy enough to get worse [snapping their fingers]. To get better, that's hard. (J., 33 years old)

The central idea that has guided the arguments presented in this book is that for psychopathology to take its place as a basic science of clinical psychology and psychiatry, it must understand the human situation in its entirety (Fukuda 2013). The *conditio humana* is the source from which the science of psychopathology should take its inspiration. It therefore makes sense to conclude it by sketching out the existential meanings by which a person can overcome substance misuse and resume their biographical development. The same notion of treatment could be extended from the analyses I have made and include an understanding of recovery as more than just giving up maladjusted, harmful behaviour (although this is a necessary step). The notion of recovery is broader than just clinical treatment in the strict sense of psychiatry or clinical psychology, since it encompasses the reconstruction of the whole of existence (Wiklund 2008). Recovery from substance misuse inevitably involves finding the indispensable conditions of possibility that allow the distortion of the biography in the present continuous and in total space to be controlled and a personal destiny to be re-established. This is what I shall do now, very briefly, since this is not within the scope of this volume.

Inevitably, the path to recovery involves confronting the existential vulnerability that appears in all substance misuse-related conditions. Temporally, these people are vulnerable to temporal instability, which leads to an indifferentiation or dedifferentiation of their biographies. Spatially, they become vulnerable to enslavement by a plenitude from which they cannot extricate themselves. Intersubjectively, their vulnerability comes either from extreme transparency and proximity to the other or from an impairment of the capacity to attune to the other and the world. Bodily, their vulnerability comes from the fossilisation of their craving like a foreign body in the field of sensations. Throughout the recovery process, substance misusers' existence is constantly at risk of being incapacitated as an autonomous and genuine

© Springer Nature Switzerland AG 2021
G. Messas, *The Existential Structure of Substance Misuse*,
https://doi.org/10.1007/978-3-030-62724-9_8

biographical development, as a person in full possession of their potentialities. Although the ultimate decision to overcome substance misuse starts from the decision-making freedom of the historical self, its realisation depends to a large extent on the construction of intersubjective supports that foster this recovery (Butler and Seedall 2006). It is these intersubjective supports that offer existential support so that personal identity can be reconstructed. Understanding recovery therefore means knowing the best ways to help an existence shattered by the collapse of its anthropological proportions face its weaknesses and re-establish its differences. It is about trying to understand what style of identity and intersubjectivity would be helpful for the resumption of the capacity to develop a personal identity. From this understanding, the clinicians can identify the positional and value senses involved in the substance misuse and help their patient make the best decisions to resume their life. I conclude this work by briefly examining the existential dilemma of recovery, based on its main dialectics.

8.1   Recovering Temporality

From what has been presented above, one important goal of the treatment of substance misusers is to help them maintain flexibility among the three dimensions of temporality (Leal and Serpa Junior 2013). Every effort should be made by the psychiatrist/clinical psychologist to prevent the patient from remaining immobile in a single state of anthropological temporal proportion, from being held captive, so to speak, by an eternal present (Moskalewicz 2016). There are three strategies that can be employed for this purpose. One way is to *reduce the intensity* of the experience of the present; another is to *substitute* the intensity caused by intoxication *with other immediate experiences*; and finally, emphasis on the dimensions of the retention and protention can be *directly increased*. All three strategies are achievable using biological (pharmacological) means, by brain stimulation and/or by psychological actions.[1] The different temporal strategies that can be employed are presented below.

Psychopharmacology is the principal means used to *reduce the intensity* of the experience of the present. It is used to reduce the intoxicating effect of psychoactive substances so they are unable to take over the patient's consciousness. This strategy therefore aims to diminish the importance attributed to the present. In the case of alcohol use, for example, naltrexone may be prescribed. By countering the action of opioid receptors, naltrexone satiates the intoxicating effects of alcohol (Nutt 2014). It does not prevent the present from being enhanced, but it does diminish this enhancement, making it less likely to have complete dominance over retention and protention. Naltrexone is also effective for curbing binge drinking (Maisel et al.

---

[1] In fact, treatments that are based on a radical reading of phenomenology make no real separation between these therapeutic dimensions (Tamelini and Messas 2019).

2013), one of the hyperpresentification-related behaviours most closely associated with health risks (Plunk et al. 2014; Schoenborn et al. 2014).

The idea that underpins *substituting* the intensity of intoxication with *other immediate experiences* is that there is little chance of completely modifying anthropological hyperpresentification, even in the absence of substance use. An illustration of this is the common association of substance misuse with extreme temperaments like novelty-seeking (Verheul 2001; Foulds et al. 2017). The frequency of this association suggests that a vulnerability to substance overuse may be mediated by existential characteristics which are susceptible to the urges of the present, leading to emphasis on or even a need for an existence that is focused on the present, ignoring or avoiding participation in retention or protention. The novelty-seeker thus inhabits a world that is full of attractions that are so enticing they end up getting lost in it. The clinician in such a case may not be able to reduce the hyperpresentification, but instead, it may be possible to find alternative ways for it to be expressed. In other words, the goal is to maintain a highly stimulated present, but filling it with healthy experiences like sports or arts, rather than harmful ones (Dunning and Waddington 2013; Landale and Roderick 2013; Soldani 2017; van Herdeen 2016).

In the *direct addition* of an experience from retention or protention to existence, the family tends to be the most significant therapeutic instrument. In fact, family involvement is often a key to success in the treatment of substance misusers (Klostermann and O'Farrell 2013; Kumpfer et al. 2003; Kemp 2014). When family relationships have been lost, outcomes tend to be less positive (Lander et al. 2013). From an anthropological perspective, this is because of the meaning the family has to the substance misuser's existence. Normally, the family is the most stable aspect of people's life; family relations have the strongest roots in existence, making them the ipso facto representatives of retention. This means they can exert an influence on the substance misuser's temporal proportions of existence, helping to expand them and overcome their tendency towards hyperpresentification. The clinician caring for a substance misuser would therefore be advised to identify which of the patient's closest friends or relations would be most able to help reinstate the past in their temporal existence.

Another way of addressing excessive participation in the present is to enhance forward-orientation and engagement with protention. This strategy can be enacted in either of two ways. One is much like the strategy for enhancing retention, although in this case, the idea is to introduce people who have *no* connection with the patient's personal history. Self-help groups are opportune for this, providing a new collective identity that the patient can turn to and depend on as they develop a new life plan (Kemp 2014; Kellogg 1993; Chappel and Dupont 1999). People inclined towards hyperpresentification may need to involve themselves in a group project like a self-help group or a therapeutic community in order to build a future, then gradually incorporate it into their personal identity (Souza 2016; Di Petta and Tittarelli 2019). Nonetheless, a person who has no future orientation may still find it hard to envisage building such a new life. As such, the group or collective relationship provides this orientation, given that it is often so hard to build a new and personal life plan alone. This obviously suggests that purely interpersonal (one-on-one) psychother-apy may not be enough in and of itself for the treatment of substance misuse (Brache 2012).

Another strategy is more aligned with the classical approach of humanistic psy-chotherapy; that is, engaging in a movement leading to the construction of a future as imagined by a free and creative subject (SAMHSA 1999). For this to work, a meaningful point of contact must be established with the patient's hyperpresentifi-cation. The idea is that the clinician acts on immediate temporality, engaging intensely and directly with the patient and responding swiftly to this interaction (Di Petta 2014). The first thing they should do is fill the patient's hyperpresent with their own presence. This should reinstate a degree of equilibrium to their anthropological proportions. Later, when this has been achieved and there is a greater presence of retention and protention in the patient, the clinician will be able to harness their regained capacity for reflection and planning to embark on the kind of existential reflections typical of traditional psychotherapy.

The immediate present is therefore the starting point for any treatment of sub-stance misuse. Interventions should first focus on reducing the degree of substance use and thereby expand the patient's temporality, which should bring about the emergence of some kind of biographical "becoming". In the early stages of treat-ment, the clinician must be available for direct contact with the patient and even provide them with physical protection. They may also intervene in the patient's life by helping them organise their social and relational resources. Or else they may help by mediating the diverse relationships capable of expanding the temporality of the patient's existence. Additionally, they may draw on their pharmacological knowl-edge to help quell the exaggerated influence of the present in the patient's existence. And finally, now in the more traditional role of the psychotherapist, they will pro-pose reflections that address the patient's existence as a whole.

8.2   Recovering Spatiality

The experience of plenitude means the contradictions inherent to existence do not have to be faced. The world appears complete and untainted by decisions and renouncements. Recovery means reinstating the capacity to experience the different perspectives that exist in each experiential act. Part of this may include developing the capacity to identify risks to third parties, especially close relatives (Fals-Stewart et al. 2003), who often pick up the pieces for substance misusers (Callinan et al. 2016). The capacity to doubt, the capacity to live in a world that is inherently com-plex, where each experience is inevitably intersubjective, is therefore all part of the route to recovery.

The intersubjective foundations of all experience are quelled under the influence of the simplified total experience that is the hallmark of existential plenitude. Either the historical self is cut off in existential abstraction and lives in a world of chimeras occupied only by itself, or it is exposed to overpowering intersubjectivity. The pathway to recovery involves reinstating a world where existential development is enabled by a more balanced intersubjective state. The social reintegration of substance misusers is not just a matter of returning to society, resuming their social activities; rather, it must burgeon from changes on a much deeper existential and ethical level: a regained capacity to experience the world as shared, where all individual experience is a proportional arrangement of the experiences of all. Therapeutic actions for substance misusers should therefore be designed to help them find a dynamic equilibrium between their own aspirations and those of the social world.

8.3 Recovering Identities – Identity Collectivisation and Suprapersonal Unification

In the collective form of intersubjectivity (see Sect. 2.3.3), there is an emphasis on the similarities between the identity experiences of the different members of a group. The collectivisation of identity means elevating the relative presence of these collective identities in relation to the singularities of a person experiencing the world. Here, collectivity is worth more than individuality and belonging is everything. What we have here is the super-personal unification of partial identities which, through the homogenisation of experiences, brings about existential cohesion.

The cohesion offered by this mode of imbalance may offer the recovering historical self, the ontological security it needs to manage its trajectory of personal renewal. The constructive impact the elevation of collectivisation has on the life of a substance misuser is patent in the words of one patient:

> My recovery is very much tied in with the fellowship I belong to...

The collective proportion of the personal identity of substance misusers can be increased by offering a professional identity, reunion with the family, membership in peer groups, joining a religious community, etc. All these forms of belonging allow the world to be experienced in the same way that many do. They enable the historical self to find the indispensable unifying force to face the dialectical tensions of all existence.

8.4 Personal Recovery and Authority

This suprapersonal unification is ultimately granted by the presence of a strong otherness throughout life, to a greater or lesser extent. Many patients report this anthropological need with dramatic clarity:

> (...) the only thing I'm afraid of, if I'm going to talk like this, is having a person in my life who doesn't have control of their emotions... *I have to be with someone who's emotionally strong,*

or

> I'm the kind of person that's no good at living alone... *I need to have someone by my side who's going to say, "come on, man, don't do that"* or *"come on, bro, why are you so uptight?* (J, 33, emphasis added)

Or even, in this more explicit exclamation:

> *I wanted a group to tell me what to do in my life post-drugs. A junkie can never do anything alone, they always ask.* And that's what I'm doing. *A guy needs some direction or he'll turn back.*

The historical self lost in the plenitude of the present continuous feels that finding what is good for them depends on the proximity of an otherness that is capable of overseeing their daily life ("*I need to have someone by my side*"), preserving the integrity of its values ("*come on, man, don't do that*"), taking responsibility for guiding its future ("*I wanted a group to tell me what to do in my life*") and ensuring its stability outside of addiction ("*a guy needs some direction or he'll turn back*").

The three quotes presented above – which are not uncommon, and indeed, explain much of the imaginary of substance misusers – reveal the authority role the extruded self-pole needs from its otherness. The role of authority in the intersubjectivity of the substance misuser is fundamental, since they will be the element capable of providing definition, clarity, differentiation, sharpness, stability, protection and identity cohesion against the existential distortion of the substance misuser. Yet, the authority of the other in recovery is loaded with ambiguity, for it is an authority which must act firmly and decisively, but also recognise that their central function, which is perhaps the noblest of all human functions, is to serve the construction of a human person. Authority in substance misuse situations must follow the original Latin meaning of the word "auctor". The *auctor* is the leader, the master, whose capacity to influence comes from their moral stature and not from their coercive power. The auctor lifts and inspires by their example and presence, helping the substance misuser find him-/herself again in the highways and byways of life. The dialectics of recovery ultimately reproduce the dilemmas of all existence. They start from the human condition and belong to us all.

References

Abettan, C. (2015). Phénoménologie et typologie dans la mélancolie: une question de méthode. In P. C. Cabestan & Jeanine (Eds.), *Mélancolie – Phénoménologie, psychopathologie, psychanalyse* (p. 208). Paris: Le Cercle Herméneutique.

Adams, B., & Sanders, T. (2011, August). Experiences of psychosis in borderline personality disorder: A qualitative analysis. *Journal of Mental Health, 20*(4), 381–391.

Addington, J., & Duchak, V. (1997). Reasons for substance use in schizophrenia. *Acta Psychiatrica Scandinavica, 96*(5), 329–333.

Adorno, R., Rui, T., Silva, S., Malvasi, P., et al. (2013). Etnografia da cracolândia: notas sobre uma pesquisa em território urbano. *Saúde & Transformação Social/Health & Social Change, 4,* 4–13.

Ambrosini, A., Stanghellini, G., & Langer, Á. I. (2011). Typus melancholicus from Tellenbach up to the present day: A review about the premorbid personality vulnerable to melancholia. *Actas Españolas de Psiquiatría, 39*(5), 302–311.

APA [American Psychiatric Association]. (2013). *Diagnostic and statistical manual of mental disorders V* (5th ed.). Arlington: American Psychiatric Publishing.

Aristotle. (1934). *Nicomachean ethics.* Cambridge, MA: Harvard University Press.

Aristotle. (1935). *Eudemian ethics.* Cambridge, MA: Harvard University Press.

Aristotle. (1957a). *Aristotelis Metaphysica.* Oxford: Clarendon Press.

Aristotle. (1957b). Problems: XXII–XXXVIII, with an English translation by W.S. Hett; Rhetorica ad Alexandrum. With an English translation by H. Rackham. (Loeb Classical Library) Cambridge & London: Harvard University Press.

Auer, R., Vittinghoff, E., Yaffe, K., Künzi, A., et al. (2016, March). Association between lifetime marijuana use and cognitive function in middle age: The Coronary Artery Risk Development in Young Adults (CARDIA) study. *JAMA Internal Medicine, 176*(3), 352–361.

Ayres, T. C., & Treadwell, J. (2011). Bars, drugs and football thugs: Alcohol, cocaine use and violence in the night time economy among English football firms. *Criminology & Criminal Justice, 12*(1), 83–100.

Baca-Garcia, E., Perez-Rodriguez, M. M. M., Basurte-Villamor, I., Fernandez Del Moral, A. L., et al. (2007, March). Diagnostic stability of psychiatric disorders in clinical practice. *The British Journal of Psychiatry, 190,* 210–216.

Bagge, C. L., & Sher, K. J. (2008, December). Adolescent alcohol involvement and suicide attempts: Toward the development of a conceptual framework. *Clinical Psychology Review, 28*(8), 1283–1296.

Baker, A. (2005). The long-term effects of parental alienation on adult children: A qualitative research study. *American Journal of Family Therapy, 33*(4), 289–302.

© Springer Nature Switzerland AG 2021
G. Messas, *The Existential Structure of Substance Misuse,*
https://doi.org/10.1007/978-3-030-62724-9

Balducci, T., González-Olvera, J. J., Angeles-Valdez, D., Espinoza-Luna, I., et al. (2018). Borderline personality disorder with cocaine dependence: Impulsivity, emotional dysregulation and amygdala functional connectivity. *Frontiers in Psychiatry, 9*, 328.

Ballerini, A. (2008). Declinazioni psichotiche dell'identità. In A. Ales Bello, A. Ballerini, et al. (Eds.), *Io e tu. Fenomenologia dell'incontro* (pp. 49–73). Rome: Edizioni Universitarie Romane.

Ballerini, A., & Di Petta, G. (2015). *Oltre e di là dal mondo: l'essenza della schizofrenia. Fenomenologia e psicopatologia*. Rome: Giovanni Fioriti Editore. 9788898991211.

Banzato, C. E. M., & Zorzanelli, R. T. (2017). Conhecimento tácito e raciocínio clínico em psiquiatria. *Psicopatologia Fenomenológica Contemporânea, 6*(2), 81–92.

Barthélémy, J.-M. (2013). Importance de l'étude structurale et évolutive des images dans l'analyse psychopathologique des phénomènes d'intoxication alcoolique et d'addiction toxicomaniaque. *Psicopatologia Fenomenológica Contemporânea, 2*(2), 88–111.

Basso, E. (2009). L'apriori nella psichiatria fenomenologica. In L. Bisin (Ed.), *Lo sguardo in anticipo. Quattro studi sull'apriori* (pp. 9–48). Milano: Edizioni di Sofia.

Baudelaire, C. (2007). *Les Paradis artificiels*. Paris: Gallimard.

Belcher, A. M., Volkow, N. D., Moeller, F. G., & Ferré, S. (2014, April). Personality traits and vulnerability or resilience to substance use disorders. *Trends in Cognitive Sciences, 18*(4), 211–217.

Bergson, H. (1889). *Essai sur les données immédiates de la conscience*. Paris: Félix Alcan.

Bilz, R. (1956). Das Belagerungserlebnis in den Alkoholhalluzinosen. Eine Untersuchung über die Situation und das Verhalten des Subjekts. *Der Nervenartz, 27*(9), 402–409.

Binder, H. (1979). Über alkoholische Rauschzustände. In K. Bash (Ed.), *Ausgewählte Arbeiten. Band I: Klinische Psychiatrie* (pp. 166–220). Bern-Stuttgart-Wien: Verlag Hans Huber.

Binswanger, L. (1922). *Einführung in die Probleme der allgemeinen Psychologie*. Berlin: Springer.

Binswanger, L. (1957). *Schizophrenie*. Günther Neske Verlag: Pfullinger.

Binswanger, L. (1960). *Melancholie und Manie. Phänomenologische Studien*. Pfüllingen: Neske.

Binswanger, L. (1965). *Wahn: Beiträge zu seiner phaenomenologischen und daseinsanalytischen Erforschung*. Verlag Günther Neske: Pfullingen.

Binswanger, L. (1992a). Drei formen misglückten Daseins: Verstiegenheit, Verschrobenheit, Manieriertheit. In M. Herzog (Ed.), *Ausgewählte werke. Band 1*. Heidelberg, Germany: Roland Asanger.

Binswanger, L. (1992b). *Traum und Existenz*. Berlin: Verlag Gachnang & Springer.

Binswanger, L. (1999). *Le problème de l'espace en psychopathologie*. Toulouse: Presses Universitaires du Mirail.

Binswanger, L. (2000). *Sur la fuite des idées*. Grenoble: Jérôme Millon.

Blankenburg, W. (1978). Grundlagenprobleme der Psychopathologie. *Nervenarzt, 49*, 140–146.

Blankenburg, W. (1981). Wie weit reicht die dialektische Betrachtungsweise in der Psychiatrie? [What are the limits of dialectic approach in psychiatry?]. *Zeitschrift für Klinische Psychologie und Psychotherapie, 29*(1), 45–66.

Blankenburg, W. (2007a). Die Verselbständigung eines Themas zum Wahn. In *Psycopathologie des Unscheinbaren: Ausgewählte Aufsätze* (pp. 25–68). Berlin: Parodos Verlag.

Blankenburg, W. (2007b). Futur-II: Perspektive in ihrer Bedeutung für die Erschließung der Lebensgeschichte des Patienten. In *Psycopathologie des Unscheinbaren: Ausgewählte Aufsätze* (pp. 235–252). Berlin: Parodos Verlag.

Blankenburg, W. (2007c). Grundsätzliches zur Konzeption einer anthropologischen Proportion. In *Psycopathologie des Unscheinbaren: Ausgewählte Aufsätze* (pp. 119–136). Berlin: Parodos Verlag.

Blankenburg, W. (2007d). Körper und Leib in der Psychiatrie. In *Psycopathologie des Unscheinbaren: Ausgewählte Aufsätze* (pp. 201–234). Berlin: Parodos Verlag.

Blankenburg, W. (2012). *Der Verlust der natürlichen Selbstverständlichkeit. Ein Beitrag zur psychopathologie symptomarmen Schizophrenen*. Berlin: Parodos Verlag.

Bleuler, E. (1950). *Dementia praecox or the Group of Schizophrenias*. New York: International Universities Press.

Bleuler, E. (2011). Les Problèmes de la schizoïdie et de la syntonie. *L'Information Psychiatrique, 87*, 37–51.

Boles, S. M., & Miotto, K. (2003). Substance abuse and violence: A review of the literature. *Aggression and Violent Behavior, 8*(2), 155–174.

Bolton, J. M., Robinson, J., & Sareen, J. (2009, June). Self-medication of mood disorders with alcohol and drugs in the National Epidemiologic Survey on Alcohol and Related Conditions. *Journal of Affective Disorders, 115*(3), 367–375.

Bonhoeffer, K. (1917). Die exogenen Reaktionstypen. *Archiv fur Psychiatrie und Nervenkrankheiten, 58*, 50–70.

Bot, S. M., Engels, R. C., Knibbe, R. A., & Meeus, W. H. (2005, June). Friend's drinking behaviour and adolescent alcohol consumption: The moderating role of friendship characteristics. *Addictive Behaviors, 30*(5), 929–947.

Bowlby, J. (1940). *Personality and mental illness: An essay in psychiatric diagnosis*. Taylor & Francis Group: UK.

Brache, K. (2012, July). Advancing interpersonal therapy for substance use disorders. *The American Journal of Drug and Alcohol Abuse, 38*(4), 293–298.

Brorson, H. H., Ajo Arnevik, E., Rand-Hendriksen, K., & Duckert, F. (2013, December). Drop-out from addiction treatment: A systematic review of risk factors. *Clinical Psychology Review, 33*(8), 1010–1024.

Buber, M. (1971). *I and thou*. New York: Touchstone.

Buchmann, S. J., Lehmann, D., & Stevens, C. E. (2019). Takotsubo cardiomyopathy-acute cardiac dysfunction associated with neurological and psychiatric disorders. *Frontiers in Neurology, 10*, 917.

Bürgy, M. (2005, November–December). Psychopathology of obsessive-compulsive disorder: A phenomenological approach. *Psychopathology, 38*(6), 291–300.

Butler, M. H., & Seedall, R. B. (2006). The attachment relationship in recovery from addiction. Part 1: Relationship mediation. *Sexual Addiction & Compulsivity, 13*(2–3), 289–315.

Callieri, B. (2001). *Quando vince l'ombra. Problemi di psicopatologia clinica*. Roma: Edizioni University Romane.

Callinan, S., Laslett, A.-M., Rekve, D., Room, R., et al. (2016). Alcohol's harm to others: An international collaborative project. *The International Journal of Alcohol and Drug Research, 5*(2), 25–32.

Carpenter, T. H., & Faraone, C. A. (1993). *Masks of dionysus*. Ithaca: Cornell University Press.

Carroll, B. J. (2012, February). Bringing back melancholia. *Bipolar Disorders, 14*(1), 1–5.

Carvalho, A. F., Stubbs, B., Vancampfort, D., Kloiber, S., et al. (2019). Cannabis use and suicide attempts among 86,254 adolescents aged 12-15 years from 21 low- and middle-income countries. *European Psychiatry, 56*, 8–13.

Ceron-Litvoc, D. (2020). Interpessoalidade na primeira infância: as possibilidades do encontro com o outro. *Psicopatologia Fenomenológica Contemporânea, 9*(1), 57–72.

Chamond, J. (2005). Binswanger et les directions de sens. In J. Chamond (Ed.), *Les directions de sens: Phénoménologie et psychopathologie de l'espace vécu: Le Cercle Herméneutique*. p.19–42

Chan, G. C., Kelly, A. B., Carroll, A., & Williams, J. W. (2017). Peer drug use and adolescent polysubstance use: Do parenting and school factors moderate this association? *Addictive Behaviors, 64*, 78–81.

Chappel, J. N., & Dupont, R. L. (1999, June). Twelve-step and mutual-help programs for addictive disorders. *The Psychiatric Clinics of North America, 22*(2), 425–446.

Charbonneau, G. (2007). *La situation existentielle des personnes hystériques: intensité, centralité et figuralité. Société d'anthropologie phénoménologique et d'Hermeneutique Générale*. Paris: Vrin.

Charbonneau, G. (2010). *Introduction à la psychopathologie phénoménologique*. Paris: MJW Fédition.

Charbonneau, G., & Legrand, J. M. (2003). *Dépressions et paradépressions. Clinique, psychopatologique et thérapeutique des manifestations paradepréssives*. Paris: Le Cercle Herméneutique.

Chong, T. W., & Castle, D. J. (2004, August). Layer upon layer: Thermoregulation in schizophrenia. *Schizophrenia Research, 69*(2–3), 149–157.

Choo, E. K., Benz, M., Rybarczyk, M., Broderick, K., et al. (2014, December). The intersecting roles of violence, gender, and substance use in the emergency department: A research agenda. *Academic Emergency Medicine, 21*(12), 1447–1452.

Clarke, M. C., Coughlan, H., Harley, M., Connor, D., et al. (2014, October). The impact of adolescent cannabis use, mood disorder and lack of education on attempted suicide in young adulthood. *World Psychiatry, 13*(3), 322–323.

Coffey, S. F., Schumacher, J. A., Baschnagel, J. S., Hawk, L. W., et al. (2011). Impulsivity and risk-taking in borderline personality disorder with and without substance use disorders. *Personality Disorders: Theory, Research, and Treatment, 2*(2), 128–141.

Colombetti, G., & Ratcliffe, M. (2012). Bodily feeling in depersonalization: A phenomenological account. *Emotion Review, 4*(2), 145–150.

Coulston, C. M., Tanious, M., Mulder, R. T., Porter, R. J., et al. (2012, June). Bordering on bipolar: The overlap between borderline personality and bipolarity. *The Australian and New Zealand Journal of Psychiatry, 46*(6), 506–521.

Crapanzano, K. A., Hammarlund, R., Ahmad, B., Hunsinger, N., et al. (2019). The association between perceived stigma and substance use disorder treatment outcomes: A review. *Substance Abuse and Rehabilitation, 10*, 1–12.

Crean, R. D., Crane, N. A., & Mason, B. J. (2011, March). An evidence based review of acute and long-term effects of cannabis use on executive cognitive functions. *Journal of Addiction Medicine, 5*(1), 1–8.

Cusinato, G. (2017). *Periagoge. Teoria della singolarità e filosofia come cura del desiderio* (2nd ed.). Verona: QuiEdit.

Cutting, J. (2012). *A critique of psychopathology* (Vol. 402, p. 9783938880517). Berlin: Parodos Verlag.

Cutting, J., & Musalek, M. (2016, March). The nature of delusion: Psychologically explicable? Psychologically inexplicable? Philosophically explicable? Part 2. *History of Psychiatry, 27*(1), 21–37.

Dahlberg, K. (2006). The essence of essences – The search for meaning structures in phenomenological analysis of lifeworld phenomena. *International Journal of Qualitative Studies on Health and Well-Being, 1*(1), 11–19.

Davis, G. P., Compton, M. T., Wang, S., Levin, F. R., et al. (2013, December). Association between cannabis use, psychosis, and schizotypal personality disorder: Findings from the National Epidemiologic Survey on Alcohol and Related Conditions. *Schizophrenia Research, 151*(1–3), 197–202.

Dearing, R. L., Stuewig, J., & Tangney, J. P. (2005, August). On the importance of distinguishing shame from guilt: Relations to problematic alcohol and drug use. *Addictive Behaviors, 30*(7), 1392–1404.

Degenhardt, L. (2018). The global burden of disease attributable to alcohol and drug use in 195 countries and territories, 1990–2016: A systematic analysis for the global burden of disease study 2016. *Lancet Psychiatry, 5*, 987–1012.

Depraz, N., Varela, F. J., & Vermersch, P. (2011). *À l'épreuve de l'expérience. Pour une pratique phénoménologique*. Bucarest: ZETA Books.

Di Petta, G. (2012). *Nel nulla esserci. Il vuoto, la psicosi, l'incontro*. Rome: Edizioni Universitarie Romane. 9788860221773.

Di Petta, G. (2014). Psychopathlogy of addictions. *Journal of Psychopathology, 20*, 471–479.

Di Petta, G. (2016). "Synthetic psychosis" by novel psychoactive substances: A psychopathological understanding of a clinical case. In G. Stanghellini & M. Aragona (Eds.), *An experiential approach to psychopathology*. Switzerland: Springer.

Di Petta, G. (2019). The world of the drug addict. In G. Stanghellini, M. Broome, et al. (Eds.), *The Oxford handbook of phenomenological psychopathology* (pp. 682–694). Oxford: Oxford University Press.

Di Petta, G., & Tittarelli, D. (2019). The "we-ness": A Dasein-analytical approach to group therapy. *Psychopathology, 52*(2), 110–116.

Dilthey, W. (1977). *Descriptive psychology and historical understanding.* Netherlands: Springer.

Dingle, G. A. (2018). Addiction and the importance of belonging. *The Psychologist, 31*(5), 36–38.

Dingle, G. A., Cruwys, T., & Frings, D. (2015). Social identities as pathways into and out of addiction. *Frontiers in Psychology, 6,* 1795.

Domínguez-Salas, S., Díaz-Batanero, C., Lozano-Rojas, O. M., & Verdejo-García, A. (2016, December). Impact of general cognition and executive function deficits on addiction treatment outcomes: Systematic review and discussion of neurocognitive pathways. *Neuroscience and Biobehavioral Reviews, 71,* 772–801.

Dörr-Zegers, O. (1995). *Psiquiatría Antropológica: Contribuciones a una psiquiatría de orientación fenomenológico-antropológica* (2nd ed.). Santiago de Chile: Editorial Universitaria. 956-11-0925-5.

Dörr-Zegers, O. (2005). Aspectos fenomenológicos y éticos del envejecimiento y la demencia. *Revista Médica de Chile, 133*(1), 113–120.

Dörr-Zegers, O. (2008, January–February). Personality disorders from a phenomenological perspective. *Actas Españolas de Psiquiatría, 36*(1), 10–19.

Dörr-Zegers, O. (2013). Fenomenología de la intersubjetividad y su importancia para la comprensión de las enfermedades endógenas. *Psicopatologia Fenomenológica Contemporânea, 3*(1), 75–90.

Dörr-Zegers, O. (2018). Space and time in the obsessive-compulsive phenomenon. *Psychopathology, 51*(1), 31–37.

Dörr-Zegers, O., Irarrázaval, L., Mundt, A., & Palette, V. (2017). Disturbances of embodiment as core phenomena of depression in clinical practice. *Psychopathology, 50*(4), 273–281.

Dunning, E., & Waddington, I. (2013). Sport as a drug and drugs in sport: Some exploratory comments. *International Review for the Sociology of Sport, 38*(3), 351–368.

EMCDDA [European Monitoring Centre for Drugs and Drug Addiction]. (2016). *Comorbidity of substance use and mental health disorders in Europe (perspectives on drugs).* Lisbon: EMCDDA.

Englebert, J. (2019). The psychopathology of psychopaths. In G. Stanghellini, M. Broome, et al. (Eds.), *The Oxford handbook of phenomenological psychopathology* (pp. 882–895). Oxford: Oxford University Press.

Fals-Stewart, W., Golden, J., & Schumacher, J. A. (2003, December). Intimate partner violence and substance use: A longitudinal day-to-day examination. *Addictive Behaviors, 28*(9), 1555–1574.

Fernandez, A. V. (2014). Reconsidering the affective dimension of depression and mania: Towards a phenomenological dissolution of the paradox of mixed states. *Journal of Psychopathology, Special Issue—Phenomenological Psychopathology and Clinical Practice: Resources for Early Career Psychiatrists, 20*(4), 414–422.

Fernandez, A. V. (2016). Phenomenology, typification, and ideal types in psychiatric diagnosis and classification. In R. Bluhm (Ed.), *Knowing and acting in medicine* (pp. 39–58). Lanham: Rowman & Littlefield International.

Fernandez, A. V. (2019). Phenomenological psychopathology and psychiatric classification. In G. Stanghellini, M. Broome, et al. (Eds.), *The Oxford handbook of phenomenological psychopathology* (pp. 1016–1030). Oxford: Oxford University Press.

Fernandez, A. V., & Køster, A. (2019). On the subject matter of phenomenological psychopathology. In G. Stanghellini, M. Broome, et al. (Eds.), *The Oxford handbook of phenomenological psychopathology* (pp. 191–204). Oxford: Oxford University Press.

Ferreira, G. M., Lee, R. S. C., Piquet-Pessôa, M., De Menezes, G. B., et al. (2020, February). Habitual versus affective motivations in obsessive-compulsive disorder and alcohol use disorder. *CNS Spectrums,* 1–8.

Figal, G. (2015). *Unscheinbarkeit: Der Raum der Phänomenologie.* Tübingen: Mohr Siebeck. 978-3161537110.

Flores, P. J. (2011). *Addiction as an attachment disorder.* United States (Maryland): Jason Aronson.

Foulds, J. A., Boden, J. M., Newton-Howes, G. M., Mulder, R. T., et al. (2017, September). The role of novelty seeking as a predictor of substance use disorder outcomes in early adulthood. *Addiction, 112*(9), 1629–1637.

Franzen, M., Sadikaj, G., Moskowitz, D. S., Ostafin, B. D., et al. (2018). Intra- and Interindividual variability in the behavioral, affective, and perceptual effects of alcohol consumption in a social context. *Alcoholism, Clinical and Experimental Research, 42*(5), 952–961.

Frías, Á., Palma, C., Farriols, N., & González, L. (2016). Sexuality-related issues in borderline personality disorder: A comprehensive review. *Personality and Mental Health, 10*(3), 216–231.

Frone, M. R. (2004). Alcohol, drugs, and workplace safety outcomes: A view from a general model of employee substance use and productivity. In J. Barling & M. R. Frone (Eds.), *The psychology of workplace safety* (pp. 127–156). American Psychological Association.

Frone, M. R. (2008). Employee alcohol and illicit drug use: Scope, causes, and consequences. In J. Barling & C. L. Cooper (Eds.), *The SAGE handbook of organizational behavior* (Micro approaches) (Vol. 1, pp. 519–540). Thousand Oaks, CA (California): Sage.

Fuchs, T. (2001). Melancholia as a desynchronization: Towards a psychopathology of interpersonal time. *Psychopathology, 34*(4), 179–186.

Fuchs, T. (2005). Corporealized and disembodied minds: A phenomenological view of the body in melancholia and schizophrenia. *Philosophy, Psychiatry & Psychology, 12*(2), 95–107.

Fuchs, T. (2007a). Fragmented selves: Temporality and identity in borderline personality disorder. *Psychopathology, 40*(6), 379–387.

Fuchs, T. (2007b). The temporal structure of intentionality and its disturbance in schizophrenia. *Psychopathology, 40*(4), 229–235.

Fuchs, T. (2010). Subjectivity and intersubjectivity in psychiatric diagnosis. *Psychopathology, 43*(4), 268–274.

Fuchs, T. (2013). Temporality and psychopathology. *Phenomenology and the Cognitive Sciences, 12*(1), 75–104.

Fuchs, T. (2018). *Ecology of the brain – The phenomenology and biology of the embodied mind.* Oxford: Oxford University Press. International Perspectives in Philosophy and Psychiatry.

Fuchs, T. (2020). Delusion, reality, and intersubjectivity: A phenomenological and enactive analysis. *Philosophy, Psychiatry & Psychology, 27*(1), 61–79.

Fuchs, T., Messas, G. P., & Stanghellini, G. (2019). More than just description: Phenomenology and psychotherapy. *Psychopathology, 52*(2), 63–66.

Fukuda, L. E. (2013). A psicopatologia na formação psiquiátrica. *Psicopatologia Fenomenológica Contemporânea, 2*(2), 51–65.

Fukuda, L. E., & Tamelini, M. G. (2016). A compreensão psicológica jasperiana revisitada sob a perspectiva da psicopatologia fenomenológica. *Psicopatologia Fenomenológica Contemporânea, 5*(2), 160–184.

Fulford, K. W. M., & Stanghellini, G. (2019). Values and values-based practice. In G. Stanghellini, M. Broome, et al. (Eds.), *The Oxford handbook of phenomenological psychopathology.* Oxford: Oxford University Press.

Fulford, K. W. M., Peile, E., & Carrol, H. (2012). *Essential values-based practice: Clinical stories linking science with people.* Cambridge: Cambridge University Press.

Gabbani, C., & Stanghellini, G. (2008). What kind of objectivity do we need for psychiatry? A commentary to Oulis's ontological assumptions in psychiatric taxonomy. *Psychopathology, 41*(3), 203–204.

Gadamer, H.-G. (1988). On the circle of understanding. In J. M. Connolly & T. Keutner (Eds.), *Hermeneutics versus science? Three german views.* Notre Dame (Indiana): University of Notre Dame Press.

Galbusera, L., & Fellin, L. (2014). The intersubjective endeavor of psychopathology research: Methodological reflections on a second-person perspective approach. *Frontiers in Psychology, 5*, 1150.

Gallagher, S., & Zahavi, D. (2008). *The phenomenological mind.* London/New York: Routledge. 9788420677958.

Giorgi, A. (1994). A phenomenological perspective on certain qualitative research methods. *Journal of Phenomenological Psychology, 25*(2), 190–220.

Giorgi, A. (2009). *The descriptive phenomenological method in psychology: A modified Husserlian approach*. Pittsburgh: Duquesne University Press.

Glaser, J. P., Van Os, J., Thewissen, V., & Myin-Germeys, I. (2010, February). Psychotic reactivity in borderline personality disorder. *Acta Psychiatrica Scandinavica, 121*(2), 125–134.

Gorostiza, P. R., & Manes, J. A. (2011). Misunderstanding psychopathology as medical semiology: An epistemological enquiry. *Psychopathology, 44*(4), 205–215.

Gozé, T., & Naudin, J. (2017). Discussing Rümke's "praecox feeling" from the clinician's experience of schizophrenic contact. *Psicopatologia Fenomenológica Contemporânea, 6*(2), 112–123.

Green, B., Young, R., & Kavanagh, D. (2005, October). Cannabis use and misuse prevalence among people with psychosis. *The British Journal of Psychiatry, 187*, 306–313.

Gregory, T. E. (2013). Alexander the great: Hero, humanitarian, or maniac? In *Exploring the European past: Texts & images* (2nd ed.). Mason: Cengage Learning.

Gunn, C., Mackus, M., Griffin, C., Munafò, M. R., et al. (2018). A systematic review of the next-day effects of heavy alcohol consumption on cognitive performance. *Addiction, 113*(12), 2182–2193.

Heidegger, M. (2006). *Sein und Zeit*. Max Niemeyer Verlag: Tübingen.

Helman, Z. (1980). *Psychopathologie structurale 3. Structure et évolution*. Hauts-de-France: Presses Universitaires du Septentrion.

Hunt, G. E., Large, M. M., Cleary, M., Lai, H. M. X., et al. (2018). Prevalence of comorbid substance use in schizophrenia spectrum disorders in community and clinical settings, 1990–2017: Systematic review and meta-analysis. *Drug and Alcohol Dependence, 191*, 234–258.

Hunt, G. E., Malhi, G. S., Lai, H. M. X., & Cleary, M. (2020, January). Prevalence of comorbid substance use in major depressive disorder in community and clinical settings, 1990–2019: Systematic review and meta-analysis. *Journal of Affective Disorders, 266*, 288–304.

Husserl, E. (1991). *On the phenomenology of the consciousness of internal time*, Netherlands: Springer. Husserliana: Edmund Husserl – Collected Works (Book 4).

Husserl, E. (2003). *Cartesian meditations*. UK: Taylor & Francis.

Janowsky, D. S., Clopton, P. L., Leichner, P. P., Abrams, A. A., et al. (1979, July). Interpersonal effects of marijuana. A model for the study of interpersonal psychopharmacology. *Archives of General Psychiatry, 36*(7), 781–785.

Jaspers, K. (1960). *Psychologie Der Weltanschauungen*. Berlin/Gottingen/Heidelberg: Springer.

Jaspers, K. (1968). The phenomenological approach in psychopathology (original 1912). *British Journal of Psychiatry, 114*, 1313–1323.

Jaspers, K. (1970). *Strindberg et Van Gogh, Swedenborg-Hölderlin – Etude Psychiatrique comparative*. Paris: Les Editions de Minuit.

Jaspers, K. (1997). *General psychopathology*. Baltimore: The Johns Hopkins University Press.

Jensen, H. H., Mortensen, E. L., & Lotz, M. (2014, November). Drop-out from a psychodynamic group psychotherapy outpatient unit. *Nordic Journal of Psychiatry, 68*(8), 594–604.

Kapfhammer, H. P. (2017, December). The concept of schizoidia in psychiatry: From schizoidia to schizotypy and cluster A personality disorders. *Neuropsychiatrie, 31*(4), 155–171.

Kawohl, W., & Rössler, W. (2008). Cannabis and schizophrenia: New findings in an old debate. *Neuropsychiatrie: Klinik, Diagnostik, Therapie und Rehabilitation: Organ der Gesellschaft Österreichischer Nervenärzte und Psychiater, 22*(4), 223–229.

Keil, G., Keuck, L., & Hauswald, R. (2016). *Vagueness in psychiatry*. Oxford: Oxford University Press. International Perspectives in Philosophy and Psychiatry.

Kellogg, S. (1993). Identity and recovery. *Psychotherapy: Theory, Research, Practice, Training, 30*(2), 235–244.

Kemp, R. (2014). Love, hate and emergence of self in addiction. *Existential Analysis, 25*(2), 257–268.

Kemp, R. (2018). Addiction as temporal disruption: Interoception, self, meaning. *Phenomenology and the Cognitive Sciences*, 1–15.

Kendler, K. S. (2016, February). The nature of psychiatric disorders. *World Psychiatry, 15*(1), 5–12.

Kienast, T., Stoffers, J., Bermpohl, F., & Lieb, K. (2014, April). Borderline personality disorder and comorbid addiction: Epidemiology and treatment. *Deutsches Ärzteblatt International, 111*(16), 280–286.

Kimura, B. (1982). The phenomenology of the between: On the problem of the basic disturbance in schizophrenia. In A. De Koonig & F. Jenner (Eds.), *Phenomenology and psychiatry*. London/Toronto/Sydney: Academic Press.

Kimura, B. (2000). *L'entre. Une approche phenomelogique de la schizophrenie* (152 p). Grenoble: Jérôme Millon.

Kimura, B. (2005). *Scritti di psicopatologia fenomenologica*. Giovanni Fioriti Editore: Rome.

Kimura, S., Sato, T., Takahashi, T., Narita, T., et al. (2000, April). Typus melancholicus and the temperament and character inventory personality dimensions in patients with major depression. *Psychiatry and Clinical Neurosciences, 54*(2), 181–189.

Klostermann, K., & O'Farrell, T. J. (2013). Treating substance abuse: Partner and family approaches. *Social Work in Public Health, 28*(3–4), 234–247.

Køster, A. (2017). Personal history, beyond narrative: An embodied perspective. *Journal of Phenomenological Psychology, 48*(2), 163–187.

Kraus, A. (1991a). Der melancholische Wahn in identitätstheoretischer Sicht. In W. Blankenburg (Ed.), *Forum der Psychiatrie. Wahn und Perspektivität* (pp. 68–80). Stuttgart: Enke.

Kraus, A. (1991b). Methodological problem with the classification of personality disorders: The significant of existential type. *Journal of Personality Disorders, 5*, 82–92.

Kraus, A. (1996a). Ambiguitätsintoleranz als Persönlichkeitsvariable und Strukturmerkmal der Krankheitsphänomene Manisch-Depressiver. In W. Janzarik (Ed.), *Persönlichkeit und Psychose*. Stuttgart: Enke.

Kraus, A. (1996b). Role performance, identity structure and psychosis in melancholic and manic-depressive patients. In H. L. Freeman (Ed.), *Interpersonal factors in the origin and course of affective disorders*. London: GASKELL – The Royal College of Psychiatrists.

Kraus, A. (1998). Der Sinn der Manie in identitätstheoretischer Sicht. In H. Csef (Ed.), *Sinnverlust und Sinnfindung in Gesundheit und Krankheit*. Würzburg Königshausen and Neumann.

Kraus, A. (2008). Relação entre Criatividade e o Círculo Maníaco Depressivo. In G. Messas (Ed.), *Psicopatologia Fenomenológica Contemporânea* (pp. 1–22). São Paulo: Roca.

Kraus, A. (2014). Die "existentielle Psychoanalyse" Jean Paul Sartre's: eine Anwendung bei Melancolischen und Hysterischen. In H. D. Lang, Pawel, & G. Pagel (Eds.), *Grenzen der Interpretation in Hermeneutik und Psychoanalyse* (pp. 137–157). Würzburg: Königshausen & Neumann.

Kretschmer, E. (2007). *Physique and Character*. London: Routledge & Kegan Paul. 978-1406744972.

Kumpfer, K. L., Alvarado, R., & Whiteside, H. O. (2003, September–November). Family-based interventions for substance use and misuse prevention. *Substance Use & Misuse, 38*(11–13), 1759–1787.

Lagache, D. (1997). *La Jalousie amoureuse*. Paris: Presses Universitaires de France.

Landale, S., & Roderick, M. (2013). Recovery from addiction and the potential role of sport: Using a life-course theory to study change. *International Review for the Sociology of Sport, 49*(3–4), 468–484.

Lander, L., Howsare, J., & Byrne, M. (2013). The impact of substance use disorders on families and children: From theory to practice. *Social Work in Public Health, 28*(3–4), 194–205.

Lane, S. P., Carpenter, R. W., Sher, K. J., & Trull, T. J. (2016, September). Alcohol craving and consumption in borderline personality disorder: When, where, and with whom. *Clinical Psychological Science: A Journal of the Association for Psychological Science, 4*(5), 775–792.

Lanteri-Laura, G. (1962). La notion de processus dans la pensée psychopathologique de K. Jaspers. *L'Evolution Psychiatrique, 4*, 459–499.

Latimer, W., & Zur, J. (2010, July). Epidemiologic trends of adolescent use of alcohol, tobacco, and other drugs. *Child and Adolescent Psychiatric Clinics of North America, 19*(3), 451–464.

Leal, E. M., & Serpa Junior, O. D. (2013). Acesso à experiência em primeira pessoa na pesquisa em Saúde Mental. *Ciência & Saúde Coletiva, 18*(10), 2939–2948.

Lee, H.-J., Bagge, C. L., Schumacher, J. A., & Coffey, S. F. (2010). Does comorbid substance use disorder exacerbate borderline personality features? A comparison of borderline personality disorder individuals with vs. without current substance dependence. *Personality Disorders: Theory, Research, and Treatment, 1*(4), 239–249.

Levinas, E. (2014). *Le temps et l'autre.* Paris: Presses Universitaires de France (PUF). Quadrige. 978-2130630296.

Levy, K. N., Edell, W. S., & McGlashan, T. H. (2007, June). Depressive experiences in inpatients with borderline personality disorder. *The Psychiatric Quarterly, 78*(2), 129–143.

Liddell, H. G., Scott, R., Jones, H. S., & McKenzie, R. (1940). *A Greek-English lexicon.* Oxford: Clarendon Press.

Lim, G. Y., Tam, W. W., Lu, Y., Ho, C. S., et al. (2018). Prevalence of depression in the community from 30 countries between 1994 and 2014. *Scientific Reports, 8*(1), 2861.

Lo Coco, G., Melchiori, F., Oieni, V., Infurna, M., et al. (2019). Group treatment for substance use disorder in adults: A systematic review and meta-analysis of randomized-controlled trials. *Journal of Substance Abuse Treatment, 99*, 104–116.

Madeira, L., Carmenates, S., Costa, C., Linhares, L., et al. (2017). Basic self-disturbances beyond schizophrenia: Discrepancies and affinities in panic disorder – An empirical clinical study. *Psychopathology, 50*(2), 157–168.

Maisel, N. C., Blodgett, J. C., Wilbourne, P. L., Humphreys, K., et al. (2013, February). Meta-analysis of naltrexone and acamprosate for treating alcohol use disorders: When are these medications most helpful? *Addiction, 108*(2), 275–293.

Mallinger, A. (2009). The myth of perfection: Perfectionism in the obsessive personality. *American Journal of Psychotherapy, 63*(2), 103–131.

Marconi, A., Di Forti, M., Lewis, C. M., Murray, R. M., et al. (2016). Meta-analysis of the association between the level of Cannabis use and risk of psychosis. *Schizophrenia Bulletin, 42*(5), 1262–1269.

Martinotti, G., Di Nicola, M., Quattrone, D., Santacroce, R., et al. (2015). Novel psychoactive substances and induced phenomena in psychopathology: The lysergic psychoma. *Journal of Psychopathology, 21*(4), 400–405.

Matthews, S., Dwyer, R., & Snoek, A. (2017, June). Stigma and self-stigma in addiction. *Journal of Bioethical Inquiry, 14*(2), 275–286.

McGilchrist, I., & Cutting, J. (1995). Somatic delusions in schizophrenia and the affective psychoses. *The British Journal of Psychiatry, 167*(3), 350–361.

Merleau-Ponty, M. (1945). *Phénoménologie de la perception.* Paris: Gallimard.

Messas, G. (2004). *Psicopatologia e transformação: um esboço fenômeno-estrutural* (1st ed., p. 210). São Paulo: Casa do Psicólogo. 85-7396-319-0.

Messas, G. (2006). *Álcool e drogas: uma visão fenômeno-estrutural.* Casa do Psicólogo: São Paulo.

Messas, G. (2007). Reação vivencial patológica. In G. Messas (Ed.), *As Formas Da Alteração Mental* (1st ed., pp. 27–62). São Paulo: Casa do Psicólogo.

Messas, G. (2010b). *Ensaio Sobre a Estrutura Vivida – Psicopatologia Fenomenológica Comparada* (1st ed.). Editora Rocca: São Paulo.

Messas, G. (2013). Sentido e limites do diagnóstico diferencial entre psicoses endógenas e exógenas. *Psicopatologia Fenomenológica Contemporânea, 2*(1), p.2–15.

Messas, G. (2014a). O sentido da fenomenologia na Psicopatologia Geral de Karl Jaspers. *Psicopatologia Fenomenológica Contemporânea, 3*(1), 23–47.

Messas, G. (2014b). On the essence of drunkenness and the pathway to addiction: A phenomenological contribution. *Journal of Addictive Behaviors Therapy & Rehabilitation, (2), 2014b.* http://dx.doi.org/10.4172/2324-9005.1000121.

Messas, G. (2014c). *Psicose e embriaguez – psicopatologia fenomenológica da temporalidade* (1st ed., 382 p). Editora Intermeios: São Paulo.

Messas, G. (2015). A existência fusional e o abuso de crack. *Psicopatologia Fenomenológica Contemporânea, 4*(1), 124–140.

Messas, G. (2015–2016). The association between substance use/abuse and psychosis: A phenomenological viewpoint. *Rivista Comprendre, 25–26*, 251–266.

Messas, G., & Andrade, T. (2018). As patologias da embriaguez na Grécia clássica: o silêncio eloquente do Corpus Hippocraticum. *Revista Internacional De Humanidades Médicas, 6*(2), 19–31.

Messas, G., & Fukuda, L. (2018). O diagnóstico psicopatológico fenomenológico da perspectiva dialético-essencialista. *Revista Pesquisa Qualitativa, 6*(11), 160–191.

Messas, G., & Tamelini, M. G. (2018). The pragmatic value of notions of dialectics and essence in phenomenological psychiatry and psychopathology. *Thaumàzein – Rivista di Filosofia, 6*, 93–115.

Messas, G., Vitucci, L., Garcia, L., Dutra, R., et al. (2016). Por uma psicopatossociologia das experiências dos usuários de drogas nas cracolândias/cenas de uso do Brasil. In *Crack e exclusão social* (pp. 163–190). Brasil: Ministério da Justiça e Cidadania. (Messas et al., 2016).

Messas, G., Fulford, K. W. M., & Stanghellini, G. (2017a, November). The contribution of human sciences to the challenges of contemporary psychiatry. *Trends in Psychiatry and Psychotherapy*. (Messas et al., 2017a).

Messas, G., Tamelini, M. G., & Cutting, J. (2017b, December). A meta-analysis of the core essence of psychopathological entities: An historical exercise in phenomenological psychiatry. *History of Psychiatry, 28*(4), 473–481. (Messas et al., 2017b).

Messas, G., Tamelini, M. G., Mancini, M., & Stanghellini, G. (2018). New perspectives in phenomenological psychopathology: Its use in psychiatric treatment. *Frontiers in Psychiatry, 9*, 466. (Messas et al. 2018).

Messas, G., Zorzanelli, R., & Tamelini, M. G. (2019a). The life-world of hysteria. In G. Stanghellini, M. Broome, et al. (Eds.), *The Oxford handbook of phenomenological psychopathology* (pp. 649–664). Oxford: Oxford University Press. (Messas et al, 2019a).

Messas, G. P., Fukuda, L., & Pienkos, E. (2019b). A phenomenological contribution to substance misuse treatment: Principles for person-centered care. *Psychopathology, 52*(2), 85–93. (Messas et al, 2019b).

Milton, J. (1976). *Paradise Lost*. Norwalk: Easton Press.

Minkowska, F. (2007). *Van Gogh – sa vie, sa maladie, son œuvr*. Paris: Editions L'Harmattan. 978-2296030930.

Minkowski, E. (1995). *Le temps vécu. Études Phénoménologiques et Psychopathologiques*. Paris: Presses Universitaires de France (PUF).

Minkowski, E. (1999a). *Traité de psychopathologie*. Le Plessis-Robinson: Institut Synthélabo.

Minkowski, E. (1999b). Vers une cosmologie. *Petite Bibliothèque Payot*.

Minkowski, E. (2000). *La Esquizofrenia: psicopatologia de los esquizóides y los esquizofrénicos*. Fondo de Cultura Económica: México, D. F.

Minkowski, E. (2002). *Ecrits Cliniques* (p. 271). Paris: Erès.

Morin, E. (1982). *Science avec conscience*. Paris: Fayard.

Moskalewicz, M. (2016). Three modes of distorted temporal experience in addiction: daily life, drug ecstasy and recovery-a phenomenological perspective. *Archive of the History of Philosophy and Social Thought, 61*(Special Issue Phenomenology and Social Sciences), 197–212.

Moskalewicz, M., & Schwartz, M. (2020a). Temporal experience in mania. *Phenomenology and the Cognitive Sciences, 2*, 19.

Moskalewicz, M., & Schwartz, M. A. (2020b). Temporal experience as a core quality in mental disorders. *Phenomenology and the Cognitive Sciences, 19*(2), 207–216.

Mueser, K. T., Nishith, P., Tracy, J. I., Degirolamo, J., et al. (1995). Expectations and motives for substance use in schizophrenia. *Schizophrenia Bulletin, 21*(3), 367–378.

Mundt, C., Backenstrass, M., Kronmiller, K. T., Fiedler, P., et al. (1997). Personality and endogenous/major depression: An empirical approach to typus melancholicus. 2. Validation of typus melancholicus core-properties by personality inventory scales. *Psychopathology, 30*(3), 130–139.

Mustonen, A., Niemelä, S., Nordström, T., Murray, G., et al. (2018). Adolescent cannabis use, baseline prodromal symptoms and the risk of psychosis. *The British Journal of Psychiatry, 212*(4), 227–233.

NIDA [National Institute on Drug Abuse]. (2018). *Common comorbidities with substance use disorders.* National Institute of Mental Health: Bethesda.

Nordgaard, J., Sass, L. A., & Parnas, J. (2013, June). The psychiatric interview: Validity, structure, and subjectivity. *European Archives of Psychiatry and Clinical Neuroscience, 263*(4), 353–364.

Nutt, D. J. (2014, January). The role of the opioid system in alcohol dependence. *Journal of Psychopharmacology, 28*(1), 8–22.

Oliva, F., Dalmotto, M., Pirfo, E., Furlan, P. M., et al. (2014, October). A comparison of thought and perception disorders in borderline personality disorder and schizophrenia: Psychotic experiences as a reaction to impaired social functioning. *BMC Psychiatry, 14*, 239.

Orsolini, L., Chiappini, S., Papanti, D., De Berardis, D., et al. (2019). The bridge between classical and "synthetic"/chemical psychoses: Towards a clinical, psychopathological, and therapeutic perspective. *Frontiers in Psychiatry, 10*, 851.

Oulis, P. (2008). Ontological assumptions of psychiatric taxonomy: Main rival positions and their critical assessment. *Psychopathology, 41*(3), 135–140.

Oumaya, M., Friedman, S., Pham, A., Abou Abdallah, T., et al. (2008, October). Borderline personality disorder, self-mutilation and suicide: Literature review. *Encephale, 34*(5), 452–458.

Oyebode, F. (2018). *Sims' symptoms in the mind: Textbook of descriptive psychopathology* (6th ed.). Netherlands: Elsevier.

Pallagrosi, M., & Fonzi, L. (2018). On the concept of praecox feeling. *Psychopathology, 51*(6), 353–361.

Pallagrosi, M., Fonzi, L., Picardi, A., & Biondi, M. (2016). Association between Clinician's subjective experience during patient evaluation and psychiatric diagnosis. *Psychopathology, 49*(2), 83–94.

Paris, J., & Black, D. W. (2015, January). Borderline personality disorder and bipolar disorder: What is the difference and why does it matter? *The Journal of Nervous and Mental Disease, 203*(1), 3–7.

Parkman, T. J., Lloyd, C., & Splisbury, K. (2015). Self-help groups for alcohol dependency: A scoping review. *Journal of Groups in Addiction & Recovery, 10*(2), 102–124.

Parnas, J., & Zahavi, D. (2002). The role of phenomenology in psychiatric diagnosis and classification. In M. Maj, W. Gaebel, et al. (Eds.), *Psychiatric diagnosis and classification.* UK: John Wiley & Sons.

Parnas, J., Licht, D., & Bovet, P. (2005). Cluster a personality disorders: A review. In M. Maj, H. S. Akiskal, et al. (Eds.), *Personality disorders*, New York: (Vol. 8). John Wiley & Sons, Ltd.

Parnas, J., Sass, L. A., & Zahavi, D. (2013, March). Rediscovering psychopathology: The epistemology and phenomenology of the psychiatric object. *Schizophrenia Bulletin, 39*(2), 270–277.

Pasche, S. (2012, June). Exploring the comorbidity of anxiety and substance use disorders. *Current Psychiatry Reports, 14*(3), 176–181.

Pieri, G. A., & Castellana, G. B. (2016). Transtorno de personalidade borderline ou transtorno afetivo bipolar? Contribuições da Psicopatologia Fenomenológica para o diagnóstico diferencial. *Psicopatologia Fenomenológica Contemporânea, 5*(2), 145–159.

Piper, B. J., Ogden, C. L., Simoyan, O. M., Chung, D. Y., et al. (2018). Trends in use of prescription stimulants in the United States and territories, 2006 to 2016. *PLoS One, 13*(11), e0206100.

Plunk, A. D., Syed-Mohammed, H., Cavazos-Rehg, P., Bierut, L. J., et al. (2014, February). Alcohol consumption, heavy drinking, and mortality: Rethinking the j-shaped curve. *Alcoholism, Clinical and Experimental Research, 38*(2), 471–478.

Potvin, S., Stip, E., & Roy, J. Y. (2003, May–June). Schizophrenia and addiction: An evaluation of the self-medication hypothesis. *Encephale, 29*(3 Pt 1), 193–203.

Poudel, A., & Gautam, S. (2017). Age of onset of substance use and psychosocial problems among individuals with substance use disorders. *BMC Psychiatry, 17*(1), 10.

Pringuey, D. (2005). Une phénoménologie de la dépendance à l'alcool. Une expérience primor-
diale de la "nostrité". *L'Evolution Pscychiatrique, 70*, 771–779.

Radhakrishnan, R., Wilkinson, S. T., & D'Souza, D. C. (2014). Gone to pot – A review of the
association between Cannabis and psychosis. *Frontiers in Psychiatry, 5*, 54.

Radoilska, L. (2013). Addiction and weakness of will: An integrated account. In L. Radoilska
(Ed.), *Addiction and weakness of will*. Oxford: Oxford University Press.

Ramey, T., & Regier, P. S. (2018, December). Cognitive impairment in substance use disorders.
CNS Spectrums, 1–12.

Randall, C. L., Thomas, S., & Thevos, A. K. (2001, February). Concurrent alcoholism and social
anxiety disorder: A first step toward developing effective treatments. *Alcoholism, Clinical and
Experimental Research, 25*(2), 210–220.

Ratcliffe, M. (2015). *Experiences of depression: A study in phenomenology* (1st ed.). Oxford: Oxford
University Press. International Perspectives in Philosophy and Psychiatry. 978-0199608973.

Ray, L. A., Mackillop, J., Leventhal, A., & Hutchison, K. E. (2009, December). Catching the alcohol buzz: An examination of the latent factor structure of subjective intoxication. *Alcoholism,
Clinical and Experimental Research, 33*(12), 2154–2161.

Richardson, T. H. (2013). Substance misuse in depression and bipolar disorder: A review of psychological interventions and considerations for clinical practice. *Mental Health and Substance
Use, 6*(1), 76–93.

Roberts, J., Gracia Canales, A., Blanthorn-Hazell, S., Craciun Boldeanu, A., et al. (2018).
Characterizing the experience of agitation in patients with bipolar disorder and schizophrenia.
BMC Psychiatry, 18(1), 104.

Rogers, J. H., Widiger, T. A., & Krupp, A. (1995, February). Aspects of depression associated with
borderline personality disorder. *The American Journal of Psychiatry, 152*(2), 268–270.

Rossi, C. D. C. (2008). A Vagueza e a Nosologia de Karl Jaspers. In G. M. Messas (Ed.),
Psicopatologia Fenomenológica Contemporânea (1st ed., pp. 91–132). São Paulo: Roca.

Rossi Monti, M., & D'Agostino, A. (2019). Dysphoria in borderline persons. In G. Stanghellini,
M. Broome, et al. (Eds.), *The Oxford handbook of phenomenological psychopathology*
(pp. 827–838). Oxford: Oxford University Press.

Rovaletti, M. L. (2001). Pour une Critique de la Raison Nosographique. *L'Information
Psychiatrique, 77*(5), 497–503.

Rovaletti, M. L. (2005). The objectivization of time in the obsessive world. In A. Tymieniecka
(Ed.), Netherlands: *Analecta Husserliana LXXXIV* (pp. 265–274).

Rovaletti, M. L. (2007). The constitution of the object in phobic experience. In Z. Loparic &
R. Walton (Eds.), *Phenomenology 2005 – Selected essays from Latin America part 2* (Vol. 2.,
cap. 22, pp. 511–525). Bucharest: Zeta Books.

Rovaletti, M. L. (2014). Melancolía y temporalidad. El planteamiento fenomenológico de
L. Binswanger. *Psicopatologia Fenomenológica Contemporânea, 3*(2), 38–56.

Roy, A. (2009). Characteristics of cocaine dependent patients who attempt suicide. *Archives of
Suicide Research, 13*(1), 46–51.

Rubio, G., & López-Ibor, J. J. (2007). Generalized anxiety disorder: A 40-year follow-up study.
Actas Psiquiat Scand, 115, 372–379.

Ruiter, M. E., Lichstein, K. L., Nau, S. D., & Geyer, J. D. (2012, October). Personality disorder features and insomnia status amongst hypnotic-dependent adults. *Sleep Medicine, 13*(9),
1122–1129.

Rümke, H. C. (1990). The nuclear symptom of schizophrenia and the praecox feeling. *History of
Psychiatry, 1*, 331–341.

SAMHSA. (1999). Brief humanistic and existential therapies. In: Substance Abuse and Mental
Health Services Administration (Ed.). *Brief interventions and brief therapies for substance
abuse* (Vol. 34). Rockville: Center for Substance Abuse Treatment.

SAMHSA. (2017). *Addressing suicidal thoughts and behaviors in substance abuse treatment*. United States of America (Maryland): Substance Abuse and Mental Health Services
Administration.

Sansone, R. A., & Sansone, L. A. (2008, September). Alcohol/substance misuse and treatment nonadherence: Fatal attraction. *Psychiatry (Edgmont), 5*(9), 43–46.

Sass, L. (2010). Phenomenology as description and as explanation: The case of schizophrenia. In D. Schmicking & S. Gallagher (Eds.), *Handbook of phenomenology and cognitive science.* Dordrecht: Springer.

Sass, L. (2014b, January). Self-disturbance and schizophrenia: Structure, specificity, pathogenesis (current issues, new directions). *Schizophrenia Research, 152*(1), 5–11.

Sass, L. (2017). *Madness and modernism: Insanity in the light of modern art, literature, and thought.* Oxford: Oxford University Press.

Sass, L. (2019). Three dangers: Phenomenological reflections on the psychotherapy of psychosis. *Psychopathology, 52*(2), 126–134.

Sass, L., & Pienkos, E. (2013). Space, time, and atmosphere a comparative phenomenology of melancholia, mania, and schizophrenia, Part II. *Journal of Consciousness Studies, 20*(7–8), 131–152.

Sass, L., & Pienkos, E. (2015). Faces of Intersubjectivity – A phenomenological study of interpersonal experience in melancholia, mania, and schizophrenia. *Journal of Phenomenological Psychology, 46*(1), 1–32.

Sawer, F., Davis, P., & Gleeson, K. (2020). Is shame a barrier to sobriety? A narrative analysis of those in recovery. *Drugs: Education, Prevention and Policy, 27*(1), 79–85.

Sayette, M. A., Creswell, K. G., Dimoff, J. D., Fairbairn, C. E., et al. (2012, August). Alcohol and group formation: A multimodal investigation of the effects of alcohol on emotion and social bonding. *Psychological Science, 23*(8), 869–878.

Schäfer, M. (2001). Die Bedeutung des Typusbegriffes in der Psychiatrie. *Fortschritte Der Neurologie – Psychiatrie, 69*(6), 256–267.

Schlimme, J. E. (2010, February). Addiction and self-determination: A phenomenological approach. *Theoretical Medicine and Bioethics, 31*(1), 49–62.

Schneider, K. (2007). *Klinische psychopathologie* (15th ed.). Stuttgart: Georg Thieme Verlag.

Schoeler, T., & Bhattacharyya, S. (2013). The effect of cannabis use on memory function: An update. *Substance Abuse and Rehabilitation, 4*, 11–27.

Schoenborn, C. A., Stommel, M., & Ward, B. W. (2014, August). Mortality risks associated with average drinking level and episodic heavy drinking. *Substance Use & Misuse, 49*(10), 1250–1258.

Schrank, B., Rumpold, T., Gmeiner, A., Priebe, S., et al. (2016, December). Parenthood among patients with psychotic disorders: Gender differences in a non-selective clinical sample. *Psychiatry Research, 246*, 474–479.

Schwartz, M. A., & Wiggins, O. P. (1987). Diagnosis and ideal types: A contribution to psychiatric classification. *Comprehensive Psychiatry, 28*, 277–291.

Shrestha, K., Rees, D. W., Rix, K. J., Hore, B. D., et al. (1985, September). Sexual jealousy in alcoholics. *Acta Psychiatrica Scandinavica, 72*(3), 283–290.

Sigmund, D. (1997). Phänomenologie der hysterischen Pseudopsychosen. *Fortschritte der Neurologie-Psychatrie, 65*, 387–395.

Silk, K. R. (2010, February). The quality of depression in borderline personality disorder and the diagnostic process. *Journal of Personality Disorders, 24*(1), 25–37.

Silverstein, S. M., Demmin, D., & Skodlar, B. (2017). Space and objects: On the phenomenology and cognitive neuroscience of anomalous perception in schizophrenia (ancillary article to EAWE domain 1). *Psychopathology, 50*(1), 60–67.

Simon, O. R., Swann, A. C., Powell, K. E., Potter, L. B., et al. (2001). Characteristics of impulsive suicide attempts and attempters. *Suicide & Life-Threatening Behavior, 32*(1 Suppl), 49–59.

Jérôme Soldani, « Ce que les régimes de temporalités peuvent nous apprendre sur les sports », Temporalités [En ligne], 25 | 2017, mis en ligne le 25 septembre 2017, consulté le 25 novembre 2020. URL. http://journals.openedition.org/temporalites/3610.

Souza, J. (2016). *Crack e exclusão social* (360 p). Ministério da Justiça e Cidadania, Secretaria Nacional de Política sobre Drogas: Brasília.

Souza, C., & Moreira, V. (2018). A Compreensão da Experiência de Depressividade na Tradição da Psicopatologia Fenomenológica. *Psicologia: Teoria e Pesquisa, 34*, e3447.

Soyka, M. (2006, June.) Alcohol hallucinosis and jealous delusion. *Fortschritte der Neurologie-Psychiatrie, 74*(6), 346–352; quiz 353–344.

Stanghellini, G. (2004). *Disembodied spirits and Deanimated bodies: The psychopathology of common sense* (Vol. 236, p. 978-0198520894). Oxford: Oxford University Press.

Stanghellini, G. (2007). The grammar of the psychiatric interview. A plea for the second-person mode of understanding. *Psychopathology, 40*(2), 69–74.

Stanghellini, G., & Ballerini, M. (2007, January). Values in persons with schizophrenia. *Schizophrenia Bulletin, 33*(1), 131–141.

Stanghellini, G., & Raballo, A. (2015, January). Differential typology of delusions in major depression and schizophrenia. A critique to the unitary concept of 'psychosis'. *Journal of Affective Disorders, 171*, 171–178.

Stanghellini, G., & Rosfort, R. (2013). *Emotions and personhood: Exploring fragility – Making sense of vulnerability.* Oxford: Oxford University Press. 9780199660575.

Stead, V. E., Boylan, K., & Schmidt, L. A. (2019). Longitudinal associations between non-suicidal self-injury and borderline personality disorder in adolescents: A literature review. *Borderline Personal Disord Emot Dysregul, 6*, 3.

Stephensen, H., & Henriksen, M. G. (2017). Not being oneself: A critical perspective on 'inauthenticity' in schizophrenia. *Journal of Phenomenological Psychology, 48*(1), 63–82.

Straus, E. (1935). *Vom sinn der sinne.* Berlin: Julius Springer.

Straus, E. (1938). Ein Beitrag zur Pathologie der Zwangserscheinungen. *Monatsschrift fir Psychiatrie und Neurologie, 98*, 63–101.

Stubbs, B., Thompson, T., Acaster, S., Vancampfort, D., et al. (2015, November). Decreased pain sensitivity among people with schizophrenia: A meta-analysis of experimental pain induction studies. *Pain, 156*(11), 2121–2131.

Subramaniam, G. A., & Volkow, N. D. (2014, September). Substance misuse among adolescents: To screen or not to screen? *JAMA Pediatrics, 168*(9), 798–799.

Subramaniam, M., Mahesh, M. V., Peh, C. X., Tan, J., et al. (2017, December). Hazardous alcohol use among patients with schizophrenia and depression. *Alcohol, 65*, 63–69.

Sweeney, C. T., Sembower, M. A., Ertischek, M. D., Shiffman, S., et al. (2013). Nonmedical use of prescription ADHD stimulants and preexisting patterns of drug abuse. *Journal of Addictive Diseases, 32*(1), 1–10.

Tamelini, M. G. (2008). Biografia e Estrutura. In G. Messas (Ed.), *Psicopatologia Fenomenológica Contemporânea* (pp. 199–213). São Paulo: Roca.

Tamelini, M. G. (2012). Cinética Estrutural na Esquizofrenia. *Psicopatologia Fenomenológica Contemporânea, 1*, 3–25.

Tamelini, M. G., & Messas, G. (2016). On the phenomenology of delusion: The revelation of its aprioristic structures and the consequences for clinical practice. *Psicopatologia Fenomenológica Contemporânea, 5*(1), 1–21.

Tamelini, M. G., & Messas, G. (2017). Phenomenological psychopathology in contemporary psychiatry: Interfaces and perspectives. *Revista Latinoamericana de Psicopatologia Fundamental, 20*(1), 165–180.

Tamelini, M. G., & Messas, G. (2019). A step beyond psychopathology: A new frontier of phenomenology in psychiatry. *Philosophy, Psychiatry & Psychology, 26*(2), 151–154.

Tatossian, A. (2002). *La phénoménologie des psychoses.* Paris: Le Cercle Herméneutique.

Tatossian, A., & Moreira, V. (2012). *Clínica do Lebenswelt: psicoterapia e psicopatologia fenomenológica* (1st ed.). São Paulo: Editora Escuta. 9788571373259.

Taylor, M. A., & Fink, M. (2008, January). Restoring melancholia in the classification of mood disorders. *Journal of Affective Disorders, 105*(1–3), 1–14.

Tellenbach, H. (1968). *Geschmack und Atmosphäre: Medien menschlichen Elementarkontaktes.* Otto Müller Verlag: Salzburg.

Tellenbach, H. (1969). Análisis psicológico-situacional del precampo en la manía endógena. In *Estudios sobre la patogénesis de las perturbaciones psíquicas* (pp. 61–78). México D.F.: Fondo de Cultura Económica.

Tellenbach, H. (1970). Dostoyevsky's prince Myshkjn: Epilepsy portrayed. In E. W. Straus & R. M. Griffith (Eds.), *Aisthesis and aesthetics* (p. 261). Pittsburgh: Duquesne University Press.

Tellenbach, H. (1983). *Melancholie Problemgeschichte Endogenität Typologie Pathogenese Klinic* (4th ed.). Berlim/Heidelberg/NovaYork/Tokyo: Springer.

Thomas, S. E., Randall, P. K., Book, S. W., & Randall, C. L. (2008, January). A complex relationship between co-occurring social anxiety and alcohol use disorders: What effect does treating social anxiety have on drinking? *Alcoholism, Clinical and Experimental Research, 32*(1), 77–84.

Thorpe, H. H. A., Hamidullah, S., Jenkins, B. W., & Khokhar, J. Y. (2020, February). Adolescent neurodevelopment and substance use: Receptor expression and behavioral consequences. *Pharmacology & Therapeutics, 206*, 107431.

Tomko, R. L., Trull, T. J., Wood, P. K., & Sher, K. J. (2014, October). Characteristics of borderline personality disorder in a community sample: Comorbidity, treatment utilization, and general functioning. *Journal of Personality Disorders, 28*(5), 734–750.

Trull, T. J., Freeman, L. K., Vebares, T. J., Choate, A. M., et al. (2018). Borderline personality disorder and substance use disorders: An updated review. *Borderline Personality Disorder and Emotion Dysregulation, 5*, 15.

van Herdeen, A. (2016). The restructuring of temporality during art making. *South African Journal of Art History, 31*(2), 187–204.

Verdejo-Garcia, A., Garcia-Fernandez, G., & Dom, G. (2019). Cognition and addiction. *Dialogues in Clinical Neuroscience, 21*(3), 281–290.

Verheul, R. (2001, August). Co-morbidity of personality disorders in individuals with substance use disorders. *European Psychiatry, 16*(5), 274–282.

Virtanen, S., Kuja-Halkola, R., Mataix-Cols, D., Jayaram-Lindström, N., et al. (2019, July). Comorbidity of substance misuse with anxiety-related and depressive disorders: A genetically informative population study of 3 million individuals in Sweden. *Psychological Medicine, 50*(10):1–10.

von Gebsattel, V. (1966a). El mundo del obsesivo. In *Antropología médica* (pp. 105–168). Madrid: Ediciones Rialp.

von Gebsattel, V. (1966b). El problema de la despersonalización. In *Antropología médica* (pp. 40–73). Madrid: Ediciones Rialp.

von Weizsäcker, V. (1950). *Der Gestaltkreis. Theorie der Einheit von Wahrnnehmen und Bewegen.* Stuttgart: Georg Thieme Verlag.

von Zerssen, D. (1988). Der Typus Manicus als gegenstück zum Typus Melancholicus in der prämorbide Persönlichkeits struktur affetkt psychotischer Patienten. In W. Janzarik (Ed.), *Persönlichkeit und Psychose* (pp. 150–171). Stuttgart: Enke.

von Zerssen, D. (1996). "Melancholic" and "manic" types of personality as premorbid structures in affective disorders. In C. Mundt, M. Goldstein, K. Hahlweg, & P. Fiedler (Eds.), *Interpersonal factors in the origin and course of affective disorders* (pp. 65–85). Gaskell: The Royal College of Psychiatrists London.

von Zerssen, D., Tauscher, R., & Pössl, J. (1994, September). The relationship of premorbid personality to subtypes of an affective illness. A replication study by means of an operationalized procedure for the diagnosis of personality structures. *Journal of Affective Disorders, 32*(1), 61–72.

Wang, P. W., & Yen, C. F. (2017, December). Adolescent substance use behavior and suicidal behavior for boys and girls: A cross-sectional study by latent analysis approach. *BMC Psychiatry, 17*(1), 392.

Welch, S. (2007). Substance use and personality disorders. *Psychiatry, Addiction Psychiatry. Part 2 of 2, 6*(1), 27–29.

WHO [World Health Organization]. (2019, April) International Classification of Diseases, 11th Revision, ICD 11.

Wiklund, L. (2008, September). Existential aspects of living with addiction - part I: Meeting challenges. *Journal of Clinical Nursing, 17*(18), 2426–2434.

Wilson, S. R., Lubman, D. I., Manning, V., & Yap, M. B. H. (2019). The impact of problematic substance use on partners' interpersonal relationships: Qualitative analysis of counselling transcripts from a national online service. *Drugs: Education, Prevention and Policy, 26*(5), 429–436.

Wycoff, A. M., Metrik, J., & Trull, T. J. (2018). Affect and cannabis use in daily life: A review and recommendations for future research. *Drug and Alcohol Dependence, 191*, 223–233.

Wyrsch, J. (1949). *Die Person des Schizophrenen. Studien zur Klinik, Psychologie, Daseinsweise.* Bern: Verlag Paul Haupt.

Yuodelis-Flores, C., & Ries, R. K. (2015, March). Addiction and suicide: A review. *The American Journal on Addictions, 24*(2), 98–104.

Zachar, P., & Jablensky, A. (2015). The concept of validation in psychiatry and psychology. In P. Zachar, D. S. Stoyanov, et al. (Eds.), *Alternative perspectives on psychiatric validation: DSM, ICD, RDoC, and beyond* (pp. 3–24). Oxford, UK: Oxford University Press.

Zahavi, D. (2018). Collective intentionality and plural pre-reflective self-awareness. *Journal of Social Philosophy, 49*(1), 61–75.

Zahavi, D. (2019). Self. In G. Stanghellini, M. Broome, et al. (Eds.), *The Oxford handbook of phenomenological psychopathology* (pp. 299–305). Oxford: Oxford University Press.

Zorzanelli, R., Dalgalarrondo, P., & Banzato, C. E. M. (2016). Realism and pragmatism in psychiatry: A debate. *Revista Latinoamericana de Psicopatologia Fundamental, 19*(3), 527–543.

Zutt, J. (1963a). Zur Anthropologie der Sucht. In *Auf dem Wege zu Einer Anthropologischen Psychiatrie* (pp. 426–438). Berlin/Gottingen/Heidelberg: Springer.

Zutt, J. (1963b). Über das Wesen der Sucht nach den Erfahrungen und vom Standpunkt des Psychiaters. In *Auf dem Wege zu Einer Anthropologischen Psychiatrie* (pp. 278–285). Berlin/Gottingen/Heidelberg: Springer.

Zutt, J. (1963c). Über den tragenden Leib. In *Auf dem Wege zu einer Anthropologische Psychiatrie.* Berlin-Heidelberg: Springer.

Zutt, J. (1963d). Über die polare Struktur des Bewußtseins. In *Auf dem Wege zu Einer Anthropologischen Psychiatrie* (pp. 55–277). Berlin/Gottingen/Heidelberg: Springer.

Index

© Springer Nature Switzerland AG 2021
G. Messas, *The Existential Structure of Substance Misuse*,
https://doi.org/10.1007/978-3-030-62724-9

Printed in the United States
by Baker & Taylor Publisher Services